A Multidisciplinary Approach to Pandemics

A Multidisciplinary Approach to Pandemics

COVID-19 and Beyond

Edited by

PHILIPPE BOURBEAU
JEAN-MICHEL MARCOUX
BROOKE A. ACKERLY

OXFORD
UNIVERSITY PRESS

OXFORD
UNIVERSITY PRESS

Great Clarendon Street, Oxford, OX2 6DP,
United Kingdom

Oxford University Press is a department of the University of Oxford.
It furthers the University's objective of excellence in research, scholarship,
and education by publishing worldwide. Oxford is a registered trade mark of
Oxford University Press in the UK and in certain other countries

Impression: 1

Published in the United States of America by Oxford University Press
198 Madison Avenue, New York, NY 10016, United States of America

British Library Cataloguing in Publication Data
Data available

Library of Congress Control Number: 2021950168

ISBN 978–0–19–289785–5

DOI: 10.1093/oso/9780192897855.001.0001

Printed and bound by
CPI Group (UK) Ltd, Croydon, CR0 4YY

Acknowledgements

We came together at the beginning of the COVID-19 pandemic to collaborate on editing a volume about the importance of multidisciplinary learning for addressing pandemics and would like to thank each other for what has turned into a healthy collaboration.

Throughout the project, even as the pandemic wore on and tested individual collaborators in different ways, each of the contributors did their part to support the success of the project. While it has always been the case that we all rely on each other, the pandemic has reminded us how important it is to stop and recognize all of the support that people give each other.

This book is partially the result of the multidisciplinary summer school 'Causes and Consequences of Pandemics' organized by the Graduate School of International Studies in May–June 2020 at the University Laval, Quebec City. We would like to offer our gratitude to all invited scholars and decision-makers who have accepted our invitation to participate in this incredible learning collaboration at such short notice. Amid the brutal new reality that COVID-19 was forcing upon all of us, these individuals agreed to set aside some time from their busy schedule to come and present their thoughts about the causes and consequences of pandemics on their jobs, responsibilities, and fields of research in front of more than 200 individuals and students.

We are grateful to those who provided funding for the elaboration of this volume, including the Mobilizing Insights in Defence and Security program of the Government of Canada. We further wish to thank the Fulbright Canada program, which brought us together through the Fulbright Canada Research Chair in International Studies at the Graduate School of International Studies, Laval University, though the pandemic itself prevented us from working together in person.

We are also grateful to the editorial team at Oxford University Press and the two anonymous reviewers for their thoughtful comments that allowed us to improve the quality of the manuscript.

We wish to thank Vanderbilt Student Government for developing and passing a land acknowledgement:

> We collectively acknowledge that Vanderbilt University occupies the ancestral hunting and traditional Lands of the Cherokee, Shawnee, Choctaw, Chickasaw, and Creek peoples. Today, these people have nation boundaries in Oklahoma, North Carolina, and Mississippi, after the Indian Removal Act of 1830 led to the forced removal of southern tribes west of the Mississippi River. In particular,

the University resides on Land ceded on November 8, 1795 in the Treaty of Hopewell. We recognize, support, and advocate for the Indigenous individuals and communities who live here now, and for those forcibly removed from their Homelands. By offering this Land Acknowledgement, we affirm Indigenous sovereignty and will work to hold Vanderbilt University more accountable to the needs of American Indian and Indigenous peoples.

Dans un esprit d'amitié et de solidarité, l'Université Laval rend hommage aux Premiers Peuples de ces lieux. Étant à la croisée du Niowentsïo du peuple Huron-Wendat, du Ndakina du peuple Wabanaki, du Nitassinan du peuple Innu, du Nitaskinan du peuple Atikmekw et du Wolastokuk Malécite, nous honorons nos relations les uns avec les autres.

Philippe Bourbeau, Quebec City, Canada
Jean-Michel Marcoux, Ottawa, Canada
Brooke Ackerly, Nashville, TN, USA

Contents

List of Figures

List of Tables

List of Contributors

Brooke A. Ackerly is Professor of Political Science at Vanderbilt University and co-Editor-in-Chief of the *International Feminist Journal of Politics* (2018–2021). In her research, teaching, and collaborations, she works to clarify without simplifying the most pressing problems of global justice, including human rights and climate change. Using feminist methodologies, she integrates into her theoretical work empirical research on activism and the experiences of those affected by injustice (grounded normative theory). Her published works include *Political Theory and Feminist Social Criticism* (Cambridge University Press, 2000), *Universal Human Rights in a World of Difference* (Cambridge University Press, 2008), *Doing Feminist Research* with Jacqui True (Palgrave Macmillan, 2010, 2019), and *Just Responsibility: A Human Rights Theory of Global Justice* (Oxford University Press, 2018).

Luc Bergeron is Adjunct Professor of Clinical Pharmacy at the Faculté de pharmacie of Université Laval and Antimicrobial Stewardship Coordinator for the CHU de Québec-Université Laval hospital. He received his bachelor's degree in pharmacy and MSc in hospital pharmacy from the Faculté de pharmacie at Université Laval. He has been a hospital clinical pharmacist since 1987 and has been actively involved in infectious diseases pharmacotherapy for over 30 years. Bergeron is recognized nationwide as an expert in the field of antibiotic therapy in Canada. He has lectured extensively on the use of antimicrobials and antimicrobial stewardship and has served as an expert on several provincial, national, and industry committees. The Canadian Society of Hospital Pharmacists recognized his expertise and influence by awarding him the title of Fellow in 2013. His primary teaching and research interests are the optimal use and safety of antimicrobials in adults and children. He has presented the results of several of his research projects at national and international conferences and has to his credit several publications in peer-reviewed journals.

Christopher Bickerton is a Reader in Modern European Politics at the University of Cambridge, Fellow at Queens' College Cambridge, and Visiting Professor at the College of Europe in Bruges. He is the author of *European Integration: From Nation-States to Member States* (Oxford University Press, 2012), which was awarded the University Association of Contemporary European Studies best book award of 2013. In 2016, he published the best-selling *The European Union: A Citizen's Guide* (Penguin). He is the author of *Technopopulism: The New Logic of Democratic Politics* (co-written with Carlo Invernizzi Accetti), which is forthcoming with Oxford University Press.

Andrea K. Bjorklund is the Associate Dean of Graduate Studies as well as a Full Professor and the L. Yves Fortier Chair in International Arbitration and International Commercial Law at McGill University Faculty of Law. In addition to serving as an adviser to the American Law Institute's project on restating the US law of international commercial arbitration, she is a member of the Advisory Board of the Investment Treaty Forum of the British Institute for International and Comparative Law. Professor Bjorklund was the inaugural International Centre for Settlement of Investment Disputes (ICSID) Scholar-in-Residence 2014–2015 and was Editor-in-Chief of the *Yearbook on International Investment Law and Policy* from 2012 to 2015. She is on the panel of arbitrators of the American Arbitration Association's International Centre for Dispute Resolution and on the roster of North American Free Trade Agreement (NAFTA) Chapter 19 arbitrators. Professor Bjorklund has widely published in investment law and dispute resolution. Before entering the academy, she was an attorney-adviser on the NAFTA arbitration team in the Office of the Legal Adviser of the US Department of State, in addition to periods at the US International Trade Commission and in private practice at Miller & Chevalier in Washington, DC. Professor Bjorklund has a JD from Yale Law School, an MA in French Studies from New York University, and a BA (with High Honors) in History and French from the University of Nebraska.

Philippe Bourbeau is the Director of the Graduate School of International Studies at the University Laval, Chairholder of the Canada Research Chair in Immigration and Security, and Professor in the Department of Political Science. His work adopts a multidisciplinary approach to international issues. His books include *On Resilience. Genealogy, Logics, and World Politics* (Cambridge University Press, 2018), *Security: Dialogue across Disciplines* (Cambridge University Press, 2015), and *The Securitization of Migration* (Routledge, 2013).

Mary-Lieta Clément is currently a doctoral student at Laval University in Quebec City, Canada. She is writing a thesis on crisis management in organizations under the supervision of Christophe Roux-Dufort. Passionate about theatre and Greek tragedy, her work focuses on the tragic part of organizational crises. She explores the inexorable, insurmountable, and irremediable nature of crises and the strategies adopted by managers when trapped in events beyond their control and their understanding. She presented the results of her research at European conferences such as Association internationale de management stratégique (AIMS) 2020, European Group for Organizational Studies (EGOS) 2020, and others. She came to her current research after obtaining a master's degree in 2016 at Montpelier Business School, an MBA in International Management at Laval University in 2017, and a short experience in logistics.

Charles-Emmanuel Côté is Full Professor at the Faculty of Law of University Laval in Quebec City and a regular member of its Graduate School of International Studies, where he teaches Public International Law, International Economic Law, and Constitutional Law. He was Associate Dean for Undergraduate Studies and Continuing Legal Education and Secretary of the Faculty of Law from 2014 to 2018. He holds a doctorate degree in law from McGill University (Dean's Honour List) and is a lawyer called at the *Barreau du Québec*. He is also a member of the board of directors of the Canadian Council on International Law (CCIL), as well as of the International Law Association (ILA) Committee on the Rule of Law and International Investment Law. Professor Côté is a member of the *Canada–United States–Mexico Agreement* (*CUSMA*) Chapter 10 panel roster for Canada, as well as of the *Canadian Free Trade Agreement* (CFTA) panel roster for Quebec. His book on the participation of private persons to the settlement of international economic disputes received an award from the International Chamber of Commerce (ICC). His current research focuses on international economic disputes settlement, investor–State dispute settlement, and the international legal aspects of federalism.

Martin Darveau is the Chief-Pharmacist of the Pharmacy Department at the CHU de Québec-Université Laval. He received his bachelor's degree in pharmacy in 1998 and a master's degree in pharmaceutical practice from the Faculty of Pharmacy of the University of Montreal. In 2005, he also obtained a second MSc in research and pharmacoeconomics. As hospital pharmacist, his primary clinical and research interests are critical care and optimal drug use. He has been involved in various peer-reviewed journal publications, both as a principal investigator or in a teaching context. Mr Darveau has also been a member of the scientific committee for the evaluation of drugs for more than 15 years at the Institut national d'excellence en santé et en services sociaux (INESSS), the institute for excellence in health and social services in the province of Quebec.

Sara E. Davies is a Professor at the School of Government and International Relations, Griffith University, Australia, and an Adjunct Associate Professor at the Gender Peace and Security Centre, School of Social Sciences, Monash University. She is an international relations (IR) scholar with a specific focus on global health governance and the women, peace, and security agenda. She has been an Australian Research Council Discovery Australian Postgraduate Award Scholar (2008–2012) and an Australian Research Council Future Fellow (2014–2018). Professor Davies's research career has been devoted to identifying the political conditions that deny humans access to civil, economic, and social human rights. Her research has focused on situations where humans face immense vulnerability: disease outbreak events, gender-based and sexual violence in conflict, and forced displacement. She is author of *Containing Contagion: Politics of Disease Surveillance in Southeast Asia* (Johns Hopkins University Press, 2019), *Global Politics of Health* (Polity, 2010), and co-author of *Disease Diplomacy* (Johns Hopkins University Press, 2015).

Jack A. Goldstone is the Virginia E. and John T. Hazel, Jr Chair Professor of Public Policy at George Mason University and a Global Fellow of the Woodrow Wilson International Center. Previously, Dr Goldstone was on the faculty of Northwestern University and the University of California and has been a visiting scholar at Cambridge University and the California Institute of Technology. He is the author of *Revolution and Rebellion in the Early Modern World* (Routledge, 2016), awarded the 1993 Distinguished Scholarly Research Award by the American Sociological Association; *Why Europe? The Rise of the West in World History* (McGraw Hill, 2009); and nine other books, as well as over 100 research articles on topics in politics, social movements, democratization, and long-term social change. His books include *Political Demography: How Population Changes are Reshaping International Security and National Politics* (Oxford University Press, 2011), and *Revolutions: A Very Short Introduction* (Oxford University Press, 2014). He has appeared on NPR, CNN, Al-Jazeera, Fox News, and written for *Foreign Policy*, *The Atlantic*, the *Washington Post*, *Al-Hayat*, and the *International Herald Tribune*. He has been a Fellow at the Center for Advanced Study at Stanford University and won fellowships from the MacArthur Foundation, the J.S. Guggenheim Foundation, the Carnegie Foundation, the US Institute of Peace, and the American Council of Learned Societies. This essay was made possible in part by a grant from the Carnegie Corporation of New York. The statements made and views expressed therein are solely the responsibility of the author.

Matthieu J. Guitton is Secretary (Vice-Dean) of the Faculty of Medicine and Full Professor at the Faculty of Medicine and at the Graduate School of International Studies of Université Laval (Quebec City, Canada), as well as Senior Researcher/Group Leader at the CERVO Brain Research Centre (Quebec City, Canada). A graduate from the University of Rouen and Université Pierre et Marie Curie—Paris VI, he obtained his PhD from the University of Montpellier (France) and was a Koshland Scholar/Postdoctoral Fellow of Excellence at the Weizmann Institute of Science (Israel). He is a Fellow of the Royal Anthropological Institute. He is the Editor-in-Chief of *Computers in Human Behavior* and *Computers in Human Behavior Reports* and serves on several other editorial boards, such as *Current Opinion in Behavioral Sciences*. He has published over 100 papers, book chapters, or editorials on subjects ranging from neuropharmacology and biomedical sciences to cyberpsychology and international security issues. His most recent works have appeared in journals such as *Computers in Human Behavior*, the *International Journal of Intelligence and CounterIntelligence*, and the *International Journal of Intelligence, Security, and Public Affairs*.

Markus Herrmann is an Associate Professor in the Department of Economics at Université Laval and researcher at the CREATE and CIREQ research centre. His research focuses on theoretical modelling of various issues in environmental and resource economics, as well as bio-economics. He holds a PhD from the Université de Montréal. In particular, he has worked on population health issues relating to antibiotic resistance in humans and on the preservation of genetic diversity to avoid pest resistance towards genetically modified crops. His current research agenda is funded by a Social Sciences and Humanities Research Council insight grant and covers the impact of habit formation and environmental consciousness among consumers on the stringency of environmental taxes. He also participates in a multidisciplinary project with Quebec's national institute of public health (INSPQ) analysing the benefits of decreased disease prevalence due to the greening of urban spaces.

Michael Hooper is an Associate Professor in the School of Community and Regional Planning at the University of British Columbia (UBC). His research focuses on the politics of housing, land use, and urbanization, with particular interest in four related themes: displacement, disasters, spatial transformation, and participatory planning. Hooper has broad geographical interests, ranging from Metro Vancouver to much further afield. Past research projects have addressed, among other topics, forced displacement in East Africa, post-disaster reconstruction in Haiti, urban densification in Mongolia, and the climate-related risks faced by unsheltered residents of US cities. Prior to joining UBC, he spent a decade teaching at Harvard University and worked with the United Nations in New York and Kenya. Hooper has been a visiting research fellow at the University of Oxford and the Nordic Africa Institute. He is a registered professional planner in Canada, the United Kingdom, and the United States.

Maripier Isabelle is an Assistant Professor in the Department of Economics at Université Laval, a researcher at the CERVO brain research centre, and chairholder of the Sentinel North Partnership Research Chair in Economics and Brain Health. She holds a PhD in economics from the University of Toronto and completed a postdoctoral fellowship at the James M. and Cathleen D. Stone Centre for the Study of Wealth Inequality at the Institut Européen d'Administration des Affaires (INSEAD). Her research addresses issues at the intersection of economic inequality, health economics, and labour economics, with a focus on questions related to brain health and mental health. She combines tools developed in economics, recent advances from research in psychiatry, and the expertise developed within the health-care system to study the causal links between changes in income distribution and individuals' health trajectories. Her work also investigates the impact of growing income and wealth inequalities on the organization and performance of health-care systems and the impact of financial incentives on the allocation of health resources and on patient care.

Kathryn H. Jacobsen, PhD, MPH, holds the William E. Cooper Distinguished University Chair and is Professor of Health Studies at the University of Richmond in Richmond, Virginia. She was previously a professor at George Mason University in Fairfax, Virginia. An epidemiologist, her research focuses on the population health transitions that occur with globalization, socio-economic development, and environmental change. Her research portfolio includes analyses of the global epidemiology of hepatitis A virus, emerging infectious diseases, adolescent risk behaviours, and other global public health concerns. She has provided technical expertise on infectious disease prevention and control to the World Health Organization and many other agencies and organizations, and she has served as a consultant on research ethics, vaccine policy, and global health education. She is the author of two widely used textbooks, *Introduction to Global Health* and *Introduction to Health Research Methods*, and more than 200 peer-reviewed scientific articles.

Sikina Jinnah is an Associate Professor of Environmental Studies at the University of California at Santa Cruz (UCSC) and an Andrew Carnegie Fellow. She is also an affiliated graduate faculty member in the UCSC Politics Department. Her first book, *Post-Treaty Politics: Secretariat Influence in Global Environmental Governance* (MIT Press, 2014) received the 2016 Harold and Margaret Sprout Award for best book in international environmental affairs from the International Studies Association. The book examines the role of international bureaucracies in managing the politics of overlapping international regimes in the areas of biodiversity, climate change, and international trade. Her second book (with Jean-Frédéric Morin), *Greening through Trade: How American Trade Policy Has Influenced Environmental Protection Abroad* (MIT Press, 2020), examines the role of preferential trade agreements in securing environmental objectives. She is also the co-author (with Jean-Frédéric Morin and Amandine Orsini) of *Global Environmental Politics: Understanding the Governance of the Earth* (Oxford University Press, 2020), and co-editor (with Simon Nicholson) of *New Earth Politics: Essays from the Anthropocene* (MIT Press, 2016). Most recently, Dr Jinnah has been working on governance of climate change engineering, arguing for immediate governance of research in this area. Her work has also been published in several scholarly journals, including *Global Environmental Politics*, *International Studies Review*, *Environmental Politics*, the *Journal of Environment and Development*, *Environmental Research Letters*, *Berkeley Journal of International Law Publicist*, *Georgetown International Environmental Law Review*, *Global Governance*, *Nature Geoscience*, and *Science*. You can learn more about Dr Jinnah's work at www.sikinajinnah.com.

Dominic D. P. Johnson received a DPhil from Oxford University in evolutionary biology, and a PhD from Geneva University in political science. Drawing on both disciplines, he is interested in the biology and evolution of human decision-making, cooperation, and conflict. His new book, *Strategic Instincts: The Adaptive Advantages of Cognitive Biases in International Politics* (Princeton University Press, 2020) argues that cognitive biases—usually assumed to be detrimental and responsible for policy failures, disasters, and wars—are adaptive heuristics that evolved because they helped us make good decisions, not bad ones. Today, they can still act as advantageous 'strategic instincts' in politics and international relations, lending a competitive edge in competition and conflict with other actors. He has published three previous books: *God Is Watching You: How the Fear of God Makes Us Human* (Oxford University Press, 2015), which examines how cross-culturally ubiquitous and ancient beliefs in supernatural punishment helped to overcome severe collective action problems in the evolution of human societies; *Overconfidence and War: The Havoc and Glory of Positive Illusions* (Harvard University Press, 2004), which argues that psychological biases to maintain overly positive images of our capabilities, our control over events, and the future play a key role in the causes of war; and *Failing to Win: Perceptions of Victory and Defeat in International Politics* (Harvard University Press, 2006), with Dominic Tierney, which examines how and why popular misperceptions commonly create undeserved victories or defeats in international wars and crises. His current work focuses on the role of evolutionary dynamics, evolutionary psychology, and religion in human conflict and cooperation.

Jean-Michel Marcoux is an Assistant Professor in the Department of Law and Legal Studies at Carleton University. He holds a PhD in Law (University of Victoria), an MA in International Studies (Institut québécois des hautes études internationales), and a BA in Public Affairs and International Relations (University Laval). Prior to joining Carleton University, he completed a postdoctoral fellowship at McGill University's Faculty of Law. Interested in international economic law and international relations theory, he is the author of *International Investment Law and Globalization: Foreign Investment, Responsibilities, and Intergovernmental Organizations* (Routledge, 2018).

Jean-Frédéric Morin is a Full Professor in the Political Science Department of Université Laval and Chairholder of the Canada Research Chair in International Political Economy. He was Professor of International Relations at the Free University of Brussels from 2008 to 2014 and researcher at McGill University from 2006 to 2008. Professor Morin's projects look at international institutions. He is particularly interested in how international institutions innovate, interact, and evolve in the fields of trade, intellectual property, and environmental governance. During the first term of his Canada Research Chair (2014–2019), he published 10 books, 28 peer-reviewed articles, 14 book chapters, and 10 policy briefs. In the same five-year period, he supervised 13 PhD students and made more than 60 presentations. His publications have appeared in journals such as *International Studies Quarterly*, *European Journal of International Relations*, *Review of International Organizations*, *International Interactions*, *Global Governance*, *Global Environmental Politics*, and *Review of International Political Economy*. Some of his publications can be downloaded from https://www.chaire-epi.ulaval.ca/en/jean-frederic-morin.

Robert Muggah is a specialist in security, migration, cities, and new technologies. He is co-founder of the Igarapé Institute—a think-and-do tank working on data-driven human, digital and climate security. He is also co-founder and principal of the SecDev Group, which is devoted to disrupting digital risk and strengthening cyber security. Muggah is also a senior adviser to McKinseys and is faculty at Singularity University. For two decades, he has advised national and municipal governments, tech companies, and international organizations on issues ranging from crime prevention to urban planning. He is (or has been) a fellow or faculty member at the University of Oxford, Princeton University, the University of San Diego, the University of British Columbia, the Catholic University of Rio de Janeiro, and the Graduate Institute in Switzerland. He is also adviser to the World Economic Forum's Council on Cities and the annual Global Risk Report. Muggah has authored eight books, most recently *Terra Incognita* (Penguin/Random House, 2020), with Ian Goldin, and over 100 peer-reviewed articles. He is a regular contributor to *The Atlantic*, BBC, CNN, *El Pais*, the *Financial Times*, *Folha de São Paulo*, *Foreign Affairs*, *Foreign Policy*, the *Guardian*, the *Economist*, the *New York Times*, *Newsweek*, *USA Today*, and *Wired*, and he gave TED Talks in 2015, 2017 and 2021. He received his DPhil from the University of Oxford.

Amandine Orsini is Professor of International Relations at the Université Saint-Louis—Bruxelles. In 2019/2020 she was visiting researcher at the European University Institute (EUI)—Robert Schuman Center on Advanced Studies. Professor Orsini has a generalist and extensive background in global environmental politics and has co-edited *Essential Concepts to Global Environmental Governance* (Routledge, 2014, 2020) and co-authored *Global Environmental Politics: Understanding the Governance of the Earth* (Oxford University Press, 2020). She also coordinates the Module POLLEN on EU environmental law and policies (Jean Monnet Module 2016–2019) and has published *EU Environmental Governance: Current and Future Challenges* (Routledge, 2020). Her research focuses on international negotiations and non-state actors in the environmental domain. She has published in peer-reviewed journals such as *Review of International Studies, Global Environmental Politics, International Studies Review, Critical Policy Studies, Global Society, Environmental Politics,* and *Business & Society*.

Richard Ouellet is Full Professor of International Economic Law at the Faculty of Law and is a member of the Graduate School of International Studies at University Laval, in Quebec City. He holds a *Diplôme d'études supérieures suisse* of the Graduate Institute of International Studies of Geneva and a doctorate degree in law from University Laval. He is a member of the Honours List of the University Laval's Faculty of Graduate and Postdoctoral Studies. He is a lawyer and member of the Quebec Bar since 1992. He is the director of the Center of Interdisciplinary Studies on International Trade and Investment (CISITI). His teachings and current research projects focus on economic integration in North America, on the new regional trade agreements, on the revival of the notion of contract-treaty in international economic law, and on the reform on the dispute settlement mechanism of the World Trade Organization. He has supervised almost 100 students at the Masters' and doctoral levels. He is the author of many conferences, chapters, and papers published in many peer-reviewed journals. He has been invited as fellow, speaker, or visiting scholar to 15 countries in America, Europe, Africa, and Asia. He is a consultant for government and non-government departments and organizations on trade and investment issues. He is a referee for peer-reviewed journals specializing in trade and investment law and in international relations. Professor Ouellet is also codirector of the journal *Études internationales*.

Geneviève Parent is a Full Professor in the Law Faculty of Laval University and holder of the Legal Research Chair in Food Diversity and Food Security. Her areas of interest are food security and national and international agri-food law. Her research focuses on national and international legal means of ensuring food diversity, the analysis of the impacts of international law on Canadian and Quebec agri-food legislation, and the search for greater consistency between international economic law and other spheres of public international law for the benefit of sustainable world food security. She has also contributed to the writing of numerous scientific works and is frequently invited to speak as an expert at various international meetings. Her expertise in agri-food law leads her to execute various consulting mandates in national and international agri-food law. Professor Parent is a part-time member of the Canada Agricultural Review Tribunal and an associate member of the Académie d'Agriculture de France.

Christophe Roux Dufort is a Full Professor of Strategic Management in the Department of Management at Laval University. He has taught crisis management in the executive MBA and international MBA programs as well as in various executive programs. Professor Roux-Dufort has also written about 30 scientific and professional articles and 5 books on crisis management. He also works as a consultant for multinational companies in France, the United States, China, and Thailand, including Michelin, Danone, Chanel, and Airbus, among others. His comments on corporate crises are regularly published in national newspapers in France and Canada. He is regularly featured in national radio broadcasts. Professor Roux-Dufort received his MBA (1990) from the University Laval and his PhD (1997) from University Paris Dauphine, France. His research interests lie in risk and crisis management, organizational learning, and the management of change. He regularly holds visiting appointments in INSEAD (France), EM LYON (France), Thammasat University (Thailand), and other universities across Europe.

Julia Smith is a Research Associate in the Faculty of Health Sciences at Simon Fraser University. She holds a PhD in Peace Studies from the University of Bradford, where she was a Rotary World Peace Fellow. Dr Smith is the author of over two dozen peer-reviewed articles on topics related to gender, global health, and human rights, as well as the book *Civil Society and the Global Response to HIV/AIDS* and numerous chapters in edited books. In addition to currently co-leading a Canadian Institutes of Health Research-funded project on understanding and mitigating the gender impacts of the response to COVID-19, she contributes to projects on the political economy of the tobacco industry and Indigenous peoples' health. She has worked with health and human rights organizations in North America, Europe, and Africa and frequently works in consultation with government actors and multilateral organizations. Dr Smith's research interests centre on the social, political, and commercial determinants of health, global health governance, gender-based analysis, human rights, participatory methods, and feminist theory.

Introduction

Pandemics, Multidisciplinarity, and Global Ethics

Brooke A. Ackerly, Jean-Michel Marcoux, and Philippe Bourbeau

Pandemics have quickly become one of the most daunting subjects of the twenty-first century. Part of the challenge in understanding a pandemic relates to its widespread nature, which is at the heart of its definition. In epidemiological terms, a 'pandemic' is defined as '[a]n epidemic occurring over a very wide area, crossing international boundaries, and usually affecting a large number of people' (Porta 2016). The widespread nature has certainly characterized previous pandemics in human history, such as the 'Spanish flu' in 1918, HIV/AIDS, and the A(H1N1) influenza in 2009. More recently, the COVID-19 outbreak has provided a prime example of how pandemics do not know any boundaries and have implications on all spheres of activity.

In addition to crossing international boundaries, it is also clear that pandemics cross boundaries between academic disciplines. To name a few, pandemics provoke a broad range of consequences in economic, ethical, geographic, legal, medical, pharmaceutical, political, and sociological terms. Moreover, the disparate impacts of pandemics on persons with disabilities, those dependent on childcare, racialized and cast minorities, Indigenous people and communities, people in poverty, and other marginalized people reveal structural injustices and the complex social political economies that sustain them.

In the introduction to this edited volume, we want to emphasize the importance of studying pandemics through a multidisciplinary dialogue. We believe that approaching the causes and consequences of pandemics on our contemporary world by relying on a single academic discipline offers a limited, narrow perspective. Moreover, reaching beyond the limits of a single discipline paves the way to an understanding of pandemics as opportunities to identify solutions that are based on principles of justice and equality. Taken as a whole, these two aspects—a multidisciplinary approach and the prospect of identifying equitable solutions—provide a common basis for the study of pandemics that animates this entire volume. We hope that this work will pave the way for multi-perspective transdisciplinary work

Brooke A. Ackerly, Jean-Michel Marcoux, and Philippe Bourbeau, *Introduction.* In: *A Multidisciplinary Approach to Pandemics.* Edited by Philippe Bourbeau, Jean-Michel Marcoux, and Brooke A. Ackerly, Oxford University Press.
 DOI: 10.1093/oso/9780192897855.003.0001

to demonstrate the role of epistemic oppression in shaping the consequences of pandemics, as well as in rendering the role of structural injustice invisible and those very consequences also invisible.

A Multidisciplinary Approach to Pandemics

The study of pandemics is not new. Pandemics and global health have been one of the paramount research themes in several disciplines, with each discipline focusing on a particular aspect of the issue. In political science, scholars have mainly investigated the 'securitization' of pandemics by the international community, state efforts to control their borders, and the role of surveillance in addressing pandemics, as well as the strengths and limitations of institutions of global governance (e.g. Davies 2008, 2010; de Bengy Puyvallé and Kittelsen 2019; Elbe 2010; Greitens 2020; Huang 2014; Kamradt-Scott and McInnes 2012; Kenwick and Simmons 2020; Lipscy 2020). Geographers have been equally active in highlighting the influence of spatial and temporal dynamics of pandemics on human geography and demography (e.g. McLafferty 2010; Welford 2018), while scholars of urban planning have underscored the relationship between urban density, housing, inequality, and pandemics (e.g. Keil and Ali 2007; Matthew and McDonald 2006). Public policy scholars address the differential impacts of pandemics on structurally disadvantaged groups (Raifman and Raifman 2020) and the problems of lack of sufficient data, for example, on persons with disabilities (Reed et al. 2020) and Indigenous people (Goha et al. 2021). Economists have studied the impacts of pandemics on monetary and fiscal policy, the unemployment rate, international trade, and the differential impacts of these (e.g. Koegh-Brown et al. 2010; Lee and McKibbin 2004). Scholars in international law have focused on the obligations of states during times of pandemic, with a particular consideration of the International Health Regulations adopted by the World Health Organization (WHO) (e.g. Fidler 1996, 2003; Halpern 2020; Heath 2020). Historians (e.g. Echenberg 2011), sociologists (e.g. Dingwall et al. 2013), pharmacists (e.g. Ford et al. 2006), and ethicists (e.g. Smith and Upshur 2019) have also shed light on particular issues. Of course, additional work from other disciplines that have contributed to the current understanding of pandemics could be added to this list.

Interestingly, one can also identify efforts to examine pandemics by integrating more than one discipline. For example, some authors have combined economics and history to analyse previous pandemics (Clay et al. 2018). Building on history and political science, some have studied how democracies and autocracies have dealt with pandemics for the past thousand years (Stasavage 2020). Others have applied international relations theory to developments in international law with a view to analysing emerging infectious diseases in the context of the globalization of public health (Fidler 1997). Still others have explicitly sought to connect the discipline of public health with international relations' expertise on diplomacy to argue that localized, regionalized health diplomacy (rather than global diplomacy) is likely to be less effective (Fazal 2020). In order to address the use of anti-viral drugs during pandemics, some authors have linked the disciplines of pharmacology, epidemiology, and health economics (Kamal et al. 2017). Pandemics have also been the subject of research in academic fields that are not defined by a traditional discipline, such as global studies (e.g. Jacobsen 2018) or gender studies (e.g. Abrahemsen 1997). While these examples are noteworthy, the overwhelming majority of work addressing the causes and consequences of pandemics are hosted within a specific academic discipline.

We might expect that interdisciplinary studies such as Indigenous studies, disability studies, gender studies, race and ethnic studies, public health, and law are well positioned to ask probing questions about the complexities of pandemics, their disparate impacts, and what these reveal about persistent structural injustices. However, the responsibility for wrestling with these questions does not rest with them alone. Yet, they provide some guidance as to the kinds of insights disciplinary scholars can offer if they develop a multidisciplinary perspective.

Given the complexities of pandemics and their impacts, there is a need to establish a dialogue across disciplines that have traditionally examined pandemics independently. It is in this regard that the present volume explicitly adopts a multidisciplinary approach, which means relying on knowledge from multiple disciplines to obtain a broader understanding of a topic (Alvargonzález 2011: 388; Long 2011: 38; Miller 2010; Thompson Klein 2017: 24). It results from ascertaining that a specific phenomenon does not neatly align with the distinctions found in academic disciplines. Limiting the analysis to the concepts, theories, and methods of a single discipline inevitably leaves gaps and offers a narrow understanding of the topic. In order to provide a comprehensive analysis, a multidisciplinary approach calls for the addition of disciplines, as well as a certain form of coordination between them.

It is also worth noting that the ambition of a multidisciplinary approach has some inherent limitations. In contrast to interdisciplinarity or transdisciplinarity, the aim of multidisciplinarity is not to combine several disciplines with a view to providing an integrated analysis (Long 2011: 40; Miller 2010; Thompson Klein 2017: 24). Rather, a multidisciplinary approach considers that a plurality of academic disciplines is relevant and that each discipline can coexist in parallel. While an interdisciplinary approach would seek to identify an integrative framework to complete the analysis, a multidisciplinary approach considers that each discipline can apply its own concepts, theories, and methods with a view to understanding a topic or solving a problem. The absence of integration that characterizes multidisciplinarity is particularly well captured in a typology provided by Thompson Klein (2017: 24): 'Juxtaposition fosters wider scope of knowledge, information, and methods. Yet, disciplines remain separate, retain their original identity, and are not questioned.'

The distinction between a multidisciplinary approach and an interdisciplinary approach can nevertheless be blurred in practice. While conceptually clear, the extent to which the 'juxtaposition' or the 'integration' of more than one discipline materializes in academic research is often difficult to fully grasp. When one seeks to adopt a multidisciplinary approach, completely avoiding the interaction among disciplines within a single work is almost impossible. Even when merely juxtaposing disciplines and maintaining their original identity, a certain form of dialogue inevitably emerges. Scholars of any discipline would be hard pressed to demonstrate that their discipline has developed in total isolation from other disciplines. This book looks for, highlights, induces, and encourages the in-between space among disciplines.

Most importantly, while the absence of integration between disciplines could be perceived as a flaw, it must be stressed that a multidisciplinary approach is relevant in its own right. By combining more than one discipline, a multidisciplinary approach plays a valuable role in expanding knowledge needed to improve our understanding (Thompson Klein 2017: 24). Even without the integration that characterizes the interdisciplinary approach, the relevance of multidisciplinarity is premised on the analytical power that results from adding multiple specialist perspectives (Long 2011: 39). One could even suggest that a multidisciplinary approach contributes to enhancing the stature of participating disciplines, given that it does not threaten their own identities (Miller 2010). Without seeking to challenge the weaknesses of each discipline, a multidisciplinary approach thus builds on their strengths to provide a broader understanding of the phenomenon at hand. A nice balance is achieved between realities, ideas, and the ways in which knowledge production is academically structured.

A multidisciplinary approach is thus a flexible means to account for several factors that must be considered in order to provide a comprehensive understanding of a phenomenon without seeking to reach an integrated paradigm that results from the combination of various disciplines. While multidisciplinarity is necessary to reach such a comprehensive understanding, a certain level of coordination is needed to avoid a form of eclecticism that would counter the benefits of the approach. To a certain extent, a cautious balance must be constantly sought.

Given that pandemics, by their very nature, are widespread and bear implications for a broad range of activities, we believe that studying their causes and consequences is best served by a multidisciplinary approach. As emphasized by Jacobsen in the context of global studies (2018: 658), '[t]he complex pathways leading to the occurrence of pandemics and the complicated responses to them cannot be understood when only one disciplinary or cultural lens is applied'. While each academic discipline can undoubtedly bring a meaningful contribution to our understanding of pandemics, juxtaposing contributions from various disciplines within a single book ensures a more comprehensive analysis of the topic at hand.

More specifically, this volume invites readers from different fields to reflect on their conceptualizations of pandemics and to consider how a multidisciplinary dialogue can stimulate and enrich our understanding of pandemics in our contemporary world. In contrast to an interdisciplinary approach, the aim is not to offer a unique paradigm upon which to conduct research on pandemics. Rather, the main objective is to explore the growing diversity of definitions, approaches, theories, causes, and consequences of pandemics. Our goal is to generate a multidisciplinary dialogue about the ontological, epistemological, paradigmatic, and normative aspects of studying pandemics.

To achieve this end, this book brings together in a single volume essays by political scientists, environmental scholars, legal scholars, clinical pharmacists, economists, scholars of urban planning, scholars in health and medicine schools, and researchers in business and management. Each author was asked to assess and analyse the central causes and consequences pertaining to the study of pandemics in their respective field of research. The authors were also asked to write for a non-specialist audience and to be mindful of how their own contribution fits within attempts to explain pandemics by relying on other disciplines. As a result of the multidisciplinary dialogue that underlies the contributions provided in this text, we believe the concrete impact they have on our understanding of pandemics is greater than the sum of the parts.

Global Ethics and Pandemics

The COVID-19 pandemic presents us with two sets of ethical imperatives. The first ethical imperative is to address preparedness, mortality, vulnerabilities, and the injustices associated with or revealed by these as they relate to the health crisis. The second is to learn from the COVID-19 pandemic the lessons that we need in order to prevent and be prepared for future pandemics. In this sense, ironically given the human tragedy of this crisis, COVID-19 poses an opportunity. COVID-19 is merely a starter pandemic. It is not as contagious as other diseases (such as measles) and not as lethal as some (such as Ebola), and it can be addressed with minor interventions—mask wearing, testing, and contact tracing. Yet, the failings of large populations to be able or willing to participate in these relatively minor interventions meant that as of September 2021, 4.5 million people had died from the disease and a more contagious variant had spread through unvaccinated populations and vaccinated populations alike. On the one hand, the complexities of pandemic preparedness, mortality, vulnerabilities, and injustice reveal that multidisciplinary analysis is necessary for revealing and addressing the threats to global justice posed by the pandemic. On the other hand, the injustices that the pandemic reveals have been latent within local and global political, economic, social, and health systems, thus posing fresh empirical questions best explored by drawing on multidisciplinary analysis.

Preparedness

Global preparedness is measured by the Global Health Security (GHS) Index in terms of anticipated ability to prevent, detect, and respond to a pandemic, the sufficiency and robustness of the health sector, the political and scientific norms for addressing pandemics, and the risks and vulnerabilities related to all of these (GHS Index 2019a).[1]

Measures of global pandemic preparedness may have been operationalizing or weighting some variables incorrectly, tracking the wrong variables, and omitting others. For example, prior to COVID-19, the United States ranked first in terms of prevention, detection, health, and norms (GHS Index 2019b). Brazil also ranked high on prevention, detection, and response (GHS Index 2019c). Both of these countries were not the country of origin of SARS-CoV-2, but they were among those leading in a number of cases of COVID-19 in 2020. By contrast, Mongolia was ranked in the bottom half of all countries on all measures except detection (GHS Index 2019d). Yet, because of strengths in detection and other variables not included in the GHS Index, as of this writing, it has had few cases, no deaths, and most importantly no internal transmission, even though their largest city is as population dense as the epicentre of the initial Italian pandemic (Samarajiva 2020). The timeline of the Mongolian response and its relative success suggests that having a response plan and the capacity to develop a response plan may be an underweighted variable in the GHS Index.

Further, the GHS Index may not be accounting sufficiently for how one measured factor affects other measured factors or how other factors not in the measure (such as dependency within the structure of the economy or interdependencies globally) affect those currently measured (such as the ability to respond). For example, India's economy has a high reliance on migratory labour, such that when the government shut down the economy to mitigate the spread of the virus, they set in motion the mobility of low-income labourers, often to destinations with relatively lower levels of health-care system capacity. Further, the GHS Index does not

[1] 'The 140 GHS Index questions are organized across six categories: 1. Prevention: Prevention of the emergence or release of pathogens; 2. Detection and Reporting: Early detection and reporting for epidemics of potential international concern; 3. Rapid Response: Rapid response to and mitigation of the spread of an epidemic; 4. Health System: Sufficient and robust health system to treat the sick and protect health workers; 5. Compliance with international norms: Commitments to improving national capacity, financing plans to address gaps, and adhering to global norms; 6. Risk Environment: Overall risk environment and country vulnerability to biological threats' (GHS Index 2019a).

account for the ways in which weakness in one aspect of pandemic preparedness cannot be compensated for by strength in another.

Moreover, there seems to have been insufficient attention to the ways that decisions in one country might affect those in another, not only in terms of prevention and detection, but also in terms of norms and managing risk. The WHO has the role of facilitating transnational communication about pandemics, yet it does not have the authority to influence national practices which are the ground game of pandemic detection, response, and health.

While not as lethal or infectious as other diseases, the ability of COVID-19 to be transmitted by asymptomatic infected people not only made detection, response, and health services relatively more important, but also raised the importance of resources to support relatively low-technology health norms (mask wearing and social distancing) for all aspects of preparedness. Thus, in addition to the havoc that COVID-19 has wrought, it has also alerted us to the range of considerations across political, scientific, medical, health, economic, and social factors and the ways that these influence each other in our national and global capacities to address pandemics.

Mortality and Exposure

Because COVID-19 is not water borne, prevention is relatively straightforward and inexpensive: behaviour (social distancing), mask wearing, testing, and tracing. (Once developed, vaccination was important, but executing large-scale global vaccination plans was neither straightforward nor inexpensive.) Yet, despite these being universally available modes of prevention, co-morbidities and variation in implementation of these within and across countries have contributed to spread and differential impacts. Moreover, for considerations of justice and inequity, these differential impacts are not random. They follow discriminatory patterns already existing in society. Gender, sexuality, disability, identity, race, ethnicity (including Indigenous people), caste, capacity, even geography (urban versus rural) and source of livelihood (caregiving) are all bases of discrimination in some contexts. When they intersect, the role of discrimination or oppression in the causal chain can become invisible. Further, these are also structural features of the political economy of most nations that resulted in some people being more likely to be exposed to the pandemic or to its impacts on their lives and livelihoods.

Of course, calculating the effect of SARS-CoV-2 on death rates is difficult due to the ambiguity around co-morbidities (Aron and Muellbauer 2020; WHO 2020). The impact on morbidity more generally is difficult to assess because of the decrease in other mortality rates (such as from transportation accidents because there are fewer people using all modes of transportation during restrictions and as a consequence of behaviour changes) and the increases in other mortalities as people defer health screenings and check-ups. However, lack of data is not evidence that there is no problem to study; it is evidence that even our structures of data collection are inadequate for understanding the impacts of the pandemic (Goha et al. 2021; Reed et al. 2020; Raifman and Raifman 2020).

Mortality due to COVID-19 varies across countries, as well as among groups within countries often by conditions of privilege. For example, economic inequality and gaps in the public health care system mean that in Peru and Bolivia, families struggle to purchase on the black-market oxygen for their sick family members, creating disparities of survival based on privilege. Moreover, considering the long-term health consequences of the disease, we anticipate high concentrations of morbidity due to COVID-19 as a pre-existing condition will be in those populations which were more vulnerable to COVID-19. Thus, there is a triple effect of vulnerability: to the disease, to co-morbidities with the disease, and to the co-morbidities created by the disease.

The ethics of these differences are complicated because while the disease does not discriminate, discriminatory background conditions such as in exposure to environmental toxins, employment patterns, and pre-existing health insecurity create patterns of exposure to the disease, as well as increased likelihood of fatality from the disease, that echo these pre-existing conditions and further expose the injustices within these conditions.

We will pick up this question in the discussion of vulnerabilities. To anticipate, there is no simple story about the demographic effects on COVID-19 mortality. In 'Necropower as a Body Project', Shatema Threadcraft (2020) argues that while biological race did not exist, we have created it. The intersection of race, gender, age, and socio-economic status make us biologically more vulnerable to SARS-CoV-2. Further, the intersection of race, gender, age, and socio-economic status make us more vulnerable to a range of political, economic, social, and health disadvantages and these unjust weaknesses in our systems further contribute to the relative differences in mortality and other health consequences. Therefore, we need a better understanding of the political, economic, social, and health disadvantages that are the background conditions of the world in which SARS-CoV-2 has so successfully thrived.

Vulnerabilities

The preceding discussion suggests that there are two considerations of vulnerabilities brought on by the pandemic: (1) the background discriminations and oppressions that make some people more vulnerable to COVID-19; and (2) the direct and indirect ways that through the social, economic, and political responses to the pandemic and getting the disease individually cause or exacerbate additional harms.

The socio-economic, political, and health background conditions vary by country, but generally follow patterns of discrimination in each country. These include: gender, sexuality, identity, race, ethnicity, caste, capacity, and even geography and source of livelihood. For understanding the impacts of these on vulnerability to COVID-19, we group these as geography (density exposure, access to health care, access to testing, and exposure to environmental toxins), employment, exploited categories (low-wage labour, gender, race, ethnicity, caste), marginalized categories (gender, sexuality, identity, race, ethnicity, caste), and the intersectional effects of these.

Some urban settings have had more access to health care and testing for SARS-CoV-2 than others. Likewise, most rural settings lack adequate health care for treatment and access to testing. These follow other conditions of poverty and affect white, African American, and Indigenous communities.

People who live in concentrated settings such as slums, low-income housing, and high-rise apartments that rely on elevators are more vulnerable to catching SARS-CoV-2. For example, during the first year of the pandemic, the most fatal zip code in New York (11239) included a subsidized housing project. Concentrated settings are not exclusively low-income settings, but they often are. Concentrated settings are not exclusively urban settings; some rural settings require people to live in concentrated ways due to the environment, geography, or availability of water, for example.

Background conditions of exposure to environmental toxins is another way that geography affects vulnerability to COVID-19. Exposure to toxins, particularly those that cause lung damage, may have left those exposed more vulnerable to mortality were they to contract the disease. Low-income, minority, marginalized, and Indigenous populations are more likely to live and work near these toxins.

Vulnerable people have to take vulnerable jobs. In most settings, the background conditions of socio-economic inequality are such that women, minorities, and marginalized groups are disproportionately employed in these vulnerable jobs.

Likewise, there are socio-economic reasons for exposure to SARS-CoV-2. Certain jobs, such as home-care work, health-care work, high-contact jobs as in some parts of the food supply chain, or any of these if they require (as most jobs do for low-wage, urban workers) public transportation in high concentration all make employees relatively more vulnerable to COVID-19. Many of these jobs, such as health care and transportation, are low-wage work deemed 'essential' and thus employees were not given the option of staying home and protecting themselves or their family members during the pandemic without risking their jobs. Other low-wage workers and informal workers such as garbage pickers and care workers continued to work though without minimal personal protective equipment. Certain industries are more vulnerable than others, certain workers are more vulnerable than others, and certain modes of employment (independent, small business, leveraged business, midsize, and large-size industry) also vary in the vulnerability of their workers.

Thus, in most settings these factors intersect. Zip code 11239 in New York has the highest percentage of people over 65, is 49.45% African American, has an unemployment rate of 14.6%, and is 61.1% female. Each of these factors individually is associated with higher vulnerability to COVID-19, but when they intersect—black and Latina women are five times as likely to contract COVID-19 as white women—the ramifications are lethal. While we see correlations between age and mortality, poverty and mortality, and race and mortality, when we look within the data to see intersections, the data tell us both that intersectional forces exacerbate the impacts on some people *and* that those same intersectional forces may obscure that differential in vulnerability. Thus, we need intersectional and multidisciplinary research in order to survive COVID-19, anticipate its created and exacerbated inequalities, and prepare for and ameliorate the impact of the next pandemic.

The vulnerabilities of COVID-19 extend further than surviving the health consequences of COVID-19. These include political, economic, and social vulnerabilities. Which factors are salient and which intersectional forms will vary by context, but a quick consideration of some concrete examples illustrates the range of necessary considerations and the import of multidisciplinary approaches to perceiving and understanding the impacts of COVID-19 on global and local justice. Notice that there are gendered and raced patterns in who is deemed an essential worker and thus not able to stay home from their job (or in the United States eligible to receive the unemployment benefit in the US stimulus packages). As with the health disparities, COVID-19 and the pandemic response have revealed chronic inequalities in vulnerabilities that existed prior to the pandemic and exacerbated these.

With variability by context, loss of employment is highly correlated with loss of access to health care (or the ability to pay for it), increased stress, decrease in nutrition, and decrease in basic health (often correlated with these other changes).

The primary mode of prevention of spread, which has been closing places of business or limiting capacities, has caused loss or suspension of low-wage service work such as taxi driving, hotel cleaning, food service, home-care work, and informal sector work more generally. These sectors not only are generally the most low-paying in an economy, but also employ the most vulnerable within populations.

In addition to environmental and economic vulnerabilities, there are also social vulnerabilities. Reporting of domestic violence against women is up. Reporting on violence against children is down because abuse of children is often identified by mandatory reporters (the teachers, doctors, and caregivers that children are seeing less of during the pandemic) (Mlambo-Ngcuka 2020). Likewise, lockdowns affected people differently and created opportunity for rights violations of others, such as through trafficking. The pandemic may create new entrants into the trafficking business and greater demand for trafficked persons (Collective 2020). Violence against Dalits is going uninterrogated by authorities in India (Gupta 2020). Likewise and additionally, the effects of the pandemic and pandemic response on people with mental illness or mental disabilities, people with certain physical disabilities, people with addictions, people in crowded housing or without housing, sexual and gender minorities, immigrant communities, seasonal migrants outside of their communities, and other vulnerable sub-populations within communities are less visible, but no less important.

Finally, health-care workers treating patients of COVID-19 and journalists covering the crises have suffered the emotional trauma of attending to and witnessing so much suffering and loss of life day after day.

Injustice and Pandemics

In sum, the injustices associated with the pandemic come from pre-existing political, economic, social, and health injustices. These are systemic in the sense that they persist in their differential impacts across a context, consistently rendering the most vulnerable relatively more vulnerable to COVID-19 and its health and economic consequences. Further, the politically and socially vulnerable are made more so by the pandemic. Multidisciplinary inquiry and intersectional analysis better enable us to identify and plan for addressing the global and local injustices of pandemics because they have the capacity to reveal the intersectional and interactive dynamics of underlying vulnerabilities across types of vulnerability, as well as how each and together these are laid bare and exacerbated by the disease and responses to it. Our methods and indices of pandemic preparedness need to keep these in mind. We need to measure them correctly, weight them significantly, and incorporate these into our analyses.

Organization of This Volume

This edited volume provides a comparative analysis of the ways in which pandemics are theorized and studied across several disciplines. It has three objectives: (1) to explore the growing diversity of theories and paradigms developed to study pandemics; (2) to initiate a multidisciplinary dialogue about the ontological, epistemological, paradigmatic, and normative aspects of studying pandemics across disciplines; and (3) to highlight the potential of pandemics to move us towards solutions based on equality and justice.

The relationship between COVID-19 and previous pandemics is a crucial one. While the COVID-19 outbreak has shed light on the need for a multidisciplinary dialogue, the edited volume does more than discuss a timely topic. It addresses the timeless (but periodic) topic of pandemics and allows us to make sense of COVID-19 in our era and into the future. It is in this context that Kathryn H. Jacobsen provides an epidemiological perspective on historic and emerging pandemics in Chapter 1. She highlights that epidemiology generates knowledge on adverse health conditions with a view to preventing new health problems. While the COVID-19 pandemic can be considered as a 'once-in-a-lifetime' event, she underscores that the response to it has drawn from previous pandemics (including cholera, SARS, influenza, HIV/AIDS and non-communicable diseases). Taken as a whole, these events have shown how a multidisciplinary field of 'pandemiology' could be a more robust and effective way to plan for and respond to pandemics.

Absorbed by the various policies and strategies deployed by governments around the world, we tend to forget that viruses are dynamic, constantly adapting, and ever evolving. To capture that dynamic, Dominic Johnson makes the case in Chapter 2 for taking an evolutionary approach to pandemics. He underscores the added value of an evolutionary perspective in making sense of the 'behaviour' of viruses, including virus strategies and mutations. Johnson also traces with unquestionable clarity what an evolutionary approach brings to our understanding of how we humans, the host, react and adapt. By exploring the cognitive challenges of the modern world (Johnson 2020; Johnson and Tierney 2019) and the cultural evolution through which humans interact, Johnson argues that several policies currently adopted might be playing into the hands of the virus. The path to success seems to be about adaptability and swiftness.

While pandemics affect every state and society, some of the consequences need to be politically and contextually analysed. In Chapter 3, Jack Goldstone asks an important yet rarely discussed question about the consequences of pandemics: can pandemics bring about political revolutions or not? Building on his previous well-recognized works on revolution (Goldstone 2001, 2014), Goldstone identifies two paths by which pandemics create pressures for political change: demographic and economic. In the current situation, and with the current knowledge about COVID-19, Goldstone contends that the disease is not severe enough to alter the trajectories of populations in any states. Yet his main argument is that it is important to distinguish among political regimes when analysing the economic impacts. Mass mobilization aimed at overthrowing the existing regime (i.e. a revolution) is only likely in authoritarian regimes, whereas a major political party realignment is only likely in democracies.

If the relationship between pandemics and revolutions is not as conclusive as some might have expected, what about the relationship between pandemics and terrorism, particularly bioterrorism? In Chapter 4, Matthieu Guitton reflects on the possibility that pandemics and bioterrorist events can become synergistic. Focusing on the ontogeny of fear in the digital age, he underscores the role played by the spread of misinformation in the perception of fear, the creation of stigmatized groups, and the possibility of biological threats (Guitton 2019). One of Guitton's arguments is that the convergence of technologies (between pandemics and bioterrorism) can lead to two types of division. The first division refers to the distinction between those who 'follow' the rules and recommendations of health authorities and those who do not trust the government. The second division relates to the creation of stigmatized groups based on socio-economic status, ethnicity, and other vectors.

In Chapter 5, Christopher Bickerton looks at the relationship between regional integration processes and pandemics. It traces several national experiences, focusing on health and economic-related measures. Bickerton shows that government responses have varied considerably—from France's restriction on internal movement, to Sweden's attempt at herd immunity, to the UK's mixed policies. Building on his previous works on European integration (Bickerton 2012; Bickerton et al. 2015), his main argument is that while the pandemic underscored the high level of financial interdependence of national economies within the European Union, it also exposed a deficit in transnational solidarity. While solidarity has been at the centre of national responses, it has largely been absent from health-related policy coordination at the European Union level.

In Chapter 6, Jean-Frédéric Morin, Sikina Jinnah, and Amandine Orsini tackle an often-invoked comparison since March 2020 of comparing pandemics and environmental crises. Drawing on previous works (Morin et al. 2020; Jinnah and Morin 2020), they offer an analysis of the underlying problem structure and the governance systems. On the first dimension, the authors describe the similarities shared by pandemics and environmental crises, including global interdependence, exponential dynamics, and disproportionate impacts. For instance, the consequences of both pandemics and environmental crises are non-linear—they increase over time. Yet the authors argue that pandemics and environmental crises present different governance systems. Among the major differences are the higher degree of centralization and the faster political response of the global health governance system. After offering some explanation for the variation, Morin and colleagues conclude with policy solutions that would improve the synergies between pandemics and environmental crises.

In Chapter 7, Michael Hooper looks at the relationship between pandemics and urban planning. Everyone is now familiar with the term 'social distancing', but many observers have pointed out that social distancing might be more difficult in some locations than in others. Hooper reviews these arguments about the role of urban density in spreading pandemics, while contrasting them with city planners' arguments that densification brings environmental, social, and economic benefits (Hooper 2019). One of Hooper's key arguments is that the relationship between urban density and pandemics is not as straightforward as some would like us to believe. One needs to inject a good dose of complexity in the analysis via the role of hard infrastructures (roads, open space, etc.), soft infrastructures (cultural activities, health-care services), city political governance systems, disaster risk preparedness, and inequality.

Charles-Emmanuel Côté, Richard Ouellet, and Jean-Michel Marcoux explore, in Chapter 8, the consequences of the several restrictionist measures implemented by states for safety reasons. By analysing the provisions allowing states to justify the adoption of these measures in international economic law, they underscore a key tension: while an extensive interpretation of concepts may ease the justification of trade and investment restrictions, the reliance on exceptions may represent an obstacle in fighting the pandemic. The authors trace the significance of exceptions in international agreements, particularly the relationship between pandemics and exceptions under the General Agreement on Tariffs and Trade and World Trade Organization law. They also discuss the links between foreign investment and exceptions in times of pandemic, highlighting the main measures implemented to fight the COVID-19 pandemic that have had an effect on foreign investors. They conclude with a warning: even if relying on exceptions suggests a step forward, it may also represent two steps backward, as some of the exceptions have not been crafted to deal with pandemics, and nationally oriented measures may impede global efforts.

Pandemics have increased gender inequality and the vulnerability of women on various fronts. In Chapter 9, Julia Smith provides a comprehensive analysis of the gender gap exposed since the outbreak of COVID-19, as well as previous pandemics. Emphasizing that the gender dimensions of pandemics are both physical and socially constructed, she applies a gender-based analysis of the gendered dimensions of pandemics and addresses the responses provided by governments and global health institutions (Wenham et al. 2020). More specifically, she focuses on the direct and indirect health impacts of outbreaks, as well as the consequences of pandemics on employment and the economy. She also argues that responses to previous pandemics have largely failed to take into consideration these gendered effects, and that gender-based responses to the ongoing COVID-19 pandemic remain piecemeal, with some notable exceptions. Overall, Smith provides a clear demonstration that pandemics entail a gender equality crisis that reaches beyond the global health crisis that is typically addressed. Her consideration of these gendered dimensions implies both an approach that is genuinely multidisciplinary and the identification of opportunities to improve global justice.

In addition to exacerbating and amplifying pre-existing inequalities, pandemics can also profoundly disrupt various aspects of globalization. One of them is organized crime. As analysed by Robert Muggah in Chapter 10, the unprecedented measures that have been adopted during the COVID-19 pandemic have caused a series of far-reaching and multifaceted effects on organized crime. The chapter thus provides an analysis of three areas where this specific pandemic has altered the opportunity structure of organized crime: (1) several shifts in criminal violence due to the imposition of lockdowns; (2) the migration of criminal actors to cyberspace; and (3) the diversification of operations with a view to rapidly responding to changes in supply and demand. Muggah also highlights how new strategies to deter organized crime have emerged as a response to these evolving changes resulting from the pandemic. In addition to strategies that have emerged under the auspices of some agencies of the United Nations and national governments, non-governmental organizations have also been particularly active in the fight against organized crime. While the COVID-19 pandemic has had an undeniable impact on organized crime, one must also expect a profound reconfiguration of enforcement efforts to counter them.

While the ambition of this book is resolutely multidisciplinary, Chapter 11 by Christophe Roux Dufort and Mary-Liéta Clément relies on an interdisciplinary approach. It provides an original understanding of crisis management as a tragedy by explicitly relying on philosophy and literature. Considering that tragedy offers new avenues to address decision-makers' behaviour in times of crisis, the authors specifically apply this analytical framework to decisions made during pandemics. More specifically, they highlight five components of tragedy that are identified in classic literature (confiscation of alternatives, duplication of reality, sacrifice, self-fulfilling decisions, and retrospective failure) and explain how these components relate to crisis management in times of pandemic. Building on this tragic reading of crisis management, Roux Dufort and Clément propose a four-stage model of the evolution and development of crises.

In Chapter 12, Sara Davies revisits the failure of international health cooperation when dealing with pandemics, particularly COVID-19. She traces the evolution of international health governance and health security going back over two decades. Davies describes the various commissions and regulatory bodies created over time, along with some of the key recommendations these institutions issued (Davies 2010). While the dominant narrative about international health governance underscores its failure and its considerable lack of cooperation, she puts forward a different narrative. Davies argues that, despite the fact that we do observe many blockades to bilateral states' health cooperation, global health governance not only continued to function, but also has in fact grown. She observes a profound transformation: global health governance during the current pandemic shifted from the traditional two-level, state-orientated system of international cooperation towards a significantly more dynamic, multilevel system of global cooperation, which includes cooperation in the domains of surveillance, human rights, and sciences.

In parallel to efforts deployed to find a vaccine during pandemics, a colossal amount of resources and work is also put into identifying promising treatments.

A comprehensive understanding of pandemics thus calls for a consideration of challenges that pharmacists must face in times characterized by a high level of uncertainty. In Chapter 13, Luc Bergeron and Martin Darveau focus on three specific aspects of the practice of pharmacy that can be significantly challenged by a pandemic. First, relying on previously developed therapeutic treatments to treat patients infected by a new disease implies some risks. The sentiment of urgency brought about by the evolving situation and the positions taken by various public figures rapidly put pharmacists at odds with their science-based training. Second, with the outbreak of a new disease, various factors can seriously affect the predictability of drug supplies to hospitals. It is in this context that a carefully crafted action plan must be implemented. Third, considering that pharmacists are not immune to developing the new disease, pandemics impose additional challenges on pharmaceutical care. When considered as a whole, these challenges offer an opportunity to review current practices in pharmacy.

In Chapter 14, Markus Herrmann and Maripier Isabelle tackle the economic determinants on which public policy decisions are made to safeguard population health, while paying special attention to the issue of income and employment losses incurred on the labour market. Their main argument is that governments should account for the social benefits in preserving the public good of population health and the costs of measures aimed at containing the pandemics. Herrmann and Isabelle discuss the key challenge associated with such an equilibrium: while policymakers do not have complete knowledge of all the variables, particularly that restrictive measures may have unevenly distributed costs across individuals and families, they nonetheless need to include these uncertainties when making a decision. By focusing on the labour market, the authors are able to underscore that vulnerable groups tend to be disproportionately hit by the virus both in terms of health inequalities and disproportionate economic impacts.

In Chapter 15, Geneviève Parent analyses the relationship between pandemics and food security. Building on the literature on food systems, she starts by describing the various food systems currently in place to show that since the mid-1990s we have witnessed the rise of an intensive and financialized agro-industrial food system of mass production. Parent then moves on to introduce the idea of food system resilience, which is characterized by three capacities: adaptive, absorptive, and transformative. These capacities encapsulate how and to what extent individuals, communities, and societies react to shocks. Parent's main argument is that the United Nations' Food Systems Summit, to be held in 2021, is the ideal opportunity to move beyond the dominant narrative of opposing global food systems with territorialized food systems in order to think about resilient and sustainable food systems.

Finally, in Chapter 16, Andrea Bjorklund focuses on the question of force majeure, a doctrine found in most municipal laws, which excuses or arrests contractual obligations because of an external event or follow-on effects that are beyond the control of the parties involved and which prevent them from fulfilling their obligations (Bjorklund 2008). Force majeure is not only invoked in domestic law; states can and have used force majeure in the context of public international law. Bjorklund explores the applicability of this use of force majeure, and, if applicable, the consequences of such in relationship to pandemics. She discusses criteria for the application of force majeure in domestic and public international law to argue that force majeure provides limited redress for parties seeking to avoid their contracts.

References

Abrahamsen, Rita. 1997. 'Gender Dimensions of AIDS in Zambia'. *Journal of Gender Studies* 6 (2): p. 177.

Alvargonzález, David. 2011. 'Multidisciplinarity, Interdisciplinarity, Transdisciplinarity, and the Sciences'. *International Studies in the Philosophy of Sciences* 25 (4): p. 387.

Aron, Janine, and John Muellbauer. 2020. 'A Pandemic Primer on Excess Mortality Statistics and Their Comparability across Countries'. *Our World in Data*, 29 June. https://ourworldindata.org/covid-excess-mortality.

Bickerton, Christopher J. 2012. *European Integration: From Nation-States to Member States*. Oxford: Oxford University Press.

Bickerton, Christopher J., Dermot Hodson, and Uwe Puetter. 2015. 'The New Intergovernmentalism: European Integration in the Post-Maastricht Era'. *JCMS: Journal of Common Market Studies* 53 (4): 703–22.

Bjorklund, Andrea. 2008. 'Emergency Exceptions to International Obligations in the Realm of Foreign Investment: The State of Necessity and Force Majeure as Circumstances Precluding Wrongfulness'. In *Oxford Handbook of International Investment Law*, edited by Peter Muchlinski and Federico Ortino, pp. 459-523. Oxford: Oxford University Press.

Clay, Karen, Joshua Lewis, and Edson Severnini. 2018. 'Pollution, Infectious Disease, and Mortality: Evidence for the 1918 Spanish Influenza Pandemic'. *Journal of Economic History* 78 (4): p. 1179.

Collective. 2020. 'Human Trafficking and Migrant Smuggling Section 2020: Impact of the COVID-19 Pandemic on Trafficking in Persons'. UN Office on Drugs and Crime. https://www.cfr.org/blog/evolution-human-trafficking-during-covid-19-pandemic.

Davies, Sara E. 2008. 'Securitizing Infectious Disease'. *International Affairs* 84 (2): p. 295.

Davies, Sara E. 2010. 'What Contribution Can International Relations Make to the Evolving Global Health Agenda?' *International Affairs* 86 (5): p. 1167.

De Bengy Puyvallée, Antoine, and Sonja Kittelsen. 2019. '"Disease Knows No Borders": Pandemics and the Politics of Global Health Security'. In *Pandemics, Publics, and Politics*, edited by Kristian Bjørkdahl and Benedicte Carlsen, pp. 59–73. London: Palgrave Macmillan.

Dingwall, Robert, Lily M. Hoffman, and Karen Staniland. 2013. 'Introduction: Why a Sociology of Pandemics?' *Sociology of Health and Illness* 35 (2): p. 167.

Echenberg, Myron. 2011. *Africa in the Time of Cholera: A History of Pandemics from 1817 to the Present*. Cambridge: Cambridge University Press.

Elbe, Stefan. 2010. 'Pandemic Security'. In *The Routledge Handbook on New Security Studies*, edited by J. Peter Burgess, pp. 163–72. London: Routledge.

Fazal, Tanisha. 2020. 'Health Diplomacy in Pandemical Times'. *International Organization* (IO COVID-19 Online Supplemental Issue): pp. 1–20.

Fidler, David P. 1996. 'Globalization, International Law, and Emerging Infectious Diseases'. *Emerging Infectious Diseases* 2 (2): p. 77.

Fidler, David. P. 1997. 'The Globalization of Public Health: Emerging Infectious Diseases and International Relations'. *Indiana Journal of Global Legal Studies* 5 (1): p. 11.

Fidler, David P. 2003. 'Emerging Trends in International Law Concerning Global Infectious Disease Control'. *Emerging Infectious Diseases* 9 (3): p. 285.

Ford, Stephen M., and John D. Grabenstein. 2006. 'Pandemics, Avian Influenza A (H5N1), and a Strategy for Pharmacists'. *Pharmacotherapy* 26 (3): p. 312.

GHS Index. 2019a. 'About'. https://www.ghsindex.org/about.

GHS Index. 2019b. '2019 GHS Index Country Profile for United States'. https://www.ghsindex.org/country/united-states.

GHS Index. 2019c. '2019 GHS Index Country Profile for Brazil'. https://www.ghsindex.org/country/brazil.

GHS Index. 2019d. '2019 GHS Index Country Profile for Mongolia'. https://www.ghsindex.org/country/mongolia.

Goha, Ahmed, et al. 2021. 'Indigenous People and the Covid-19 Pandemic: The Tip of an Iceberg of Social and Economic Inequities'. *Journal of Epidemiology and Community Health* 75 (2): p. 207.

Goldstone, Jack A. 2001. 'Toward a Fourth Generation of Revolutionary Theory'. *Annual Review of Political Science* 4 (1): pp. 139–87.

Goldstone, Jack A. 2014. *Revolutions: A Very Short Introduction*. Oxford: Oxford University Press.

Greitens, Sheena. 2020. 'Surveillance, Security, and Liberal Democracy in the Post-COVID World'. *International Organization* (IO COVID-19 Online Supplemental Issue): pp. 1–22.

Guitton, Matthieu J. 2019. 'Manipulation through Online Sexual Behavior: Exemplifying the Importance of Human Factor in Intelligence and Counterintelligence in the Big Data Era'. *International Journal of Intelligence, Security, and Public Affairs* 21 (2): p. 117.

Gupta, Rudrani. 2020. 'Hatras Gang Rape Was Not the First. There Is a List of Heinous Crimes against Dalit Women'. *Shethepeople*, 30 September. https://www.shethepeople.tv/news/hathras-gang-rape-crimes-against-dalit-women.

Halpern, Michaela S. 2020. 'State Obligations under Public International Law during Pandemics'. *Emory International Law Review* 35: p. 1.

Heath, J. Benton. 2020. 'Pandemics and Other Health Emergencies'. In *The Oxford Handbook on the International Law of Global Security*, edited by Robin Geiss and Nils Melzer, pp. 585-605. Oxford: Oxford University Press.

Hooper, Michael. 2019. 'When Diverse Norms Meet Weak Plans: The Organizational Dynamics of Urban Rubble Clearance in Post-Earthquake Haiti'. *International Journal of Urban and Regional Research* 43 (2): pp. 292–312.

Huang, Yanzhong. 2014. 'Pandemics and Security'. In *Routledge Handbook of Global Health Security*, edited by Simon Rushton and Jeremy Youde, pp. 83–91. London: Routledge.

Jacobsen, Kathryn H. 2018. 'Pandemics'. In *The Oxford Handbook of Global Studies*, edited by Mark Juergensmeyer, Saskia Sassen, Manfred B. Steger, and Victor Faessel, pp. 647–62. Oxford: Oxford University Press.

Jinnah, Sikina, and Jean-Frédéric Morin. 2020. *Greening through Trade: How American Trade Policy Is Linked to Environmental Protection Abroad*. Cambridge: MIT Press.

Johnson, Dominic. 2020. *Strategic Instincts: The Adaptive Advantages of Cognitive Biases in International Politics*. Princeton, NJ: Princeton University Press.

Johnson, Dominic, and Dominic Tierney. 2019. 'Bad World: The Negativity Bias in International Politics'. *International Security* 43 (3): pp. 96–140.

Kamal, Mohamed A., et al. 2017. 'Interdisciplinary Pharmacometrics Linking Oseltamivir Pharmacology, Influenza Epidemiology and Health Economics to Inform Antiviral Use in Pandemics'. *British Journal of Clinical Pharmacology* 83: p. 1580.

Kamradt-Scott, Adam, and Colin McInnes. 2012. 'The Securitisation of Pandemic Influenza: Framing, Security and Public Policy'. *Global Public Health* 7 (S2): p. S95.

Keil, Roger, and Harris Ali. 2007. 'Governing the Sick City: Urban Governance in the Age of Emerging Infectious Disease'. *Antipode* 39 (5): p. 846.

Kenwick, Michael, and Beth Simmons. 2020. 'Pandemic Response as Border Politics'. *International Organization* (IO COVID-19 Online Supplemental Issue): pp. 1–23.

Keogh-Brown, Marcus R., Simon Wren-Lewis, W. John Edmunds, Philippe Beutels, and Richard D. Smith. 2010. 'The Possible Macroeconomic Impact on the UK of an Influenza Pandemic'. *Health Economics* 19: p. 1345.

Lee, Jong-Wha, and Warwick J. McKibbin. 2004. 'Globalization and Disease: The Case of SARS'. *Asian Economic Papers* 3 (1): p. 113.

Lipscy, Phillip Y. 2020. 'COVID-19 and the Politics of Crisis'. *International Organization* (IO COVID-19 Online Supplemental Issue): pp. 1–30.

Long, David. 2011. 'Interdisciplinarity and the Study of International Relations'. In *International Studies: Interdisciplinary Approaches*, edited by Pami Aalto, Vilho Harle, and Sami Moisio, pp. 31–65. London: Palgrave Macmillan.

Matthew, Richard A., and Bryan McDonald. 2006. 'Cities under Siege: Urban Planning and the Threat of Infectious Disease'. *Journal of the American Planning Association* 72 (1): p. 109.

McLafferty, Sara. 2010. 'Placing Pandemics: Geographical Dimensions of Vulnerability and Spread'. *Eurasian Geography and Economics* 51 (2): p. 143.

Miller, Raymond C. 2010. 'Interdisciplinarity: Its Meaning and Consequences'. In *Oxford Research Encyclopedia: International Studies*, edited by Renée Marlin-Bennett, online version. Oxford: Oxford University Press.

Mlambo-Ngcyka, Phumzile. 2020. 'Violence against Women and Girls: The Shadow Pandemic'. *UN Women*, 6 April. https://www.unwomen.org/en/about-us/about-un-women.

Morin, Jean-Frédéric, Amandine Orsini, and Sikina Jinnah. 2020. *Global Environmental Politics*. Oxford: Oxford University Press.

Porta, Miquel. 2016. 'Pandemic'. In *A Dictionary of Epidemiology*, edited by Miquel Porta (6th edn). Oxford: Oxford University Press.

Raifman, Matthew A., and Julia R. Raifman. 2020. 'Disparities in the Population at Risk of Severe Illness from Covid-19 by Race/Ethnicity and Income'. *American Journal of Preventive Medicine* 59 (1): p. 137.

Reed, Nicholas S., Lisa M. Meeks, and Bonnielin K. Swenor. 2020. 'Disability and Covid-19: Who Counts Depends on Who Is Counted'. *The Lancet* 5 (8): e423.

Samarajiva, Indi. 2020. 'COVID Underdogs: Mongolia—the Best COVID-19 Response in the World'. *Medium*, 18 May. https://medium.com/indica/covid-underdogs-mongolia-3b0c162427c2.
Smith, Maxwell, and Ross Upshur. 2019. 'Pandemic Disease, Public Health, and Ethics'. In *The Oxford Handbook of Public Health Ethics*, edited by Anna C. Mastroianni, Jeffrey P. Kahn, and Nancy E. Kass, pp. 797–809. Oxford: Oxford University Press.
Stasavage, David. 2020. 'Democracy, Autocracy, and Emergency Threats: Lessons for COVID-19 from the Last Thousand Years'. *International Organization* (IO COVID-19 Online Supplemental Issue): pp. 1–17.
Thompson Klein, Julia. 2017. 'Typologies of Interdisciplinarity: The Boundary Work of Definition'. In *The Oxford Handbook of Interdisciplinarity*, edited by Robert Frodeman, Julie Thompson Klein, and Roberto C.-S. Pacheco, pp. 21–34 (2nd edn). Oxford: Oxford University Press.
Threadcraft, Shatema. 2020. 'Necropower as a Body Project'. Work in progress.
Welford, Mark. 2018. *Geographies of Plague Pandemics: The Spatial–Temporal Behavior of Plague to the Modern Day*. London: Routledge.
Wenham, Clare, Julia Smith, and Rosemary Morgan. 2020. 'COVID-19: The Gendered Impacts of the Outbreak'. *The Lancet* 395 (10227): p. 846.
World Health Organization (WHO). 2020. 'Estimating Mortality from COVID-19'. Scientific Brief, 4 August. https://www.who.int/news-room/commentaries/detail/estimating-mortality-from-covid-19.

1
An Epidemiological Perspective on historic and Emerging Pandemics

Kathryn H. Jacobsen

Defining Pandemics

Epidemiologists are public health scientists who quantify the various health issues that affect populations; identify the social, environmental, and other factors that cause those adverse health conditions; and then apply that knowledge to the prevention of new public health problems and the resolution of existing ones. In the language of epidemiology, a pandemic is a worldwide or widespread epidemic of a disease that causes a substantial number of people to become ill (Porta 2016). When determining whether a pandemic is occurring, epidemiologists usually consider geography, frequency, and severity. Together, these three dimensions are used to evaluate whether an event is global, epidemic, and a threat to population health.

To meet the geographic requirement for classification as a pandemic, a disease must adversely affect multiple world regions at one time (Card 2012). The word 'pandemic' conveys a sense of risk and urgency (Doshi 2011), but the 'pan-' prefix means all (or everyone) and is not derived from root words related to panic. An outbreak of a deadly infectious disease that devastates affected communities but remains contained within one world region is not a pandemic event. A pandemic only happens when local transmission of a pathogen is occurring simultaneously on several continents or in several world regions (Kelly 2011).

The difference between a global public health concern and a pandemic is illustrated by the way the World Health Organization (WHO) changed its classification of the novel coronavirus that was first identified in Wuhan, China, in the final weeks of 2019. The WHO declared the newly identified SARS-CoV-2 coronavirus to be a public health emergency of international concern (PHEIC), an official categorization based on criteria in the International Health Regulations (IHR), on 30 January 2020, after several thousand confirmed cases had occurred in China and a few dozen cases had occurred in other countries among travellers from China and their close contacts (WHO, 2020a). The WHO did not designate COVID-19,

Kathryn H. Jacobsen, *An Epidemiological Perspective on Historic and Emerging Pandemics.* In: *A Multidisciplinary Approach to Pandemics.* Edited by Philippe Bourbeau, Jean-Michel Marcoux, and Brooke A. Ackerly, Oxford University Press. © Oxford University Press (2022). DOI: 10.1093/oso/9780192897855.003.0002

the disease caused by infection with SARS-CoV-2, as a pandemic until 1 March 2020, after thousands of locally acquired cases were diagnosed in the Republic of Korea, Iran, and Italy and community transmission had been observed in dozens of other countries (WHO, 2020b).

An epidemic is a time period in which new cases of an adverse health condition are occurring at higher-than-expected rates (Barreto et al. 2006). The statistic that is most often used to quantify the frequency of new cases of an infectious disease in a population is the incidence rate, which is the number of new diagnoses in a selected time period, such as a day or a week, divided by the population at risk of the infection during that time period. Individuals who are already immune to an infectious disease because of current or prior infection or vaccination are removed from the denominator because they are not at risk of new infection. The high incidence rates for SARS-CoV-2 infection in many countries during 2020 were documented by laboratory-confirmed case counts, which were known to underestimate the true burden from coronavirus, especially in places with limited laboratory capacity, and by tallies of suspected cases who met clinical case definitions for COVID-19 based on signs and symptoms rather than laboratory tests.

Because the incidence rates for most adverse health conditions vary by place and time, there is no rule that an epidemic is declared when the incidence rate doubles from baseline or increases by some other preselected multiplier or when case counts exceed a predetermined number of cases per 100,000 residents per week. If a disease routinely occurs in a population, the status of the disease in that population changes from endemic to epidemic when the incidence rate spikes to a value that is qualitatively deemed to be higher than normal. Emerging infectious diseases have an expected incidence rate of zero, but they may shift from being classified as outbreaks when only sporadic cases are occurring to being classified as epidemics when there is sustained local transmission in human populations.

Severity is often considered to be the most nebulous of the three criteria for a pandemic. Traditional epidemiologic definitions may omit this component, focusing on spatial distribution and case counts rather than subjective deliberations about whether a global epidemic should be prioritized for public health action (Porta 2016). There is no set case fatality rate (measured in units such as deaths per 1,000 cases) or mortality rate (measured in units such as deaths per 100,000 total population members) that must be exceeded for a disease to be classified as severe. At the individual level, a disease that causes serious illness, long-term disability, or death is severe. At the population level, severity is a function of the number of people who develop severe disease and the psychological, social, political, and financial hardships that are caused by widespread illness or by the public health interventions used to prevent importation and limit local transmission.

Scientists knew soon after the detection of SARS-CoV-2 in Wuhan that the virus had a relatively low case fatality rate in most age groups but posed a high risk to older adults and individuals with a variety of comorbidities. Because the virus was so contagious and caused moderate to severe disease in a substantial proportion of infected adults, the novel coronavirus was quickly determined to be a significant threat to individual-level and population-level health in affected places. The severity of COVID-19 was confirmed by reports that many places experiencing SARS-CoV-2 epidemics had hospitalization rates and all-cause mortality rates that far exceeded the expected rates based on typical seasonal and demographic patterns and by evidence of a global economic slowdown caused by coronavirus-related restrictions on mobility and commerce. Many countries closed workplaces, schools, restaurants, and public venues for weeks or months to slow the rates of community transmission of SARS-CoV-2. Some of those nations had incidence rates that were relatively low compared to the hardest-hit areas, but they still experienced economic shocks and major disruptions to normal daily routines.

Emerging infectious diseases usually have greater pandemic potential than existing ones because novel pathogens can spread quickly through populations that have no immunological protection against them from prior infections or vaccines. Local SARS-CoV-2 epidemics were quickly established in new countries and world regions in the early months of 2020 as international travel introduced the virus into immunologically naïve populations. While the COVID-19 pandemic was a 'once-in-a-century' event, the response to it drew on the lessons learned from prior pandemics, including the cholera pandemics of the nineteenth century.

Cholera and SARS: Pandemics and International Health Regulations

A series of devastating cholera pandemics occurred in quick succession during the height of the colonial era. The first wave began in Asia and then spread across the globe through the shipping industry between 1817 and 1823. Subsequent pandemics occurred in 1826–1838, 1839–1855, 1863–1874, 1881–1896, and 1899–1923 (Lee 2001). *Vibrio cholerae* bacteria cause severe diarrhoea that can rapidly lead to death from dehydration. Tens of millions of people died as cholera spread across Asia and the Middle East, moved into Europe and North Africa, and was eventually transported to the Americas (Lee and Dodgson 2000). Quarantines of incoming ships and sailors had been somewhat effective in limiting the spread of plague, a bacterial infection (*Yersinia pestis*) transmitted to humans through the bites of fleas that live on rats and other rodents, but they were not effective against an infection that was transmitted through contaminated water. The discharge of ballast water from ships into harbours could cause outbreaks of cholera at ports of call long before quarantined sailors were allowed to come onshore (Ruiz et al. 2000).

Scientific experimentation methods for identifying effective disease control interventions were available even before John Snow linked an outbreak of cholera in London in 1854 to a public water pump on Broad Street. Snow's discovery provided evidence that cholera was acquired through ingestion of faeces-contaminated water, countering the widespread miasma theory that blamed febrile diseases on exposure to foul-smelling airs. However, there was little incentive to apply Snow's finding to international shipping during an era in which the economic benefits of international commerce tended to be seen as far outweighing the health risks of cross-border travel (Huber 2006). A series of International Sanitary Conferences that were held with delegates from European countries and several other nations between 1851 and 1911 aimed to limit slowdowns of international trade during cholera epidemics and pandemics. Haphazard binational agreements were replaced with more robust multinational ones that sought to protect public health, but also restricted the limitations that signatories could place on international trade during epidemics (Lee and Dodgson 2000).

Recent pandemics have similarly raised anxiety about global integration, while reminding businesses and consumers of the benefits of global trade and the inconveniences associated with disruption to the exchanges of goods and people (see Chapter 8 by Côté et al. and Chapter 14 by Herrmann and Isabelle in this volume). The International Sanitary Regulations (ISR) developed during the International Sanitary Conferences of the nineteenth century to improve information sharing and transportation safety during epidemics were the foundation for the WHO's initial communicable disease rules enacted in 1951, shortly after the organization's founding in 1948 (Fidler 2005). In 1969, the ISR were renamed the International Health Regulations (IHR), and the list of notifiable diseases was updated to include cholera, plague, relapsing fever, smallpox, typhus, and yellow fever. Modifications made in 1973 and 1981 reduced the number of reportable diseases to just cholera, plague, and yellow fever, calling for 'maximum security' against pandemics but emphasizing 'minimal interference' with world travel and trade (Fidler 2005).

The emergence of severe acute respiratory syndrome (SARS) early in the twenty-first century revealed some major limitations in global pandemic preparedness (Heymann 2004). The first cases of SARS were identified in Guangdong, China, in November 2002. In March 2003, SARS spread to Hong Kong, an outbreak occurred in Toronto, Canada, and several other countries reported cases in international travellers. The affected countries were able to contain their SARS epidemics by isolating patients and quarantining their contacts (Lipsitch et al. 2003), and in July 2003 the WHO announced that the global outbreak was contained. SARS ended up being a 'mini pandemic' that caused about 8,000 cases and 800 deaths (Cherry 2004). Fears that this coronavirus disease would cause a devastating pandemic or become endemic with seasonal epidemics were not realized (see Chapter 12 by Davies in this volume). However, this scare revealed the limitations of a short list of notifiable diseases, disincentives for countries to communicate openly about non-reportable diseases, and the limited ability of the WHO and its member nations to enforce compliance with reporting mandates and with limiting responses to outbreaks in other countries to recommended WHO actions rather than more restrictive ones (Kamradt-Scott and Rushton 2012).

The 2005 revision of the IHR mandates that the governments of all United Nations member nations notify the WHO immediately about any outbreaks of infectious diseases that could become international public health emergencies. Mandatory reporting now applies to influenza, viral haemorrhagic fevers, and all other emerging infectious diseases that have the potential to become pandemic. The increased focus on global health security includes enhanced requirements for conducting continuous routine public health surveillance, communicating with the WHO about population health status, and coordinating response efforts with the WHO and other entities (Hoffman 2010).

The 2005 IHR created a new classification system for infectious diseases with pandemic potential. A PHEIC can be declared by the WHO when an infectious disease that causes severe illnesses is likely to, or has already, spread to other countries and requires a coordinated global response (Bennett and Carney 2017). Several events have been declared to meet the PHEIC criteria: the 2009–2010 H1N1 influenza pandemic, the outbreak of the Ebola virus in West Africa in 2014–2016, a resurgence of polio that began in 2014, the spread of Zika virus in the Americas in 2016, the spread of Ebola virus in the Democratic Republic of the Congo in 2019–2020, and the COVID-19 pandemic that began in 2020 (Wilder-Smith and Osman 2020). PHEIC status enables the WHO to provide technical, financial, and other support for epidemic control efforts in exchange for affected countries accepting and following through on the policy and practice guidelines issued by the WHO.

The responses to both cholera and SARS had to balance national and international security goals with the realities of a globalized system of commerce (McCloskey et al. 2014). Countries can attempt to isolate from the rest of the world to keep harmful pathogens from crossing into new geographic areas, but closing borders to raw materials, manufactured goods, and other imported products can wreak havoc on economies and the workforce, as was so clearly observed during the various waves of the COVID-19 pandemic. (As highlighted by Herrmann and Isabelle in Chapter 14 of this volume, the integration of economies and supply chains have both shaped the geography of contamination and magnified the cost of inaction and of protective measures deployed during pandemics).

Influenza and Pandemic Preparedness

Influenza is a major concern of epidemiologists and public health emergency planners because influenza viruses are airborne pathogens that can be easily transmitted between humans, influenza infections can cause severe illness and death in a sizable proportion of infected individuals, and the viruses undergo frequent mutations that can generate highly contagious and virulent new strains (Eccleston-Turner et al. 2019). An emergent influenza virus can quickly circle the globe. The first truly global influenza pandemic is likely to have occurred in 1510, soon after global shipping began linking the Americas with the rest of the world (Kamradt-Scott 2012). Subsequent pandemics of influenza, or at least influenza-like diseases, occurred in the 1730s, 1760s, 1780s, 1830s, 1840s, 1890s, and several times thereafter (Morens and Fauci 2007).

The 'Spanish flu' pandemic that began in 1918 is likely to have originated either in China or on pig farms in Kansas, in the United States, before spreading globally (Palmer 2010). Spain was not heavily affected by the pandemic, but Spain was a neutral country during the First World War and did not censor reports of cases, unlike neighbouring European countries, which did not want reports of mass casualties from infections to be in the news. Spanish reporting about the pandemic unfairly led to the flu being regarded as a Spanish phenomenon by other countries, even as Spain referred to the virus as 'French flu' (Palmer 2010). The pandemic caused tens of millions of deaths, with the highest rates of excess mortality occurring in South Asia, sub-Saharan Africa, and East Asia (Murray et al. 2006).

Typical influenza strains cause seasonal outbreaks, with peak incidence in the northern hemisphere between November and March and peak incidence in the southern hemisphere between April and September (Newman et al. 2018). Those seasonal strains typically have the highest fatality rates among neonates, adults of advanced age, and people with weak immune system responses due to chronic illnesses or the side effects of medical treatments. Novel influenza pathogens do not follow seasonal patterns, and they do not always affect the typical at-risk populations. The new influenza strain that emerged in 1918 caused the highest death rates among young adults in their twenties and thirties (Murray et al. 2006).

The configuration of two of the proteins on the surface of influenza A viruses are used to classify influenza types: hemagglutinin (H) and neuraminidase (N). Pandemics in the 1800s were probably caused primarily by H2N2 and H3N8 strains (Neumann and Kawaoka 2019). The strain that emerged in 1918 was an H1N1 influenza. H1N1 remained the dominant influenza virus circulating in human populations for several decades after 1918. H2N2 became the dominant strain after a pandemic in 1957–1960, then was replaced by an H3N2 strain after a pathogen that was first diagnosed in Hong Kong caused a pandemic in 1968–1972 (Glezen 1996). In April 2009, about 90 years after the H1N1 pandemic of 1918–1920 wreaked havoc globally, the first cases of a novel H1N1 virus were diagnosed in Mexico and the US state of California.

Various influenza viruses affect birds, pigs, humans, and a variety of other animals. New vaccine formulations are developed every year to account for minor mutations called antigenic drift. More dramatic changes called antigenic shift occur when two very different types of influenza viruses, typically from two different animals, merge and form a novel strain of influenza. The 2009 H1N1 strain was a 'human swine influenza A' that had originated in pigs, before mutating in ways that enabled it to be transmitted easily between humans. Although influenza viruses are spread through the air and pigs were not part of the chain of transmission for the new human strain, the name 'swine flu' incorrectly implied that pigs and pork products were dangerous (Schein et al. 2012). Alternative names like 'Mexican flu' and 'North American flu', based on the locations where the first cases were identified, led to unfair stigmatizing of Mexicans (Schein et al. 2012).

Even though scientists determined early on that the 2009 strain did not cause severe disease in most people who contracted it, the virulence of the 1918 strain raised concern about the potential for a novel H1N1 strain to cause millions of deaths among young adults (Girard et al. 2010). On 25 April 2009, soon after H1N1 was shown to be spreading between humans, the WHO declared H1N1 to be a PHEIC. This was the first-ever PHEIC declaration since that designation was created by the 2005 revisions to the IHR, and it triggered mandated H1N1 surveillance, reporting, and communication by all United Nations member nations.

Because of the persistent threat of a pandemic influenza event, the WHO uses a six-phase classification to recommend the planning, monitoring, communication, and other actions that member nations should implement at various times. Phases 1–3 describe times when animal influenza viruses are causing no more than sporadic cases of human disease. On 27 April 2009, the WHO designated H1N1 as a phase 4 situation after human-to-human infections were confirmed. Two days later, on 29 April, the pandemic shifted into phase 5 when outbreaks were confirmed in two countries within one world region. By 11 June, sustained local outbreaks were confirmed to be occurring in a second world region, and H1N1 had reached phase 6, the highest level on the WHO's pandemic influenza scale (Dupras and Williams-Jones 2012).

Although the six phases describe geographic spread rather than indicating the severity of the disease caused by an influenza strain, the language of a highest-phase pandemic created significant anxiety in many places (Chew and Eysenbach 2010). Public health officials quickly advised against non-essential international travel, and several countries quarantined or banned travellers from North America (Katz and Fischer 2010). Officials in lower-income countries recommended social distancing, while high-income countries stockpiled antivirals, even though there was uncertainty about whether existing drugs would be effective against the new strain (Shetty 2009). Some schools in some countries were temporarily closed to slow transmission of the virus, but this was not a widely used preventative method (Cauchemez et al. 2014).

Case reports can only be submitted to the WHO by countries that have the epidemiological and laboratory capacity to track cases and test for circulating pathogens. During the early months of the 2009 H1N1 pandemic, countries that were unable to test for H1N1 were left off the map of confirmed cases. Much of the African continent looked like an H1N1-free zone, even though countries in the region were almost certainly experiencing influenza epidemics. The distribution of cases on the world map filled in as more countries were able to test for H1N1, and by December 2009 cases had been reported by more than 200 countries (Girard et al. 2010). By that time, however, H1N1 was no longer considered to be a major threat to global public health because worldwide death totals were in the thousands rather than the millions expected from a severe influenza pandemic (Dawood et al. 2012). On 10 August 2010, the WHO declared that the H1N1 pandemic was over.

The governmental, media, and public responses as the COVID-19 pandemic widened its geographic reach in 2020 ended up being similar to both the 1918–1920 and 2009–2010 influenza pandemics: early confusion over what to call the pathogen, followed by intentional use of politically pejorative terms such as 'China virus' after the strain was officially named according to international scientific protocols; severe undercounting of cases in low-income countries due to limited laboratory capacity; disparities in the distribution of medical supplies (including personal protective equipment, medications, and then vaccines) and media attention, with high-income countries benefitting from greater resources than low-income countries; and a mishmash of recommended preventative actions that varied significantly by country, did not always align with scientific evidence, changed over time at unpredictable junctures rather than being directly linked to scientific advances, and were often communicated poorly.

There are still few good options available for slowing or stopping the spread of novel respiratory viruses. (And, as discussed in Herrmann and Isabelle in Chapter 14 in this volume, these measures come at a cost and the institutional and individual incentives to implement such measures do not always align). Simple public health measures such as testing, isolation of cases, and contact tracing generally remain the best options for early containment of epidemics with pandemic potential. Travel bans typically delay the onset of an epidemic in a country that closes its borders by only a few weeks (Ferguson et al. 2006). Widespread use of antiviral medication can substantially reduce the influenza attack rate during an outbreak if the circulating strain happens to be susceptible to the drug rather than being resistant to it (Ferguson et al. 2006), but novel strains of influenza, coronaviruses, and other emerging infections may not be tamed by existing medications. Vaccines are often effective in slowing the spread of seasonal influenza, but even the most optimistic timelines still require months to develop, test, manufacture, and distribute a vaccine for a novel pathogen. Vaccines that protect against COVID-19 were made available in record time, but the rollout of vaccines was still very slow in most countries, even in high-income areas, one year after the pandemic began.

Given the timing between past influenza pandemics, the world could be said to be 'overdue' for a bad one. An H7N9 influenza virus that is highly pathogenic in poultry caused several human infections in 2013 (Gao et al. 2013), and sporadic human cases of other H7N9 strains have occurred in the subsequent years (Ma et al. 2019). Sporadic human infections with H5N6, H5N8, and H9N2 viruses that were circulating in bird populations have also been detected in recent years (EFSA 2021). Further mutations of H5N1, H7N9, another type of 'bird flu', or another type of influenza virus that is not currently circulating in human populations may trigger the next influenza pandemic. The IHR encourage greater financial and technical support for pandemic prevention, detection, and response, especially in lower-income countries, but many countries continue to fall short of the IHR standards for pandemic preparedness (Kandel et al. 2020). There is an urgent need to continue to improve global pandemic preparedness and communication before the next emergent event (see Chapter 2 by Johnson in this volume).

HIV/AIDS and Non-communicable Diseases: Modern Pandemic Rhetoric

Phylogenetic analyses of human immunodeficiency virus (HIV) suggest that the virus is likely to have first moved into human populations in Central Africa early in the twentieth century (Sharp and Hahn 2011), but the acquired immunodeficiency syndrome (AIDS) that the virus causes was not recognized until a series of cases were diagnosed in the United States in the early 1980s. Many well-resourced countries invested significant funds in HIV research, prevention, and treatment, but the absence of a coordinated global response was one of many factors that enabled the virus to spread into new populations. The number of people living with HIV increased to nearly 10 million by 1990 (UNAIDS 2020). By 2000, more than 20 million people were living with HIV and nearly 20 million had already died from the infection (Piot et al. 2001).

Although HIV is not a highly contagious virus and is not spread through the air, food, water, or casual contact, AIDS was characterized early on as a uniquely devastating infectious disease (Smith and Whiteside 2010). AIDS was first identified in the gay community, but cases were soon diagnosed in other population groups, including people with haemophilia and pregnant women who had received blood transfusions before blood products were routinely screened for HIV, and heterosexual transmission and injecting drug use spread the virus into additional populations. By the mid-1990s, when HIV began devastating communities in both urban and rural sub-Saharan Africa, there was widespread agreement that HIV/AIDS had become a global disease (Benatar 2002).

In 2001, the United Nations created a new global strategy for coordinating prevention efforts, increasing access to testing and treatment, and reducing the stigma associated with HIV and AIDS (Piot and Coll Seck 2001). The international health models of the latter half of the twentieth century had typically involved high-income countries funding child health and nutrition programmes and combatting tropical diseases in selected low-income countries that the donor nations viewed as strategic partners for business and security (Koplan et al. 2009). In the new era of global health that emerged as a result of the global response to HIV/AIDS, there is a greater emphasis on multinational, multilateral initiatives (Brandt 2013). The Global Fund to Fight AIDS, Tuberculosis and Malaria and several other global health partnerships were launched around the turn of the twenty-first century to address HIV/AIDS and other global health crises, and these groups continue to be major funders and implementers of HIV initiatives today (IHME 2020). They now operate alongside global health partnerships devoted to newer world priorities, such as the Coalition for Epidemic Preparedness Interventions (CEPI), which was founded in 2016 to coordinate development of, and access to, new vaccines for emerging infectious diseases (Gouglas et al. 2019).

Although HIV/AIDS remains a high-priority global health issue, the outlook is quite different now than it was 20 years ago (GBD Health Financing Collaborator Network 2020). Improved access to highly effective antiretroviral therapy (ART) has transformed HIV from a rapidly fatal infection to a chronic disease that often can be successfully managed for many years, or even decades. The number of people with HIV worldwide who are taking ART increased from less than 8 million in 2010 to about 26 million by 2020; the percentage of people with HIV who were receiving treatment increased from about 25% of the 31 million people who were living with HIV in 2010 to about 67% of the 38 million people who were living with HIV in 2020 (UNAIDS 2020). The growing prevalence of HIV infections was a direct result of more people with HIV gaining reliable access to affordable life-extending medications (UNAIDS 2020).

HIV met the typical definition of a pandemic by the late 1980s, less than a decade after AIDS was first recognized. Transmission was occurring in every world region and most countries, which met the geographic requirement for a pandemic. The incidence rate was high in some populations and much higher than the zero expected cases before the AIDS crisis was recognized, which fulfilled the frequency requirement for a pandemic. And there was worldwide concern about the severe impacts of HIV/AIDS on health systems and vulnerable communities.

However, the term 'pandemic' has not been consistently used to describe HIV. The Joint United Nations Programme on HIV/AIDS (UNAIDS) prefers to use the term 'global epidemic' rather than pandemic. This language is intended to emphasize that there is considerable variation by country and region in which populations are most at risk (UNAIDS 2011). Framing HIV as a series of concurrent and overlapping epidemics with unique characteristics rather than a single pandemic makes it easier to explain why prevention, diagnosis, and treatment interventions must be tailored to national and local conditions. Avoiding words like 'pandemic' that are associated with fear is also a way to destigmatize HIV (Prins 2004).

It could also be reasonable to argue that HIV has transitioned from an epidemic state to an endemic one. Endemicity occurs when an adverse health condition is always present in a population and incident cases occur at a relatively constant rate. The global HIV incidence rate remains far too high at nearly 1.7 million new cases per year, but there has been a gradual downward trend in incidence since the peak of about 2.8 million new cases in 1998 (UNAIDS 2020). HIV is now treated as a chronic disease that is managed with long-term therapies. Current global HIV initiatives have a goal of eventually reducing new cases of HIV infection to zero, but more resources are allocated to providing long-term ART treatment for people living with HIV than to non-pharmaceutical prevention methods (UNAIDS 2014). If HIV/AIDS has transitioned towards being in an endemic phase rather than an epidemic one, then it would no longer meet the epidemiological definition of a pandemic.

Pandemics are most likely to occur when there is widespread vulnerability to a disease in human populations and the causative agent for the disease is highly contagious, but there is no firm epidemiological requirement that a pandemic be caused by an infectious pathogen (Morens et al. 2009). Some researchers and advocacy groups have opted to use the word 'pandemic' to describe global public health concerns that are not infectious diseases because this term draws attention to their causes (Allen 2017). Using the popular connotation of a pandemic as a life-threatening and urgent threat to population health is one way to communicate the need for expanded funding and programming for emerging non-communicable diseases (NCDs) and other non-infectious conditions (Jönnson 2014).

Obesity was one of the first non-communicable conditions that was described as a pandemic (Egger and Swinburn 1997). Obesity may be considered to meet the traditional definition of a pandemic because obesity affects populations in every country, it is increasing in frequency (NCD-RisC 2017), and it is associated with increased health risks (Field et al. 2001). Some researchers have described obesity as 'contagious' because weight gain clusters within social networks (Powell et al. 2015). However, obesity is generally considered to be a risk factor for adverse health outcomes rather than a disease in and of itself (Heshka and Allison 2001), so obesity may not meet the definitional requirement that a pandemic causes disease in human populations. This same limitation applies to behavioural risk factors that have been described as pandemic, such as physical inactivity (Kohl et al. 2012) and tobacco use (Warner and MacKay 2006).

Type 2 diabetes occurs worldwide and is recognized as a disease that is associated with serious complications if blood sugars are not managed carefully, including neuropathy, blindness, cardiovascular disease, and kidney failure. About

80% of people with type 2 diabetes today live in low-income or middle-income countries (Chan et al. 2020), and the disorder is becoming more prevalent even after adjusting for population growth and aging (NCD-RisC 2016). Complications of diabetes are expensive for patients, caregivers, and health systems, with direct health expenditures worldwide already exceeding $760 billion annually (Williams et al. 2020). Because diabetes is a disease of global concern that is increasing in frequency and is severe for affected individuals and for populations, it could meet the traditional definition of a pandemic (van Dieren et al. 2010). However, the frequency of diabetes is typically measured by the prevalence of total existing cases at a selected point in time rather than by the incidence of new cases. Individuals develop type 2 diabetes gradually, typically over years, so populations experience gradual increases in diabetes prevalence rather than spikes in incidence.

There is no consensus about whether a disease with a slow onset (measured at the population level by prevalence) rather than an acute onset (measured at the population level by incidence) meets the definition for an epidemic. This same limitation would apply to other NCDs, including cardiovascular diseases, cancers, neurological conditions such as Parkinson's Disease (Dorsey et al. 2018), and many other common causes of disability and death.

A New Science of 'Pandemiology'?

The evolving use of the word 'pandemic' within the health sciences and beyond may require a rethinking of the traditional epidemiological definition of a pandemic that focuses on geography, frequency, and severity (Jacobsen 2018). The development of a new multidisciplinary field of 'pandemiology' might provide the most robust and useful answers to important questions about how we recognize, categorize, plan for, respond to, and interpret pandemics.

Since a pandemic is a global epidemic, one set of questions for 'pandemiologists' to answer focuses on how to define epidemics. What incidence rate or magnitude of increase in incidence counts as an epidemic? How quickly must a situation be emerging to count as an epidemic? Is it useful to conceive of slow-motion global public health crises like climate change as pandemics, or would that dilute the intended meaning of the word (see the Introduction to this volume by Ackerly et al.)?

A second set of questions focuses on which adverse health conditions are appropriate to describe as pandemics. Should the term 'pandemic' be reserved for contagious diseases? Should it apply both to rapid-onset, short-lasting, acute infections and to gradual-onset, long-lasting, infectious diseases? Would it be useful to global public health to use 'pandemic' to describe increasing population health burdens from NCDs, mental health disorders, violence, and other injuries? Would it be useful to use 'pandemic' to describe behavioural risk factors and the various social and environmental determinants of health that are becoming more widespread? Will it be useful to classify the anticipated adverse effects of global climate change on population health as a pandemic (see Chapter 6 by Morin et al. in this volume)?

A third set of questions relates to whether severity should be solidified as a defining characteristic of a pandemic along with a widespread distribution and a higher-than-expected number of cases. Should pandemics be interpreted narrowly as applying only to diseases with high fatality rates, or interpreted broadly as including any health-related condition that meets the geographic and frequency parts of the definition of a pandemic?

'Pandemiology' could seek to better define pandemics; understand how globalization and other complex human and environmental factors generate pandemics; identify the types of pandemics that may become human security threats in the coming decades; and form an evidence base of effective and cost-effective interventions for preventing, responding to, and recovering from pandemics. The prevention and containment of future pandemics—however they are defined—will demand improved global preparedness strategies and global responses (Jacobsen 2020). The process of negotiating these shared plans, communicating about emergent events, navigating cooperative interventions, and implementing other critical responses to pandemics will work best if all involved parties understand the basic science of pandemics and are skilled at collaborating across disciplines, professions, and sectors.

References

Allen, Luke. 2017. 'Are We Facing a Noncommunicable Disease Pandemic?' *Journal of Epidemiology and Global Health 7* (1): pp. 5–9.

Barreto, Mauricio L., Maria Glória Teixeira, and Eduardo Hage Carmo. 2006. 'Infectious Disease Epidemiology'. *Journal of Epidemiology and Community Health 60* (3): pp. 192–5.

Benatar, Solomon R. 2002. 'The HIV/AIDS Pandemic: A Sign of Instability in a Complex Global System'. *Journal of Medicine & Philosophy 27* (2): pp. 163–77.

Bennett, Belinda, and Terry Carney. 2017. 'Public Health Emergencies of International Concern: Global, Regional, and Local Responses to Risk'. *Medical Law Review 25* (2): pp. 223–39.

Brandt, Allan M. 2013. 'How AIDS Invented Global Health'. *New England Journal of Medicine 368* (23): pp. 2149–52.

Card, Alan J. 2012. 'Pandemicity and Severity Are Separate Constructs'. *American Journal of Public Health 102* (7): e12.

Cauchemez, Simon, Maria D. Kerkhove, Brett N. Archer, et al. 2014. 'School Closures during the 2009 Influenza Pandemic: National and Local Experiences'. *BMC Infectious Diseases 14*: p. 207.

Chan, Juliana C. N., Lee-Ling Lim, Nicholas J. Wareham, et al. 2020 'The Lancet Commission on Diabetes: Using Data to Transform Diabetes Care and Patient Lives'. *The Lancet 396* (10267): pp. 2019–82.

Cherry, James D. 2004. 'The Chronology of the 2002–2003 SARS Mini Pandemic'. *Pediatric Respiratory Reviews 5* (4): pp. 262–9.

Chew, Cynthia, and Gunther Eysenbach. 2010. 'Pandemics in the Age of Twitter: Content Analysis of Tweets during the 2009 H1N1 Outbreak'. *PLoS One 5* (11): e14118.

Dawood, Fatima S., A. Danielle Iuliano, Carrie Reed, et al. 2012. 'Estimated Global Mortality Associated with the First 12 Months of 2009 Pandemic Influenza A H1N1 Virus Circulation: A Modelling Study'. *Lancet Infectious Diseases 12* (9): pp. 687–95.

Dorsey, E. Ray, Todd Sherer, Michael S. Okun, and Bastiaan R. Bloem. 2018. 'The Emerging Evidence of the Parkinson Pandemic'. *Journal of Parkinson's Disease 8* (S1): pp. S3–8.

Doshi, Peter. 2011. 'The Elusive Definition of Pandemic Influenza'. *Bulletin of the World Health Organization 89* (7): pp. 532–8.

Dupras, Charles, and Bryn Williams-Jones. 2012. 'The Expert and the Lay Public: Reflections on Influenza A (H1N1) and the Risk Society'. *American Journal of Public Health 102* (4): pp. 591–5.

Eccleston-Turner, Mark, Alexandra Phelan, and Rebecca Katz. 2019. 'Preparing for the Next Pandemic—the WHO's Global Influenza Strategy'. *New England Journal of Medicine 381* (23): pp. 2192–4.

Egger, Gary, and Boyd Swinburn. 1997. 'An 'Ecological' Approach to the Obesity Pandemic'. *British Medical Journal 315* (7106): pp. 477–80.

European Food Safety Authority (EFSA). 2021. 'Avian Influenza Overview December 2020–February 2021'. *EFSA Journal 19* (3): e06497.

Ferguson, Neil M., Derek A. T. Cummings, Christophe Fraser, James C. Cajka, Philip C. Cooley, and Donald S. Burke. 2006. 'Strategies for Mitigating an Influenza Pandemic'. *Nature 442* (7101): pp. 448–52.

Fidler, David P. 2005. 'From International Sanitary Conventions to Global Health Security: The New International Health Regulations'. *Chinese Journal of International Law 4* (2): pp. 325–92.

Field, Alison E., Eugenie H. Coakley, Aviva Must, et al. 2001. 'Impact of Overweight on the Risk of Developing Common Chronic Diseases during a 10-Year Period'. *Archives of Internal Medicine 161* (13): pp. 1581–6.

Gao, Rongbao, Bin Cao, Yunwen Hu, et al. 2013. 'Human Infection with a Novel Avian-Origin Influenza A (H7N9) Virus'. *New England Journal of Medicine 368* (20): pp. 1888–97.

Girard, Marc P., John S. Tam, Olga M. Assossou, and Marie Paule Kieny. 2010. 'The 2009 A (H1N1) Influenza Virus Pandemic: A Review'. *Vaccine 28* (31): pp. 4895–902.

Glezen, W. Paul. 1996. 'Emerging Infections: Pandemic Influenza'. *Epidemiologic Reviews 18* (1): pp. 64–76.

Global Burden of Disease (GBD) Health Financing Collaborator Network. 2020. 'Health Sector Spending and Spending on HIV/AIDS, Tuberculosis, and Malaria, and Development Assistance for Health: Progress Toward Sustainable Development Goal 3'. *The Lancet* 396 (10252): pp. 693–724.

Gouglas, Dimitrios, Mario Christodoulou, Stanley A. Plotkin, and Richard Hatchett. 2019. 'CEPI: Driving Progress toward Epidemic Preparedness and Response'. *Epidemiologic Reviews 41* (1): pp. 28–33.

Heshka, S., and David. B. Allison. 2001. 'Is Obesity a Disease?' *International Journal of Obesity 25* (10): pp. 1401–4.

Heymann, David L. 2004. 'The International Response to the Outbreak of SARS in 2003'. *Philosophical Transactions of the Royal Society of London, Series B (Biological Sciences) 359* (1447): pp. 1227–9.

Hoffman, Steven J. 2010. 'The Evolution, Etiology and Eventualities of the Global Health Security Regime'. *Health Policy and Planning 25* (6): pp. 510–22.

Huber, Valeska. 2006. 'The Unification of the Globe by Disease? The International Sanitary Conferences on Cholera, 1851–1894'. *Historical Journal 49* (2): pp. 453–76.

Institute for Health Metrics and Evaluation (IHME). 2020. *Financing Global Health 2019: Tracking Health Spending in a Time of Crisis*. Seattle: IHME.

Jacobsen, Kathryn H. 2018. 'Pandemics'. In *Oxford Handbook of Global Studies*, edited by Mark Juergensmeyer, Saskia Sassen, Manfred B. Steger, and Victor Faessel, pp. 647–62. Oxford: Oxford University Press.

Jacobsen, Kathryn H. 2020. 'Will COVID-19 Generate Global Preparedness?' *The Lancet 395* (10229): pp. 1013–4.

Jönnson, Kristina. 2014. 'Legitimation Challenges in Global Health Governance: The Case of Non-Communicable Diseases'. *Globalization 11* (3): pp. 301–14.

Kamradt-Scott, Adam. 2012. 'Changing Perceptions of Pandemic Influenza and Public Health Responses'. *American Journal of Public Health 102* (1): pp. 90–8.

Kamradt-Scott, Adam, and Simon Rushton. 2012. 'The Revised International Health Regulations: Socialization, Compliance and Changing Norms of Global Health Security'. *Global Change, Peace and Security 24* (1): pp. 57–70.

Kandel, Nirmal, Stella Chungong, Abbas Omaar, and Jun Xing. 2020. 'Health Security Capacities in the Context of COVID-19 Outbreak: An Analysis of International Health Regulations Annual Report Data from 182 Countries'. *The Lancet 395* (10229): pp. 1047–53.

Katz, Rebecca, and Julie Fischer. 2010. 'The Revised International Health Regulations: A Framework for Global Pandemic Response'. *Global Health Governance 3* (2): pp. 1–18.

Kelly, Heath. 2011. 'The Classical Definition of a Pandemic Is Not Elusive'. *Bulletin of the World Health Organization 89* (7): pp. 540–1.

Kohl, Harold W., Cora Lynn Craig, Estelle Victoria Lambert, et al. 2012. 'The Pandemic of Physical Inactivity: Global Action for Global Health'. *The Lancet 380* (9838): pp. 294–305.

Koplan, Jeffrey P., T. Christopher Bond, Michael H. Merson, et al. 2009. 'Towards a Common Definition of Global Health'. *The Lancet 373* (9679): pp. 1993–5.

Lee, Kelley. 2001. 'The Global Dimensions of Cholera'. *Global Change and Human Health 2* (1): pp. 6–17.

Lee, Kelley, and Richard Dodgson. 2000. 'Globalization and Cholera: Implications for Global Governance'. *Global Governance 6* (2): pp. 213–36.

Lipsitch, Marc, Ted Cohen, Ben Cooper, et al. 2003. 'Transmission Dynamics and Control of Severe Acute Respiratory Syndrome'. *Science 300* (5627): pp. 1966–70.

Ma, Mai-Juan, Yang Yang, and Li-Qun Fan. 2019. 'Highly Pathogenic Avian H7N9 Influenza Viruses: Recent Challenges'. *Trends in Microbiology 27* (2): pp. 93–5.

McCloskey, Brian, Osman Dar, Alimuddin Zumla, and David L. Heymann. 2014. 'Emerging Infectious Diseases and Pandemic Potential: Status Quo and Reducing Risk of Global Spread'. *Lancet Infectious Diseases 14* (10): pp. 1001–10.

Morens, David M., and Anthony S. Fauci. 2007. 'The 1918 Influenza Pandemic: Insights for the 21st Century'. *Journal of Infectious Diseases 195* (7): pp. 1018–28.

Morens, David M., Gregory K. Folkers, and Anthony S. Fauci. 2009. 'What Is a Pandemic?' *Journal of Infectious Diseases 200* (7): pp. 1018–21.

Murray, Christopher J. L., Alan D. Lopez, Brian Chin, Dennis Feehan, and Kenneth H. Hill. 2006. 'Estimation of Potential Global Pandemic Influenza Mortality on the Basis of Vital Registry Data from the 1918–20 Pandemic: A Quantitative Analysis'. *The Lancet 368* (9554): pp. 2211–18.

Neumann, Gabriele, and Yoshihiro Kawaoka. 2019. 'Predicting the Next Influenza Pandemics'. *Journal of Infectious Diseases 219* (Suppl 1): pp. S14–20.

Newman, Laura P., Niranjan Bhat, Jessica A. Fleming, and Kathleen M. Neuzil. 2018. 'Global Influenza Seasonality to Inform Country-Level Vaccine Programs: An Analysis of WHO FluNet Influenza Surveillance Data between 2011 and 2016'. *PLoS One* 13 (2): e01932363.

Non-Communicable Disease (NCD) Risk Factor Collaboration (NCD-RisC). 2016. 'Worldwide Trends in Diabetes since 1980: A Pooled Analysis of 751 Population-Based Studies with 4.4 Million Participants'. *The Lancet 387* (10027): pp. 1513–30.

NCD Risk Factor Collaboration (NCD-RisC). 2017. 'Worldwide Trends in Body-Mass Index, Underweight, Overweight, and Obesity from 1975 to 2016: A Pooled Analysis of 2,416 Population-Based Measurement Studies in 128.9 Million Children, Adolescents, and Adults'. *The Lancet 390* (10113): pp. 2627–42.

Palmer, Roxanne. 2010. 'A Disease—or Gene—By Any Other Name Would Cause a Stink'. *Nature Medicine 16* (10): p. 1059.

Piot, Peter, Michael Bartos, Peter D. Ghys, Neff Walker, and Bernhard Schwartländer. 2001. 'The Global Impact of HIV/AIDS'. *Nature 410* (6831): pp. 968–73.

Piot, Piot, and Awa Marie Coll Seck. 2001. 'International Response to the HIV/AIDS Epidemic: Planning for Success'. *Bulletin of the World Health Organization 79* (12): pp. 1106–12.

Porta, Miquel, ed. 2016. *A Dictionary of Epidemiology* (6th edn). Oxford: Oxford University Press.

Powell, Katie, John Wilcox, Angie Clonan, et al. 2015. 'The Role of Social Networks in the Development of Overweight and Obesity among Adults: A Scoping Review'. *BMC Public Health 15*: p. 996.

Prins, Gwyn. 2004. 'AIDS and Global Security'. *International Affairs 80* (5): pp. 931–52.

Ruiz, Gregory M., Tonya K. Rawlings, Fred C. Dobbs, et al. 2000. 'Global Spread of Microorganisms by Ships'. *Nature 408* (6808): pp. 49–50.

Schein, Rebecca, Sand Bruls, Vincent Busch, Kumanan Wilson, Larry Hershfield, and Jennifer Keelan. 2012. 'A Flu by Any Other Name: Why the World Health Organization Should Adopt the World Meteorological Association's Storm Naming System as a Model for Naming Emerging Infectious Diseases'. *Journal of Health Communication 17* (5): pp. 532–45.

Sharp, Paul M., and Beatrice H. Hahn. 2011. 'Origins of HIV and the AIDS Pandemic'. *Cold Springs Harbor Perspectives in Medicine 1* (1): a006841.

Shetty, Priya. 2009. 'Preparation for a Pandemic: Influenza A H1N1'. *Lancet Infectious Disease 9* (6): pp. 339–40.

Smith, Julia H., and Alan Whiteside. 2010. 'The History of AIDS Exceptionalism'. *Journal of the International AIDS Society 13*: p. 47.

United Nations Programme on HIV/AIDS (UNAIDS). 2011. 'UNAIDS Terminology Guidelines—Revised Version: October 2011'.

UNAIDS. 2014. 'Fast-Track: Ending the AIDS Epidemic by 2030'.

UNAIDS. 2020. 'AIDS by the Numbers 2020'.

van Dieren, Susan, Joline W. J. Beulens, Yvonne. T. van der Schouw, Diederick E. Grobbee, and Bruce Neal. 2010. 'The Global Burden of Diabetes and Its Complications: An Emerging Pandemic'. *European Journal of Cardiovascular Prevention and Rehabilitation 17* (Suppl 1): pp. S3–8.

Warner, K. E., and J. MacKay. 2006. 'The Global Tobacco Disease Pandemic: Nature, Causes, and Cures'. *Global Public Health 1* (1): pp. 65–86.

Wilder-Smith, Annalies, and Sarah Osman. 2020. 'Public Health Emergencies of International Concern: A Historic Overview'. *Journal of Travel Medicine 27* (8): p. 227.

Williams, Rhys, Suvi Karuranga, Belma Malanda, et al. 2020. 'Global and Regional Estimates and Projections of Diabetes-Related Health Expenditure: Results from the *International Diabetes Federation Diabetes Atlas*, 9th edition'. *Diabetes Research and Clinical Practice 162*: 108072.

World Health Organization (WHO). 2020a. 'Statement on the Second Meeting of the International Health Regulations (2005) Emergency Committee Regarding the Outbreak of Novel Coronavirus (2019-nCoV)'. 30 January.

WHO. 2020b. 'WHO Director-General's Opening Remarks at the Media Briefing on COVID-19'. 11 March.

2

What Viruses Want

Evolutionary Insights for the Covid-19 Pandemic and Lessons for the Next One

*Dominic D. P. Johnson**

Introduction: The Utility of a Biological Approach

Politics and international relations used to be the domain of philosophers, historians, and social scientists. But in the twenty-first century, the life sciences are becoming increasingly indispensable disciplines for both the study and practice of political life. Biology in particular represents a crucial area of knowledge for political leaders to understand, and to inform policy. Why so?

First, *major global challenges are increasingly biological or ecological in nature*, notably climate change, environmental stress, biodiversity loss, resource management, population pressures, biomedical technology, global health and—not least—pandemics such as COVID-19 (see Chapter 6 by Morin et al. in this volume). Biology and other scientific disciplines are essential to understanding such problems and their effects, and to devising technical solutions.

Second, human health and behaviour themselves are increasingly understood to have important *genetic, biological, and cognitive underpinnings*, which are crucial to understanding the impacts on, and the reactions of, individual human beings (citizens and leaders alike) and the population in response to contemporary political and global challenges. We need to better understand our own biology and behaviour to meet these challenges effectively.

While insights from the life sciences are numerous and varied, they are also unified under a single, overarching theoretical framework: evolution. Evolution

* I am hugely grateful for excellent comments and suggestions on the chapter draft from Andrea Bjorklund, Dan Blumstein, Philippe Bourbeau, Edmund LeGrand, Jean-Michel Marcoux, and Terence Taylor.

Dominic D. P. Johnson, *What Viruses Want.* In: *A Multidisciplinary Approach to Pandemics.*
Edited by Philippe Bourbeau, Jean-Michel Marcoux, and Brooke A. Ackerly, Oxford University Press.
 DOI: 10.1093/oso/9780192897855.003.0003

explains all life on Earth, its origins, variation, adaptations, and interactions. Indeed, as Theodosius Dobzhansky observed, 'nothing in biology makes sense *except* in the light of evolution' (Dobzhansky 1973). Evolutionary biology therefore allows one to start from first principles in addressing a given problem by drawing on a common theoretical grounding and a vast empirical record that spans billions of years and millions of organisms, among which humans are just one. This broader picture allows us to see patterns, causes, and consequences in the dynamics of many contemporary challenges, as well as in our own species, that standard social science approaches cannot (Barkow 2006; Lederberg 2000; Sagarin 2012; Sagarin et al. 2010; Sagarin and Taylor 2008; E. O. Wilson 1999). Evolutionary approaches thus bring novel insights for a variety of topics in politics and international relations, but especially for one of the most important global challenges of the century: pandemic disease outbreaks such as COVID-19.

The Problem: Non-Rational Actors and Dynamic Threats

One might think that, while obviously needing biology (and subfields such as genetics and epidemiology) to understand virus outbreaks and develop treatments and vaccines, managing a global pandemic itself is largely a problem to be dealt with by economic and political tools. However, the COVID-19 pandemic has revealed serious flaws in that view. Prior to the crisis, the United Kingdom and the United States were judged to be among the best prepared for a global pandemic. The 2019 Global Health Security Index (GHSI) had ranked the UK and the US as first and second out of 195 countries, both for overall preparedness and specifically in their capacity for 'rapid response to and mitigation of the spread of an epidemic' (Roberts 2020: 17–18). At the time of writing, in the grip of the pandemic, they stand among the worst in the world (by cases or by deaths per population).[1] Evidently, our expectations for the state apparatus that would be needed to deal with a global pandemic and who is best placed to implement it were wrong. Surprisingly, responses even from apparently well-resourced nations were too little, too late, and ineffective. Many poorer countries have managed to keep infection rates significantly lower. Different countries have varied widely in their experience and strategies, and have performed well or badly at different times and in different respects. But in general, political leaders (among others) have demonstrated a familiar tendency to underestimate the threat and overestimate their ability to deal with it (Johnson 2004; Sharot 2011a).[2]

[1] See Johns Hopkins University of Medicine Coronavirus Resource Center (https://coronavirus.jhu.edu).

[2] Successful pandemic responses clearly did not depend on the ideal of a western democratic political system, since some democracies have fared relatively poorly and some autocracies have fared relatively well. Rather, other factors seem to have proven more important for the effectiveness of pandemic

An evolutionary perspective can help to understand these failures and why a pandemic virus is so hard to defeat. If humans and states were rational actors facing a static threat, we could follow the data and the scientific advice and governments could respond to a global pandemic with effectiveness and coordination.[3] We would still have a major problem to deal with, but it would be easier to solve than the one we actually have, which is responding to a *rapidly changing* threat with a population that is *far from the ideal of rational actors*, waylaid by a variety of evolved dispositions and cognitive biases. Of course, great uncertainty means it is hard for anyone to know just how aggressively one 'should' fight the virus, given that every extra effort imposes costs and sacrifices opportunities. But the uncertainty also means that there is greater room for big mistakes, and thus greater weight on applying the precautionary principle—to err on the side of caution (Johnson et al. 2013).

Worse still, leaders themselves have struggled to understand and communicate the scientific data and advice. Of course, they have a difficult balancing act to trade off multiple competing demands and stakeholders—not least keeping the economy afloat while, at the same time, severely curtailing people's freedoms. But it is hardly uncontroversial to say that they have recurrently got a lot about COVID-19 wrong. Even well-informed opinion leaders and policymakers, who may have seen things clearly themselves, still evidently expected *other* people to behave rationally and for a long time continued to treat the virus as a *static* threat. Meanwhile, some leaders blatantly failed to recognize the gravity of the situation. Adam Roberts lamented US President Donald Trump's actions as 'serially gormless involvements in the COVID-19 crisis' (Roberts 2020: 31).

By virtue of evolution, humans are not rational actors but instinctive biological ones, with varied and contingent responses, and viruses are not a static threat but a dynamic and changing one. We need to think more about our own evolution as well as the evolution of viruses to effectively address pandemics. Politics obviously remains central, but an evolutionary perspective can help.

Plan of the Chapter

This chapter focuses on two broad insights from evolution: (1) the biology and evolution of viruses; and (2) the biology and evolution of the host—us. As for the first, *evolutionary biology* provides a framework for considering what viruses 'want', that is, the selective pressures that cause them to operate the way they do,

mitigation efforts, regardless of regime type, such as past experience, crisis leadership, and flexible institutions (Roberts 2020).

[3] As discussed by Herrmann and Isabelle in Chapter 14 of this volume, the fact that rational agents can have heterogenous initial preferences, and the externalities linked to individuals' choices and behaviours, would nevertheless make this a complex task, of course.

their adaptations, strategies, mechanisms of spread, severity, lethality, and (not least) their rapid genetic mutation and the evolution taking place right now—the evolutionary 'arms race' that underlies viruses' and hosts' strategies to outwit and stay ahead of each other.

As for the second, an evolutionary perspective also helps us understand the *hosts*—human beings—and our behaviour and responses to disease. Sometimes our biology and behaviour seems puzzling or irrational, but it can make more sense under the lens of evolution. For example, *evolutionary medicine* provides a framework for thinking about why the human body succumbs and reacts the way it does to disease and treatment. This includes, for example, how and why pathogens manipulate our biology in order to spread more effectively, and why the body's reaction—often itself an overreaction—to infection rather than the infection itself can be crucial to the consequences of disease (Wrotek et al. 2020). In addition, *evolutionary psychology* helps to explain common *behavioural* responses to disease, as evolved heuristics that, today, can have 'adaptive' or 'maladaptive' consequences. Depending on the context, such heuristics include the manifestation of over-optimism and ill-preparedness for disasters, the 'negativity bias' underlying apparent overreaction and fear, and the conflicts between self-interest and the public good. Finally, *gene-culture co-evolution* sheds light on the interaction between human evolution and the environment, and how selection pressures acting on human biology are in part shaped by the cultural traits and environment we have ourselves created. This means that changing physical and social environments have, in turn, impacted our genetic adaptations, not least in relation to disease and our responses to them.

This chapter gives an overview of these various evolutionary insights. Each is a rather different set of ideas, even representing different subdisciplines in themselves (e.g. biology, genetics, medicine, psychology, anthropology). But they are united by the common underlying theoretical framework of evolution. In taking a brief look at them all, this chapter aims to advance the broader goal of the book in exploring how different disciplinary approaches can bring new ways of thinking about problems in politics and international relations (see the Introduction by Ackerly et al.). Evolution raises a range of new questions, and often novel solutions, which are unique to an evolutionary approach. One could write such a chapter at any time and focusing on any number of topics. But COVID-19 starkly highlights the importance of biology in the future of the globe (and the field), as well as the importance of humans not just as political actors but also as biological organisms with an evolutionary legacy and part of a complex evolving ecosystem that we ignore at our peril. Arguably, we have not appreciated the danger of our biological vulnerabilities in a newly globalized world until it was too late.

The Pathogen: An Evolutionary Perspective on Viruses

The Biology of Viruses

Viruses have been around for millions of years and long predate humans—we are a mere blip in the story. However, we haven't known about them for long. As the smallest biological entities, around 50 times smaller than bacteria (varying from just 20 to 300nm), they cannot be seen with a light microscope and eluded identification altogether until the advent of electron microscopy in the 1930s. Before that, they remained mysterious agents of disease in plants and other organisms, earning them the name 'virus'—the latin word for poison (Campbell 1993; Green et al. 1990).

Though simple, or precisely because of their simplicity, viruses are remarkable entities. Comprising just a small amount of genetic material and a protein casing, they are able to hijack a host organism's cellular machinery and turn it over to exclusively serve their own purposes. Following infection, proteins on the virus's exterior (such as the now famous 'spike protein' in SARS-CoV-2—the virus giving rise to COVID-19) bind to receptors on the host cell surface and then fuse with or inject their genetic material directly into the cell. Once inside, the host's DNA is deactivated and the cell starts producing the building blocks of more virus particles instead, replicating multiple new copies of their genetic material and synthesizing more encasing proteins. Viruses have the property of 'self-assembly', meaning that after production of the new components, the virus genes and protein casings automatically snap back together to form complete virus particles. Finally, the new viruses burst from the cell, going on to infect new cells in the same or new hosts. In a final trick, some viruses actually take on a coat of the host cell's own membrane as they escape, so that the virus looks to other host cells like one of its own. Viruses are masters of disguise and this makes them particularly hard for hosts to detect and defeat.

The clinical effects of viruses are highly variable. Some damage or kill the cells they use to replicate, others release toxins, others trigger the body's own defences to go into overdrive in fighting the virus. (The immune response can be seen as an emergency trade-off that puts the body at risk, e.g. with high fever, but in order to better fight the virus (Wrotek et al. 2020).) The damage done depends on the extent to which the host tissue is able to regenerate. Influenza virus affects the epithelial lining of the respiratory tract, the cells of which regenerate by normal cell division. Thus, an infected person can recover fully. By contrast, the polio virus infects nerve cells, which never divide and thus cannot be replaced, rendering the damage permanent.

The Evolution of Viruses

As well as understanding how viruses work, biology also sheds light on how viruses first emerged and evolved—and importantly, how they continue to evolve today. Since viruses rely on host cells to replicate, they cannot have predated other forms of life; rather, they must have evolved *from* existing organisms. They are thought to have originated as breakaway genetic material (initially like other naturally occurring 'mobile genetic elements', such as plasmids and transposons), which then acquired an independent ability to parasitize the machinery of host cells to create more copies of themselves. One tell-tale sign of viruses' origins is that they often tend to be more genetically similar to their hosts than they are to other viruses (indeed, many virus genes are more or less identical to those of their hosts), betraying an original shared ancestry with the hosts themselves (Campbell 1993; Green et al. 1990). The evolution of viruses and host organisms are deeply intertwined so that, in genetic terms, many viruses have become part of the make-up of hosts, just as hosts are part of the make-up of viruses (Ryan 2009; Villarreal 2005).

This origin also accounts for viruses' 'host range'—the number and types of different species that a given virus can infect. This depends largely on the recognition of binding proteins on the virus exterior and corresponding receptors on the host cell surface. Sometimes, common receptors found in different cells allow infection by the same virus of multiple species. Swine flu, for example, can infect both pigs and humans. Rabies, similarly, can infect rodents, dogs, and humans. Other viruses have a much narrower range, and may be limited not merely to a single species but to *specific cells* within that species. The common cold virus, for example, only affects cells of the upper respiratory tract, and ignores others. SARS-CoV-2 appears to have originated in bats, and then jumped to humans, probably via an intermediate host, such as a pangolin (Burki 2020).

One can argue about whether viruses represent 'living' things. With no cells or cellular machinery of their own (which all other living organisms have), they are 'obligate parasites' that are not able to reproduce without the help of the cells of another organism. Unlike bacteria, which can live and grow on a petri dish, viruses are inert and *cannot* replicate unless they infect a host cell. However, they have genetic material written out in the 'universal language of life' (as DNA or RNA), which contain the instructions for reproducing more copies of themselves (Campbell 1993: 354). This means that viruses evolve.

Whenever organisms replicate, mutations inevitably arise in the copying of their genetic code from one generation to the next (every time DNA or RNA is copied, there is a chance that mutations occur). Often, these mutations have no significant effect (and are thus 'neutral mutations'), or may actually be damaging to the organism (deleterious mutations). But sometimes these mutations bring novel advantages for replicating even more effectively. If so, carriers will do better than the original form and spread, along with the novel mutation. This is the engine of evolution, and confers the ability to generate novel adaptations and, ultimately, speciation. The same is true for viruses, both in their origin and their subsequent development. SARS-CoV-2, for example, must have undergone a mutation that allowed a virus formerly confined to animal hosts to 'jump' to human hosts. The COVID-19 pandemic, therefore, is not due to a pre-existing virus as such, but to its *evolution*. As discussed later, it has evolved, and will evolve again.

On the one hand, these small changes in the genetic code are helpful for global mitigation efforts—without the accumulation of copying errors in the virus's genetic code (most of which are neutral mutations), scientists would not have been able to build a genetic family tree of how the virus has changed over time, which allows them to trace its origins and track its spread. On the other hand, mutations among pathogens represent a special danger of their own because they generate new variants to fuel an arms race of pathogen effectiveness and host defences (Dawkins and Krebs 1979; Ridley 1994). If and how—and how fast—the virus mutates ultimately affects our ability to avoid it, as well as to develop immunity and successful vaccines, and for these to stay effective for a reasonable period of time. Natural or induced immunity to the virus now does not guarantee continued immunity in the future against a virus that is changing all the time. This is why we have to develop new seasonal flu vaccines every year, which vary in their effectiveness.

What Viruses 'Want': An Evolutionary Lens on Virus Strategies

Of course, viruses don't 'want' anything, in the sense in which that word is commonly used and understood by most people. But as shorthand for how organisms are adapted to survive and reproduce by doing things that help them do so, it is a useful way of thinking about things. It allows us to think through the biology and behaviour of any organism to identify how the strategies they employ—even, or especially, if initially puzzling—may in fact be functional, biological adaptations that aid the organism in achieving its ends. It focuses our attention on the evolutionary rationale for why organisms have adapted to do the things they do. How does their biology or behaviour succeed in getting more copies of themselves into the next generation? This differentiates potentially functional characteristics from mere accidents, random noise, or empirical but unexplained trends.

We can engage the same logic for viruses. They seem nasty, vindictive pathogens because they make people ill and sometimes kill them. But viruses are biological organisms that are just doing what they do in order to survive and reproduce. In fact, their entire mode of replication is a remarkable evolutionary innovation. From the gene's eye view, as famously espoused by Richard Dawkins, viruses are notable in that they have figured out a way to escape the confines of 'orthodox' replication, in which genes have to share their passage to the future with groups of many other genes in the chromosomes of sperm and egg, combining to transmit genes from one body to another once per generation (Dawkins 1976). Instead, virus genes bypass having to wait around for the painfully slow process of host reproduction altogether because their genetic material literally floats independently through the air to travel directly from body to body. This means that they can replicate much faster than other organisms, and without having to make all the adaptive compromises with other genes that have other priorities and duties in the body. Viruses have found a much more efficient method of replication.

This evolutionary perspective is important because it helps us to make sense of the often surprising biology and 'behaviour' of viruses, to understand the conditions that might be conducive to spreading or mitigating them, and the conditions under which they are likely to evolve in benign or harmful ways. Below are some examples, before we apply the approach to COVID-19.

In their efforts to increase the probability that they get passed on and replicated, many pathogens have evolved mechanisms to change not only their own behaviour, but also to change the behaviour of their hosts. For example, while coughing or sneezing might be seen as 'annoying byproducts of the virus's activities', in fact, they are highly adaptive consequences that help to transmit the virus and can be considered as 'deliberately engineered by the virus to help it to travel from one host to another' (Dawkins 1976: 246). Viruses are more likely to survive if they have traits that facilitate their spread among people, and common symptoms of viral diseases such as coughing, sneezing, and diarrhoea greatly enhance the transmissibility of the virus, as they forcefully expel them into the environment where other people can pick them up (Ewald 1997).

Similar dynamics are at play in other viruses, such as rabies. The rabies virus is transmitted by saliva, and thus requires infected animals coming into close contact with others and biting them. That can happen via normal animal interactions, but they don't bite each other all the time. However, rabies actually changes the behaviour of an infected animal in several ways that greatly increase the probability of transmission. Symptoms of rabies include (1) foaming at the mouth, which increases the amount and readiness of saliva to infect others; (2) restless roaming behaviour, taking infected animals far beyond their normal home range; and (3) an increase in aggressiveness that makes what are 'normally peaceful and friendly animals become ferocious biters' (Dawkins 1976: 247). A rabid dog becomes unafraid and aggressive. While we think of the virus as primarily afflicting the individual dog, it also drastically alters the host's biology and behaviour to help itself get into more dogs, and thereby replicate and spread more copies of the virus. Interestingly, a corollary is that the virus does not 'want' the dog to die; rather, it wants the dog to go around infecting as many other individuals as possible before it does so. A similar logic applies to other viruses. A smart virus should not kill its host. If anything, it should devise ways to be able to infect them again in the future.

As Rafe Sagarin put it, what 'the virus wants more than anything is stability . . . like a businessman trying to maintain a steady clientele' (Sagarin 2012: 156).

The Evolution of SARS-CoV-2: Genetic Mapping

Knowledge of the biology of SARS-CoV-2 has obviously been vital in developing clinical treatment of the virus and vaccines, as well as in forming policies of prevention and mitigation. What is perhaps less obvious is the importance of the *evolution* of the virus in mitigation efforts and the development of policy responses.

First, there is good news. An evolutionary approach is indispensable because it has allowed what would otherwise be an impossible study of how the virus spreads. Because mutations in the virus's genetic code occur at a regular rate, the cumulative history of gradual changes can be used as a molecular clock, leaving trails of breadcrumbs behind each new lineage as it spreads around the world. As the virus accumulates slight variations over time as a result of these copying errors (most of which have little effect but, nevertheless, build up cumulative fingerprints), we can build a genealogy of the virus. This allows one to trace, via the number and pattern of mutations, the branches of the 'family tree' and the common ancestors of emerging variants of the virus. The technique has long been used to track other virus pandemics, as was done, for example, with swine flu (H1N1) (Smith et al. 2009), and there has now been a vast scientific effort to trace the changing genomes of SARS-CoV-2 worldwide (see the Global Initiative for Sharing All Influenza Data (GISAID) database, https://www.gisaid.org, and Nextstrain, https://nextstrain.org).

One important insight is that it gives an estimate of when the virus *first emerged* among humans in China—and this date is estimated to be mid-to-late November 2019 or early December (Bedford et al. 2020). Why is this important? Because there are hugely significant political questions (and conspiracies) about the origins of COVID-19 and cover-ups about the first incidences of the virus in China and other countries, and whether it might have been man-made (Burki 2020). Evolutionary biology has been crucial in putting to rest some potentially inflammatory politics, quite apart from helping to deal with the virus. It is equally vital, of course, for political leaders and influential voices to understand this biology accurately.

Another important insight is that genetic sequencing allows us to tell how the virus has *spread*—from which points of origin, between which countries and among which people, and when these occurred. Then, in combination with other data, this can reveal what interventions have been more or less successful (or unsuccessful) in permitting the spread of particular strains. For example, the spread of one early variant of COVID-19, dubbed 20A.EU1, from Spain to the

UK during the summer of 2020 is evidence that the country-to-country travel restrictions in place at the time failed to contain the virus (a combination of states' permissive travel policies and people's eagerness to continue travelling). Evolutionary geneticist Emma Hodcroft, involved in the tracking project, pointed out that one obvious policy implication is the ability to distinguish local transmission (within country) to imported transmission (from other countries), which can be crucial to effective containment, as well as when to ease lockdown restrictions in the future (Cookson and Bott, 2020).

The Evolution of SARS-CoV-2: Virus Strategies

But what about the role of evolution in the strategies that the virus employs? How good is SARS-CoV-2 in this evolutionary arms race of cat and mouse? One feature that sets it apart from other viruses is its level of deceptiveness. In other flu viruses, people tend to become noticeably sick before they become particularly infectious (with the SARS outbreak in 2003, for instance, there were no cases of people spreading infection until after the onset of symptoms; see www.cdc.gov). This made mitigation efforts relatively straightforward because infected people can be easily identified and isolated before they infect others. That radically slows onward infection. But with COVID-19, the viral load hits a peak around, or even before, people first feel unwell (He et al. 2020). That means that people are likely to have already passed the virus on before they even realize they have it. The virus can be replicating away in the body's cells without generating any symptoms at all, and without even alerting our own immune system to its presence. In the words of virologist Paul Lehner, 'This virus is brilliant, it allows you to have a viral factory in your nose and feel completely well' (Gallagher 2020). It does this by deactivating the release of interferons that usually signal the presence of an infection to the rest of the body. Applying our gene's eye view, this, of course, is highly adaptive because transmission of the virus is much more 'successful' if you are not aware you are sick and carry on going about your normal business—and thus more effectively spread it to others. It is an unusual but understandable feature of SARS-CoV-2, as Lehner highlights: 'This is a really brilliant evolutionary tactic—you don't go to bed, you go out and have a good time.' Even laboratory observation of infected cells do not reveal that the virus is there, despite tests showing they are 'screaming with virus', which Lehner calls one of the virus's 'joker cards'.

This adaptive characteristic has, of course, been one of the enduring problems of COVID-19 pandemic mitigation, as well as the reason for the need for strict self-isolation measures if one has been in contact (even unknowingly) with an infected, or possibly infected, person. As well as developing clinical treatments, we have had to devise ways to clamp down on potential hosts and detect virus cases before people develop symptoms and to track down all potential contacts even if they were fleeting contacts with strangers. This has proven to be an immense technical, social, and political challenge. In this respect, the virus is well ahead of us in the evolutionary arms race. The stealthy infection and spread of COVID-19, arguably the greatest challenge of the global pandemic response, is—from an evolutionary perspective—exactly what the virus wants.

This biological property of COVID-19 also accounts for much of the public and political discontent about the lockdowns. It seems fundamentally illogical to stop people who *seem* well from doing things, and can still feel harsh even if one understands the problem. But this is precisely how the virus is spreading. The hidden diffusion of invisible agents among apparently healthy people is hard to grasp, yet essential to act upon if we are to achieve effective prevention. Unfortunately, it means the restriction of civil liberties of asymptomatic people, which makes for unpopular policy and public discontent. Notably, the relatively low mortality rate of COVID-19 makes this dilemma worse. The balance of risk and associated fear and responses (Blumstein 2020) would likely be different in a more dangerous virus outbreak.

Virus Mutations: The Next-Generation Threat

The SARS-CoV-2 virus that leads to COVID-19 is damaging and deadly enough as it is, but the much scarier possibility has always been that it mutates to become even better at what it does: more infectious, stealthier, or more deadly. Viruses, like all organisms, are under the pressure of natural selection, which favours variants that reproduce more effectively at the expense of variants that reproduce less effectively. Thus, any mutation that increases the virus's ability to reproduce or pass on more copies of itself will spread, regardless of any other consequences for the host.

Evolutionary geneticists often tend to express a word of caution here—as noted above, most mutations are neutral or deleterious to the virus. They thus tend to lead to ineffective viruses or merely lay down an additional marker for our tracing of their spread, but rarely result in a suddenly more dangerous form (e.g. because of increased transmissibility or severity). Early on in the pandemic, that may have seemed unlikely or even far-fetched. However, it has become perhaps the single most important problem, especially in a novel global pandemic with a vast susceptible population of billions of people, and a danger that an evolutionary approach has forced us to pay attention to (Korber et al. 2020; Van Egeren et al. 2020). Here's why it matters.

First, remember that a mutation can occur every time genetic material is copied in the process of replication. For humans, that occurs once a generation. For viruses, this happens millions of times even within a single infected individual—in days (it is estimated that at peak infection a single person has 10^9–10^{11} individual virions in their body; Sender et al. 2020). The capacity for mutation (and thus evolution) is operating at a *much* faster speed than it is for humans and other animals that are confined to biological reproduction. The same is true of bacterial pathogens, which is why we are constantly losing the arms race against them in the widespread problem of antibiotic resistance—the time frame for the evolution of bacteria resistant to a new antibiotic 'is often frighteningly short' (Gluckman et al. 2011: 257). It is also important to recognize one very important thing: the selection pressure on the virus will *increase*, rather than decrease, once it is faced with vaccination programmes and an accumulating herd immunity that start fighting it directly (Van Egeren et al. 2020). The greatest danger in the arms race may be yet to come. In the 'war' against the virus so far, we have mainly been running away (in avoiding and averting it). Only now are we starting to shoot back.

Second, as mentioned earlier, mutations of the virus genome are what allowed it to move from animals to humans in the first place. It was formerly a virus that had a host range limited to other animal species (mainly bats) but was not infectious to humans. But then, there was a mutation, or a set of mutations, that together allowed it to 'jump' to humans (Burki 2020). That was not an inconsequential mutation for the human population. More such evolutionary leaps by other as yet unknown viruses lie in the future.

Third, new mutations of the virus *since* that origin have already emerged. We saw above that many of these are just small alterations that help us trace different strains, but do not necessarily change how the virus operates. But other mutations (or combinations of several mutations) represent new variants of the virus that can have different characteristics. And these are not just minor details. For example, it is estimated that the 20A.EU1 variant of coronavirus that emerged in Spain over the summer of 2020 underlay the second wave in Europe (in the autumn of 2020). It accounted for more than 80% of UK cases (at the time of first drafting in October 2020), probably in large part because of holidaymakers who travelled to Spain over the summer and brought it home with them (Hodcroft et al. 2020). Of course, since the original drafting of this chapter, we have seen a steady stream of additional new variants that are proving much more significant (to which I will return shortly).

Fourth, the virus can jump around again between species. In Denmark, coronavirus jumped from humans to mink, of which there were millions in farms sustaining the largest fur-trading industry in the world (Milne and Cookson 2020). But this is not just a problem for the animals. The virus mutated into a different strain within the mink population, and then jumped *back* to humans again. It was feared that this new variant may spread more widely among the human population and render vaccines under development less effective. The Danish government sought emergency powers to exterminate all 17 million mink in the country (the Netherlands had already eliminated their entire population). This is the kind of danger that mutations can pose when the virus becomes exposed to large and interacting populations of people and other animals.

Implications of an Evolutionary Approach

If new variants of the virus are not too different from previous ones, then immune responses among recovered (or vaccinated) individuals may remain effective even against new variants. But this is not necessarily the case. That is, of course, why the virus evolves. It does not 'want' to be recognized or defended by hosts' immune systems, and new variants that avoid detection and defences will do better than older variants to which herd immunity is building. Plus, most importantly of all, as well as merely posing a challenge to levels of immunity, new variants may be more infectious or more harmful than their ancestors. The 20A.EU1 variant mentioned above did not seem to be more infectious. But at least three other variants quickly emerged that did appear to be becoming more infectious. The first, variant D614G, emerged quite early on in February 2020, and already was suggested to be more infectious and to lead to higher viral loads than original forms of the virus (Korber et al. 2020; Volz et al. 2020). While there was debate about the extent to which it was more transmissible (Grubaugh et al. 2020), it is clear that after emergence it spread rapidly around the world, replacing and coming to dominate in even well-established populations of former variants, suggesting that it had been subject to a process of positive selection (Korber et al. 2020). It was also of concern because the variant was an amino acid change in the spike protein, which is exactly what vaccines were targeting. Fortunately, early variants still appeared to be susceptible to vaccines under development (Weissman et al. 2020). However, modelling suggests that subsequent mutations are likely to give rise to resistance in an 'evolutionary escape' (or 'vaccine escape') that will be subject to greater levels of positive selection with the roll out of vaccines and accumulating levels of recovered immunity in the population (Van Egeren et al. 2020). Korber et al. (2020) developed an 'early warning' system to closely monitor spike protein evolution as the pandemic develops.

They did not have to wait long before something more sinister came along. In December 2020, a H69/V70 variant rapidly spread to become the dominant form of the virus in the South-East of the UK, spreading quickly around the country and plunging it into a third severe lockdown (European Centre for Disease Prevention and Control 2020). Sometimes, new variants can come to dominate accidentally via founder effects (new variants spread more because they happen to emerge in areas with high rates of social mixing and transmission). However, it is believed that this variant was indeed up to 70% more transmissible than prior forms of the virus, making finely balanced disease control restrictions suddenly inadequate. Also, the mutations again related to changes in the virus spike protein, raising concerns about the efficacy of new vaccines just being rolled out and the antibodies from people who formerly had COVID-19. At the time, it was thought that the current vaccines would remain effective, as they attack several different parts of the virus. Even if not, they can be adjusted to work on similar variations (as are the seasonal flu vaccines).

Finally, of even greater concern was the 501.V2 variant that emerged in South Africa. This one had more significant changes to the spike protein, and thus could pose problems for the vaccines being deployed. Antibodies to previous COVID-19 infections may not be able to recognize new virus variants as easily. No doubt, by the time of publication things will have moved on further (at the time of copy-editing, we are again in the grip of yet another new variant—Omicron). But the point should be clear: viruses are evolving entities that do not just present a static challenge to 'solve', but a race in which it is vital to stay in for the long haul and keep up. Public policy has many demands, but an evolutionary perspective presses home that it is imperative to rapidly quash the virus to manageable levels before it can evolve into an even greater problem.

With such a large and vulnerable population with no prior immunity, there is much scope for the virus not only to spread, whether quickly, or in a long 'slow burn', but either way to evolve rapidly along the way. This is unlike other viruses to which there has been at least some prior immunity in the population, and which thus spread more slowly and to a more limited group. Even with past novel viruses such as swine flu, it was similar enough to extant viruses that people already had at least some protection from previous exposure. COVID-19 is entirely new, and no one had any prior immunity, which is why it was constantly on the verge of ripping through unprotected populations like wildfire, in an exponential increase.[4] The greater the population infected, the greater the sheer number of virus replications taking place and thus the greater number of mutations that will occur and, consequently, the higher the probability of more virulent forms emerging.

Policy Implications

For all the intense public and political discussion of COVID-19, what was striking is that the role of virus *evolution* was largely overlooked—at least here in the UK—until the rapid spread of the H69/V70 variant forced the issue (and sharply reversed government policy). An evolutionary perspective raises troubling policy questions of its own. Until that point, many people seem to have assumed a static threat which was waiting patiently for us to attack it when we were able—with treatments, vaccines, and other measures. But the reality is that the virus has always been changing and we need to think about its ongoing and future evolution as well as its current state. In weighing up options for how to deal with the virus, how might our own actions and policies impact the course of its evolution? This important question seems to be rarely, if ever, discussed (at least in the media and among

[4] There is some indication that, while we do not have antibodies, prior cold virus T cells may help fight COVID-19 (Doshi 2020).

politicians). If we could click our fingers and eradicate the virus, there would be no further evolution. The problem with a slow war is that it gives time for evolution to take place. The existence of multiple animal–human–animal jumps and numerous emerging variants suggest that this remains a significant risk. If we maintain partial and rolling lockdowns, allowing a slow burn of the virus through the global population, the potential for further evolution of the virus will stay high over a longer period of time. As well as minimizing hospitalizations and deaths and getting back to normal life and economic recovery, another important reason to move hard and fast with lockdowns and vaccination programmes is to smother the virus to manageable levels as quickly as possible before it can evolve into something different, or worse. This might even arguably be the *most* important rationale for draconian policies and infringements of civil liberties. A constant evolution of viruses happens already with seasonal flu viruses, and we are likely to face a new (but harder) ongoing battle with SARS-CoV-2 for years to come. One piece of good news is that the underlying rate of genetic change in SARS-CoV-2 is actually relatively slow compared to some other viruses (such as HIV or flu; although, of course, the problem is still the sheer number, rather than rate, of opportunities for COVID-19 infections in a population of billions). One article cautioned, back in April 2020: 'Although surveillance has not shown any mutations that would affect its transmissibility or virulence, scientists are watching closely in case they appear' (Cookson and Bott 2020). This has now happened multiple times, and evolutionary theory suggests we should not be surprised.

There is also a further problem to consider, and which governments and public health services need to remain vigilant about. As Van Egeren et al. (2020) warn, the virus will only really come under significant evolutionary selection pressure when we have mass vaccinations and the accumulation of immunity fighting back. Until recently, the virus has enjoyed a vast sea of susceptible individuals with no immunity to counter its spread. The rise of vaccinated and recovered people in populations around the world will make the virus's environment for replication much tougher, and any new potentially beneficial mutations correspondingly more advantageous relative to existing forms. Indeed, in a vaccinated world, mutations will become key to virus survival. The toughest part of the arms race may be yet to come.

The Host: An Evolutionary Perspective on Human Responses to Disease

Evolutionary Medicine

Beyond the direct application of evolutionary principles to understand and fight pathogens themselves, evolutionary theory has also given rise to a wholesale rethink of medicine at the level of the *host*—how humans succumb and respond to disease. 'Evolutionary medicine' is a relatively new field that brings its own brand of insights for clinical medicine and public health (Gluckman et al. 2009; Nesse and Williams 1995; Williams and Nesse 1991). To simplify the story, much of medicine has treated the human being as a machine which, when it develops a fault, needs fixing. Instead, evolutionary medicine focuses on how the machine was built by natural selection in the first place, how the types of 'fault' have developed and changed over time, and how the machine might best behave and be treated to avoid them. Looking at health and disease from an evolutionary perspective—that is, in the context of the evolutionary history of human beings and our exposure to changing environments and prevailing diseases—generates different sorts of questions and novel responses. These are not instead of, but complementary to the normal mechanistic identification of causes, symptoms, and treatments, and an approach that is becoming an important part of medical training (Nesse et al. 2010; Nesse and Stearns 2008). The insights from evolutionary medicine can be classed into three main categories.

First, evolutionary medicine's 'core principle' is that *natural selection acts to promote biological fitness, not health or longevity* (Gluckman et al. 2011: 251). This is a vital nuance because, while counter-intuitive to the casual observer, after reproductive age natural selection has little interest in (there is less 'selection pressure') keeping us alive. This explains why we become so vulnerable to certain diseases as we age and why our responses to them weaken. For example, genes that promote growth in early life to become strong and resilient may have been favoured by natural selection, but later in life the same genes can contribute to obesity, diabetes, and cardiovascular disease—a phenomenon called 'agonistic pleiotropy' (Gluckman et al. 2011: 255). Selection is often absent, or not strong enough to mitigate the detrimental effects later on because if we are no longer producing offspring there are no (or lesser) consequences for our genes in subsequent generations. One implication for viruses such as COVID-19 is the susceptibility of older people to infection and severe symptoms. Long-lived individuals can sometimes have an advantage, in having built up immunity to numerous different disease pathogens over their lifetimes. However, when faced with a novel virus to which we have no prior immunity, older people are at a physiological disadvantage because they produce less varied T cells, making it harder for them to develop immunity to new pathogens by trial and error.[5]

Second, *evolutionary legacy affects our susceptibility to disease in different environments*. For example, scurvy is a debilitating and potentially fatal disease that occurs on long sea voyages or during famines, when one fails to obtain vitamin C

[5] On the other hand, and in a different domain, older people also accumulate long memories that include rare but catastrophic events that most people—including political leaders—have never experienced before and may thus discount too readily. Sometimes, elders see dangers and hardships that others cannot imagine and this biological store of knowledge could be one reason why natural selection has kept humans alive after reproduction as long as it has. Thanks to Ed LeGrand for this point.

from fresh fruit and other natural sources. Like many animals, human ancestors used to be able to synthesize vitamin C themselves. But at some point in our ancestral past, we lost the necessary enzyme for making this crucial part of our diet (probably through random neutral mutations) when fruit was a plentiful part of our environment and we didn't need to make vitamin C of our own. Other examples include short-sightedness, which is much more common today as a result of our increasingly indoor life focusing on close objects in artificial light, which distorts the growth of our eyes in childhood. The rise in mental illness is also thought to be partly a result of navigating a novel social environment that isolates us from the close and extensive family and social groups that were ever-present in our evolution (Dunbar 2003; Gluckman et al. 2011). As one example applied to the COVID-19 pandemic, imposed periods of isolation and the prevention of social and physical contact are precisely the kinds of novelty that can be psychologically harmful for a social animal like us.

Third, *evolutionary mismatch* describes the problems that can arise given that the contemporary world is very different from the one in which we evolved. Our biological and behavioural mechanisms are adaptations designed for the conditions of our past, not the present. Notably, for most of our evolutionary history, 'we largely lived in small social groups, survived on very different diets and were exposed to a much lower density of pathogens and toxins' (Gluckman et al. 2011: 252). This leads to a potential *mismatch* between the environment in which (and for which) our bodies and brains evolved and the very different social and physical environments in which we now live. This often plays havoc with the way we behave in relation to our current environment and our biological responses to it. A classic example is our taste for sugar, salt, and fat. This is an evolved disposition that was highly adaptive when such commodities were rare in our evolutionary past (and, indeed, long before that for all vertebrate species) and it was adaptive to seek them out, but in today's world of plentiful junk food the same disposition contributes to heart disease and diabetes which kill, for example, half a million Americans a year (www.cdc.gov/nchs/fastats, 2020).

Obvious insights from this evolutionary perspective for COVID-19 include, first, the shift to living in extremely large, dense, and globally interconnected groups, through which diseases can spread easily and rapidly into new susceptible populations. Human biology and social organization have a long history of cohabitation with disease (Lederberg 2000; Roberts 2020), but we are not so well equipped to deal with the novelty and scale of new global pandemics. Second, population expansion has led to large numbers of people settling in formerly natural areas in many parts of the world, increasing exposure to wild animals and the consequent emergence of zoonotic diseases. Wild animals tend to be the source of most major influenza virus pandemics, and in the future animal-to-human transmissions are expected to increase over time with burgeoning populations and declining alternative habitats, with an inevitable encroachment into wildlife areas and an increased probability of exposure to (and evolution of) new pathogens.

One might ask why it is that, after all the millions of years of evolution, the human body seems so vulnerable to so many different kinds of disease. But the answer itself also comes from evolutionary biology. First, pathogens are evolving too, so there is an arms race in which the evolution of our defences has to constantly adapt to counter the evolving strategies of disease pathogens, or when we move into novel environments (as with the constant battle to develop a new seasonal flu vaccine each year). Second, natural selection can't solve every problem, and must make trade-offs in which susceptibility to a given disease may be a necessary risk of pursuing some other important evolutionary function (such as sickle-cell anaemia reducing the blood's oxygen-carrying capacity, but at the same time providing protection against malaria). Third, since selection does not maximize health and longevity, but rather maximizes reproduction, many diseases result from a sacrifice of resources that might otherwise have been allocated to greater defence and countermeasures against pathogens.

Evolutionary Psychology

An important question arising from an evolutionary perspective is the extent to which we are adapted to deal not just with the *biological* challenges of the modern world, but also with the *cognitive* challenges of the modern world. The basic story here is that, ideally, we would act as rational actors, but we don't. One might expect general intelligence and rational thinking to be able to observe a problem accurately, evaluate the evidence in an even-handed manner, and act accordingly to minimize harms and maximize returns. However, a large research literature now shows that, empirically, humans fail to conform to this rational actor model of behaviour in numerous ways (Fiske and Taylor 2013; Gilovich et al. 2002; Kahneman 2011). Instead, even when the information we have is accurate, we are subject to a host of evolved cognitive heuristics and biases that lead us to make decisions that violate, sometimes quite radically, the expectations of rational choice. There are long lists of such biases, which have been identified and replicated under controlled conditions in the lab, as well as observed at work in the real world, where they contribute to significant decision-making failures from financial and policy disasters to crises and wars (Jervis 1976, 2017; Tetlock 1998, 2005). One important application is to think through how cognitive biases may affect our responses to the current and future pandemics. Cognitive biases are especially prominent when we face a blizzard of conflicting or confusing information (as we have about so many aspects of COVID-19 and governmental advice) and have to rely on our gut instincts instead of perfect information and calculation.

Before we come to specific examples, if these biases are such a liability, why do we have them? This is where evolutionary psychology comes in. Human physiological and psychological traits evolved to deal with the adaptive problems of our evolutionary past, not with the often very different kinds and scale of problems that we experience today, especially those that occur in international relations and events such as global pandemics (Barkow et al. 1992; Buss 2005; Pinker 2002; Wright 1994). The human lineage spent 99% of its history in a Pleistocene environment of small kin groups of hunter-gatherers, and only 1% in the post-agricultural environment of large, urbanized societies with sophisticated institutions and technologies. As a result, we should not necessarily expect evolved psychological mechanisms to trigger in appropriate circumstances, or to cause their intended effects. (In fact, many human dispositions extend much further back in the evolution of not just humans, but also *ancestral* species that preceded us many millions of years ago, cementing them into our, and many other, vertebrate physiological systems (Blumstein 2020).) Even when they *are* triggered by an appropriate stimulus (i.e. an evolutionarily relevant one), in modern settings the behaviour they give rise to may nevertheless cause inappropriate or costly outcomes (since the prevailing costs and benefits of the consequences of our behaviour have also changed). This phenomenon helps to explain, for example, the stubborn persistence of self-interest, nepotism, status seeking, addiction, and crimes of passion, even when those behaviours will come back to bite us and we know it (Burnham and Phelan 2001; Frank 1988; Giphart and van Vugt 2018; Kenrick and Griskevicius 2013).

Unfortunately, many of our evolved cognitive mechanisms appear to have been severely detrimental to efforts to mitigate the COVID-19 pandemic, both among the public and among political leaders as well—first in recognizing the danger, second in responding to it, and third in coordinating activities to fight it.

First, human brains are arguably ill suited to fully grasp the *threat* itself and the consequent implications of a global pandemic. As the virus initially spread in China and on to other regions, it is remarkable to think back to the slow reactions among governments around the world. They could have been even worse, of course, but national responses were widely regarded as having been complacent and slow. Historically, this turns out to be quite a common phenomenon. States repeatedly fail to recognize and prepare for impending dangers, especially novel dangers with which they are unfamiliar (Betts 1983; Johnson and Madin 2008; Sagarin 2012).[6] Several cognitive biases contribute to doubt or disbelief about the severity of new dangers, such as the widespread 'optimism bias' (Sharot 2011b), 'cognitive dissonance' (Cooper 2007; Festinger 1957), and the 'exponential-growth prediction bias', which, in the case of COVID-19, means that people fundamentally fail to appreciate the potential rapidity of its spread (Banerjee et al. 2020).

[6] Although, of course, states can sometimes be overly fearful as well; see Thrall and Cramer (2009).

There also seems to be a survivorship bias when it comes to addressing diseases, as we 'tend to underestimate past threats and disasters because we know that humankind survived them' (Roberts 2020: 8). In short, several important cognitive biases appear to have been at work in hindering our ability to act quickly.

Second, people's *responses* to the virus have also been hampered by common cognitive biases. The UK government (among others) set up a behavioural insights team specifically to anticipate how people would likely respond to the pandemic and restrictions on freedom, and how policy could be developed to counter common biases and maximize compliance (www.bi.team/our-work/covid-19). The major dynamic among afflicted populations has, fortunately, been a general acceptance of the problem and cooperation with government lockdowns and restrictions on behaviour. But such draconian rules have not always been agreed with or followed, and there have been multiple and sustained breaches, as well as organized protests and resistance. Much of the violations (and compliance) are due to people's perfectly rational assessment of their own level of risk, and making corresponding trade-offs in deciding what they can and cannot (or should and should not) do. The primary problem with that has been that people—especially younger ones—are assessing their *own* immediate risk (perhaps correctly), but not the risk that their behaviour poses to others, the longer-term consequences of sustained risk-taking, or the cumulative risk if everyone does the same thing. We tend to discount others and the future. At least part of the problem in achieving and enforcing lockdown rules, therefore, has been a natural disinclination, amplified by self-interest and cognitive dispositions, to change one's behaviour because of invisible agents—especially if one feels fine.

In ancestral environments, we were subject to lower and fewer novel pathogen loads, within a much lower population, at a lower density, and with more activity outdoors. While diseases were common, we are not well adapted to perform and sustain the kinds of behaviours necessary to fight a global pandemic (when completely novel diseases were introduced into susceptible populations in history, such as by Spanish conquistadors in South America, the consequences were catastrophic). The need for constant social distancing, perhaps most notably, especially with close friends and family, is not just inconvenient but flies in the face of our instinctive social nature.[7] Moreover, the agents of disease themselves are intangible. While we have deeply ingrained natural disgust mechanisms that react to obvious signs of unsanitary or infected objects, people, and food (Curtis et al. 2011), we do not have an evolved repulsion for invisible agents of disease such as viruses. George Murdock surveyed 186 Indigenous societies around the world and found all of them to attribute illness not to the work of microscopic pathogens, but

[7] For an animal behaviourist perspective on this exact point, see Daniel T. Blumstein. "Banning Sociality Is Costly Our obligate sociality makes us vulnerable to necessary pandemic controls." Psychology Today, 29, 2020.

rather to the malicious work of supernatural agents (Murdock 1980). We have to fight against the grain of human nature to prevent ourselves from engaging in social contact and conceiving of biological agents of disease. People go about their business—often seeking out contact and without masks—appearing remarkably unafraid, perhaps itself an adaptive characteristic but one that carries new dangers in unusual times (Sharot 2011a).

Third, there is a severe problem of *coordination and cooperation*. An effective population response requires subordinating one's self-interest for the greater public good. Despite (or sometimes precisely because of) government policies, there are strong incentives for individuals to continue moving around and meeting people to maintain their welfare and livelihoods, avoid losing their job or their clients, and see and help friends and family, not to mention having fun and doing the things they want to do. This is a classic collective action problem. While the virus would most effectively be stamped out if everyone put their self-interests aside and contributed 100% to the public good, people have strong incentives acting in the opposite direction. This is exacerbated if one sees others violating the rules or enjoying exceptions. The collective action problem is already a 'problem' as it is because, as well as the uncertainty about whether the collective goal will be achieved at all, the decision to participate oneself means that one may end up wasting time, effort, or resources in contributing to a lost cause. Moreover, having contributed, one is also left in a worse position compared to others who did not expend any of their time, effort, or resources (Olson 1965; Ostrom 1990). Of course, this is why leadership and rules become vital in such cases to ensure or enforce cohesion, rather than to merely expect or hope for it. But it doesn't always succeed. Especially in times of crisis like this one, 'Trust in leadership is essential because struggles against infectious diseases necessitate a degree of individual sacrifice for the social good' (Roberts 2020: 32). Pandemic restrictions in particular need to be perceived as clear, having a solid rationale, and working towards a definite goal. If they don't, self-interest prevails. In short, while we can see the logic of coordinated action and how it would be more effective if everyone commits to it, at the same time, we have powerful dispositions to look after ourselves and our families first. These are not just random psychological tendencies; they are deeply entrenched aspects of our evolved psychology (Lieberman et al. 2007; Pinker 2002). Rational logic and politicians imploring us to follow the rules only goes so far in a deeply social animal.

Before ending this section, it is worth highlighting three important corollaries. First, all of the above tended to imply cognitive biases acting among the public at large. However, cognitive biases apply just as much to leaders and policymakers as they do to everyone else. As well as cognitive biases affecting public reactions and compliance, therefore, they also contribute to explaining the policies (or the lack of policies) of state decision-makers (see, e.g. Jervis 2017; Sears et al. 2003; Tetlock 2005). As one obvious example, several high-profile politicians in multiple countries came under fire or had to step down because they breached the very lockdown rules their own governments had imposed (top English, Scottish, and New Zealand lawmakers travelled to be with family in violation of lockdown restrictions). Human instincts are a powerful force and evolved incentives often override our more rational side, whether consciously or not (T. D. Wilson 2004). This applies to us all.

Second, some biases can work in opposition. For example, above I suggested that people are primarily self-interested. But, of course, there are also strong dispositions that, under certain circumstances, make humans remarkably prosocial as well (Cronk and Leech 2013; McCullough 2020; Ridley 1996). This means we must be careful to identify the *conditions* that give rise to one bias rather than another. Above, I mentioned overconfidence as a potential contributor to ill-preparedness in the face of the pandemic. But in other respects we also suffer from a 'negativity bias', which can explain instances of overreaction and fear (Baumeister et al. 2001; Tierney and Baumeister 2019). Therefore, we need to consider the different contexts and conditions under which each bias emerges, and how they may interact. Positive and negative biases, for example, can apply simultaneously but with respect to different objects: optimism bias appears to be prominent in evaluations of the *self* or one's future prospects, whereas the negativity bias tends to come to the fore when people are evaluating *others'* behaviour or the environment—including especially the risk of disease and contagion (Rozin and Royzman 2001). When both biases arise in combination, this can be a recipe for disaster, for example, inflating the threat of some external agent but, at the same time, overestimating our own ability to overcome it (Johnson and Tierney 2019). This may help to explain instances of both fear and complacency surrounding the pandemic response.

Third, many of the biases mentioned above are well known in social psychology and behavioural economics. One could thus accept their role without invoking any evolutionary origin. What exactly does an evolutionary perspective add? An evolutionary perspective is helpful because it sheds light on why we have these biases in the first place (their ultimate causes), what the biological mechanisms and triggers for the biases are (their proximate causes), and thus the physical and social conditions under which we can expect them to be amplified or reduced, and—consequently—how they can best be mitigated. Furthermore, an evolutionary perspective also forces us to consider the adaptive significance of our cognitive biases. What are they *for*? Applying an evolutionary lens reminds us that cognitive biases should not always be seen as detrimental. After all, they evolved because they helped us make good decisions, not bad ones. Thus, in the right (evolutionarily relevant) contexts they may, in fact, steer us to make more effective decisions rather than disastrous ones, especially in fast-moving situations when we have to act with poor information under uncertainty, without the luxury of time or resources to wait on perfect decision-making. Instead, we have to rely on instinct (Gigerenzer and Brighton 2009; Haselton et al. 2009; Johnson 2020). Arguably, for example, the negativity bias may have been helpful in the COVID-19 pandemic because, by making at least some people *overly* fearful of contagion, even if irrational, it increased the efficacy and compliance of social distancing and national lockdowns.

Cultural Evolution

Up until now, I have focused on aspects of virus or human behaviour that have evolved by biological natural selection. However, humans and human societies are not bound merely by genetics. For many thousands of years, humans have also adapted to their physical and social environment through *cultural* adaptations (such as tools, clothes, rituals, social institutions, and so on). While these are 'cultural' phenomena, over time they nevertheless undergo the same dynamics of Darwinian selection as do genetic adaptations—it is just that, rather than genes being differentially selected, it is *ideas* and *innovations* that are differentially selected, with beneficial ones spreading at the expense of less effective ones (Creanza et al. 2017; Mesoudi 2011). Of course, like genes, sometimes new cultural traditions are neutral and have no positive or negative effect, and just remain in the population through drift (a lack of counter-selection). But the point is that cultural adaptations can also often exert an important positive impact on survival and reproduction (as well as feeding back to create new environments for subsequent *genetic* adaptations; Diamond 2005). The major difference between biological and cultural evolution is that cultural adaptations can arise and spread much faster, passing from mind to mind on the scale of days, compared to genetic adaptations, which have to wait many years for each new biological generation to turn over (and only then be tested by selection).

Because regional environments and local ecologies are so different around the world (from arctic tundra and desert to mountains and rainforest), different populations have evolved many cultural as well as genetic differences in their responses to the prevailing challenges of health and disease. Just as many diseases only (or mainly) occur in some parts of the world, so some *genetic* adaptations to diseases are more prevalent in some populations rather than others. There are many examples, from the distribution of malaria and sickle cell anaemia (the latter protects from the former) to lactose intolerance and the domestication of cattle (this inability to digest lactose in milk occurs in the absence of the latter tradition).[8] But many *cultural* characteristics have also arisen in response to disease, from permitted or

[8] Populations that domesticated cattle in Europe and Africa significantly changed their nutritional environment and developed genetic mutations to digest lactose, but populations that did not domesticate cattle did not. In traditional medicine, lactose intolerance was seen as an 'abnormality' or 'syndrome', but an evolutionary perspective sees it as a perfectly normal biological state in populations that did not domesticate cattle (Gluckman et al. 2011).

banned types of food and rituals of food preparation, to social norms surrounding illness and cleanliness (Murdock 1980; Murdock and Wilson 1978).

One set of recent studies suggests that cultural variation in social organization is itself an adaptation to local levels of disease pathogens, which may have relevance (at least as one interesting hypothesis to explore) to different populations' susceptibility or responses to COVID-19. Researchers have long noted systematic and consistent differences across cultures in their levels of 'collectivism' versus 'individualism'. This was a general distinction made in early comparisons of cultures by Max Weber, and collectivism–individualism was later explicitly developed as a cross-cultural variable by Geert Hofsteder and others, and has become, according to some advocates, 'a paradigmatic element of culture that, in the eyes of many social scientists, is fundamental to any understanding of cross-cultural differences' (Fincher et al. 2008: 1283; Hofstede 1980; Triandis 1995). The basic idea is that collectivist cultures (such as Brazil, India, Russia, and Japan) are more likely to emphasize the in-group over out-groups. By contrast, individualist cultures (such as the United States, the UK, France, and Germany) Of course, there is much variation within countries and among individuals, but the collectivist–individualist distinction captures a broad trend (Triandis 1995: 2).[9] (Ma-Kellams et al. 2011) still do this as well, but to a lesser extent, elevating instead individual interest and out-group opportunities.

But *why* does collectivism and individualism vary among cultures? A variety of theories have emerged, tending to focus on the sociological consequences of different regional practices, such as the legacies of farming wheat versus rice, for example. But Thornhill and colleagues suggest that it may also be a social response to disease. He and his colleagues see the collectivist–individualist dimension of

[9] Triandis defines *collectivism* as:

> a social pattern consisting of closely linked individuals who see themselves as parts of one or more collectives (family, co-workers, tribe, nation); are primarily motivated by the norms of, and duties imposed by, those collectives; are willing to give priority to the goals of these collectives over their personal goals; and emphasize their connectedness to members of these collectives.
>
> (Triandis 1995: 2)

Note that collectivism is similar but not identical to ideological conservatism, although the latter is itself is also known to be strongly associated with conformity and out-group hostility (Jost et al. 2003). By contrast, *individualism* is defined as:

> a social pattern that consists of loosely linked individuals who view themselves as independent of collectives; are primarily motivated by their own preferences, needs, rights, and the contracts they have established with others; give priority to their personal goals over the goals of others; and emphasize rational analyses of the advantages and disadvantages to associating with others.
>
> (Triandis, 1995: 2)

Scholars have challenged whether it represents a simplistic continuum or is multi-dimensional (Singelis et al. 1995; Taras et al. 2014). Nevertheless, while the terms themselves 'are used by many people in different parts of the world and are given different meanings', in cross-cultural psychology a large body of research identifies a number of factors that distinguish between these two broad types of orientation across cultures (Nisbett 2003; Oyserman et al. 2002).

behaviour as a 'species-typical, evolved sensitivity to information inputs from the immediate environment' (Fincher et al. 2008: 1284). In other words, genetic dispositions combined with developmental plasticity allow human psychological and behavioural mechanisms to tune their level of collectivism–individualism to match the demands of their environment (and in other work, they show that this seems to be associated with the types of political systems and religions that have emerged as well). However, what demands of the environment are we talking about? Thornhill has found that the strongest statistical predictor of collectivism–individualism around the world is the prevalence of disease pathogens in the local environment. In short, the stronger in-group/out-group bias of collectivist cultures may have arisen, at least in part, as a defence mechanism to avoid the transmission of diseases from other groups in areas of high pathogen prevalence.

The idea that the in-group/out-group bias serves as an adaptation to reduce the risk of disease transmission has been theorized for some time (e.g. Haselton and Nettle 2006), and Thornhill's studies have suggested some empirical support. The same adaptive logic that groupish behaviour may have evolved (or may now serve) to avoid disease transmission is well supported in biology more generally, as it occurs across many taxonomic groups. This suggests that, along with many other species, over our evolutionary history we have been subjected to significant disease risks that, when severe enough, 'select social animals, like humans, for an adaptive xenophobia' (Rozsa 2000: 396). Above, we considered the conflict between self-interest and group-interests undermining lockdown restrictions in the global pandemic, and to some extent the same tension has arisen between different groups within and between countries. In times of crises, when people are threatened, the in-group/out-group bias becomes stronger. They are more likely to look out for themselves and their families, but also for members of their in-group with which they identify and often rely on to thrive and survive, and to become especially wary of out-groups (Hewstone et al. 2002; Inglehart et al. 2006).

While somewhat speculative, it is interesting that the poor performance of the pandemic response among some notable rich, western individualist countries, such as the United States and the UK, falls into line with this thesis—it was arguably harder for them to restrict individual liberties and close down their people and trade to the outside world. Meanwhile, many collectivist countries fared better, as measured by deaths per population (WHO COVID-19 Dashboard, https://covid19.who.int, January 2021). Broader statistical analyses conducted so far also support this association (Jiang et al. 2020).

Conclusions: Using Evolution to Help Us

Without evolutionary biology, we would be seriously in the dark about important questions on COVID-19, including: how did the virus emerge, how has it spread, how is it changing, and how might it best be countered? This is all the more important in a global pandemic, where global networks, international travel, and a vast susceptible population means rapid analyses of the virus geneology are vital to understanding how it is spreading and how it can best be stopped. But there is a dark side too. An evolutionary perspective suggests that many of our policies in the global mitigation efforts are playing into the hands of the virus. Evolution teaches us that organisms are always evolving and adapting, and we are not in a static fight but a dynamic one that we need to win quickly because it will get harder

Table 2.1 Some implications for pandemic mitigation efforts involving (a) the virus and (b) the host (and note these are considerations, not policy recommendations).

Target	Issue area	Political approach	Evolutionary approach
(a) Virus	**Restrictions**	Limit (to keep the economy going)	Maximize (not just to reduce spread but to reduce the opportunity for further mutation)
	Speed	Measured (to balance competing demands)	As fast as possible (to reduce positive feedback in spread and mutation)
	Travel	Lax (allow travel corridors and holidays where possible)	Strict (danger not just of spread, but also of seeding of new variants across borders)
(b) Host	**Assessment**	Implicit expectation of rational decision-making and behaviour (and thus that people will accept and follow information, advice, and guidelines)	No expectation of rational decision-making and behaviour (rather, a persistence of overconfidence, risk-taking, and other cognitive and behavioural biases)
	Social behaviour	People should follow social distancing if the logic is explained	People are unlikely to comply strictly with social distancing, given our intensely social nature (thus, augment other measures to compensate)
	Culture	Societal responses largely determined by wealth, resources, and regime type	Societal responses also determined by cultural characteristics (individualistic, rather than collectivist societies may need to act differently to achieve similar results)

Note: The insights above are not always unique or exclusive to an evolutionary perspective (they may arise from other disciplinary approaches as well), but the point is that an evolutionary perspective *emphasizes their importance* beyond what it already is. Moreover, in combination they suggest a new way of approaching the problem.

the longer the fight goes on and the greater the opportunity for the evolution of new virus variants—which will get stronger, not weaker. If the virus does not mutate too quickly, does not evolve into more virulent forms, and remains vulnerable to vaccines, then we will get away with a lot of political blundering. But we are not only fighting the consequences of evolution for the virus, we are also fighting the consequences of evolution for ourselves.

We have often been puzzled by our own responses. Not least, our slow and grudging recognition of the problem in the first place, our underestimation of its impact and our overestimation of our ability to avoid it or deal with it, our ill-adaptedness to lockdown restrictions, and the impediments to collective action. If we were rational actors, those would indeed be a puzzle. But the puzzle evaporates when we recognize humans not as rational actors, but instead as the products of natural selection with an evolutionary legacy of our own, which has given rise to an array of evolved dispositions that powerfully influence the way we think and behave. These manifest themselves differently in different cultural and political contexts, giving rise to a range of responses and successes and failures. But some fundamental traits appear to present some common dangers for us all. This may explain why we have been here before. Effective responses to global disasters—and pandemics in particular—require considerable preparation, monitoring, scale, and speed, well beyond the levels needed to address more quotidian challenges and threats. As Rafe Sagarin lamented long before COVID-19, 'By the time new diseases are visible to most health programs, and they marshal the resources to respond, it's too late' (Sagarin 2012: 75).

Many times during the crisis, people have pointed to critical things that need to be in place for an effective response, whether better leadership, more information, greater economic bail outs, deeper international cooperation, and so on. But to a large extent, and ever more so as the virus changes over time (we are at the beginning of a marathon, not the end of a sprint), we also need to apply an evolutionary lens to make sense of the peculiarities of both the virus and its host, and to understand its spread and the responses of human bodies and minds (Table 2.1 captures some key policy insights of this evolutionary approach). To paraphrase Dobzhansky (1973), much about the pandemic—in the behaviour of both the virus and its host—does not make sense except in the light of evolution.

References

Banerjee, Ritwick, Joydeep Bhattacharya, and Priyama Majumdar. 2020. 'Exponential-Growth Prediction Bias and Compliance with Safety Measures in the Times of COVID-19'. *arXiv*: 2005.01273.

Barkow, Jerome. H. 2006. *Missing the Revolution: Darwinism for Social Scientists*. Oxford: Oxford University Press.

Barkow, Jerome. H., Leda Cosmides, and John Tooby, eds. 1992. *The Adapted Mind: Evolutionary Psychology and the Generation of Culture*. Oxford: Oxford University Press.

Baumeister, Roy F., Ellen Bratslavsky, Catrin Finkenauer, and Kathleen D. Vohs. 2001. 'Bad Is Stronger Than Good'. *Review of General Psychology 5* (4): pp. 323–70.

Bedford, Trevor, Richard Neher, James Hadfield, Emma Hodcroft, Misja Ilcisin, and Nicola Müller. 2020. 'Genomic Analysis of nCoV Spread: Situation Report'. 30 January. https://nextstrain.org/narratives/ncov/sit-rep/2020-01-30.

Betts, Richard 1983. *Surprise Attack: Lessons for Defense Planning*. Washington, DC: Brookings Institution Press.

Blumstein, Daniel T. 2020. *The Nature of Fear: Survival Lessons from the Wild*. Cambridge, MA: Harvard University Press.

Burki, Talha 2020. 'The Origin of SARS-CoV-2'. *The Lancet 20* (9): pp. 1018–19.

Burnham, Terence, and Jay Phelan. 2001. *Mean Genes: From Sex to Money to Food, Taming Our Primal Instincts*. New York: Penguin.

Buss, David M., ed. 2005. *The Handbook of Evolutionary Psychology*. New York: Wiley.

Campbell, Neil A., ed. 1993. *Biology* (3rd edn). Redwood City, CA: Benjamin Cummings.

Cookson, Clive, and Ian Bott. 2020. 'Mutations Map Holds the Key to Bringing Coronavirus under Control'. *Financial Times*, 21 April.

Cooper, Joel 2007. *Cognitive Dissonance: 50 Years of a Classic Theory*. New York: Sage.

Creanza, Nicole, Oren Kolodny, and Marcus W. Feldman. 2017. 'Cultural Evolutionary Theory: How Culture Evolves and Why It Matters'. *Proceedings of the National Academy of Sciences (PNAS) 114* (30): pp. 7782–9.

Cronk, Lee, and Beth L. Leech. 2013. *Meeting at Grand Central: Understanding the Social and Evolutionary Roots of Cooperation*. Princeton, NJ: Princeton University Press.

Curtis, Valerie, Michael D. Barra, and Robert Aunger. 2011. 'Disgust as an Adaptive System for Disease Avoidance Behaviour'. *Philosophical Transactions of the Royal Society B 366* (1563): pp. 389–401.

Dawkins, Richard 1976. *The Selfish Gene*. Oxford: Oxford University Press.

Dawkins, Richard, and John R. Krebs. 1979. 'Arms Races between and within Species'. *Proceedings of the Royal Society of London B 205*: pp. 489–511.

Diamond, Jared 2005. *Collapse: How Societies Choose to Fail or Succeed*. New York: Penguin.

Dobzhansky, Theodosius 1973. 'Nothing in Biology Makes Sense Except in the Light of Evolution'. *American Biology Teacher 35* (3): pp. 125–9.

Doshi, Peter 2020. 'Covid-19: Do Many People Have Pre-Existing Immunity?'. *British Medical Journal 370*: m3563.

Dunbar. Robin I. M. 2003. 'The Social Brain: Mind, Language, and Society in Evolutionary Perspective'. *Annual Review of Anthropology 32*: pp. 163–81.

European Centre for Disease Prevention and Control (ECDC). 2020. 'Rapid Increase of a SARS-CoV-2 Variant with Multiple Spike Protein Mutations Observed in the United Kingdom'. Stockholm: ECDC.

Ewald, Paul W. 1997. *Evolution of Infectious Disease*. Oxford: Oxford University Press.

Festinger, Leon 1957. *A Theory of Cognitive Dissonance*. Stanford, CA: Stanford University Press.

Fincher, Corey L., Randy Thornhill, Damian R. Murray, and Mark Schaller. 2008. 'Pathogen Prevalence Predicts Human Cross-Cultural Variability in Individualism/Collectivism'. *Proceedings of the Royal Society B 275* (1640): pp. 1279–85.

Fiske, Susan T., and Shelley E. Taylor. 2013. *Social Cognition: From Brains to Culture* (2nd edn). New York: McGraw-Hill.

Frank, Robert H. 1988. *Passions within Reason: The Strategic Role of the Emotions*. New York: Norton.

Gallagher, James 2020. 'COVID: Why Is Coronavirus Such a Threat?' *BBC News*, 22 October. https://www.bbc.com/news/health-54648684.

Gigerenzer, Gerd, and Henry Brighton. 2009. '*Homo Heuristicus*: Why Biased Minds Make Better Inferences'. *Topics in Cognitive Science 1*: pp. 107–43.

Gilovich, Thomas, Dale Griffin, and Daniel Kahneman, eds. 2002. *Heuristics and Biases: The Psychology of Intuitive Judgment*. Cambridge: Cambridge University Press.

Giphart, Ronald, and Mark van Vugt. 2018. *Mismatch: How Our Stone Age Brain Deceives Us Every Day (And What We Can Do About It)*. London: Little, Brown Book Group.

Gluckman, Peter D., Alan S. Beedle, and Mark A. Hanson, eds. 2009. *Principles of Evolutionary Medicine*. Oxford: Oxford University Press.

Gluckman, Peter D., Felicia M. Low, Tatjana Buklijas, Mark A. Hanson, and Alan S. Beedle. 2011. 'How Evolutionary Principles Improve the Understanding of Human Health and Disease'. *Evolutionary Applications 4* (2): pp. 249–63.

Green, Nigel P. O., G. Wilfred Stout, and Dennis J. Taylor, eds. 1990. *Biological Science* (2nd edn). Cambridge: Cambridge University Press.

Grubaugh, Nathan D., William P. Hanage, and Angela L. Rasmussen. 2020. 'Making Sense of Mutation: What D614G Means for the COVID-19 Pandemic Remains Unclear'. *Cell 182* (4): pp. 812–27.

Haselton, Martie G., Gregory A. Bryant, Andreas Wilke, D. A., et al. 2009. 'Adaptive Rationality: An Evolutionary Perspective on Cognitive Bias'. *Social Cognition 27*: pp. 733–63.

Haselton, Martie G., and Daniel Nettle. 2006. 'The Paranoid Optimist: An Integrative Evolutionary Model of Cognitive Biases'. *Personality and Social Psychology Review 10* (1): pp. 47–66.

He, Xi, Eric H. Y. Lau, Peng Wu, et al. 2020. 'Temporal Dynamics in Viral Shedding and Transmissibility of COVID-19'. *Nature Medicine 26*: pp. 672–5.

Hewstone, Miles, Mark Rubin, and Hazel Willis. 2002. 'Intergroup Bias'. *Annual Review of Psychology 53*: pp. 575–604.

Hodcroft, Emma B., Moira Zuber, Sarah Nadeau, et al. 2020. 'Emergence and Spread of a SARS-CoV-2 Variant through Europe in the Summer of 2020'. *medRxiv*. https://doi.org/10.1101/2020.10.25.20219063.

Hofstede, Geert. 1980. *Culture's Consequences: Comparing Values, Behaviors, Institutions and Organizations Across Nations*. Beverly Hills, CA: Sage.

Inglehart, Ronald F., Mansoor Moaddel, and Mark Tessler. 2006. 'Xenophobia and In-Group Solidarity in Iraq: A Natural Experiment on the Impact of Insecurity'. *Perspectives on Politics 4* (3): pp. 495–505.

Jervis, Robert. 1976. *Perception and Misperception in International Politics*. Princeton, NJ: Princeton University Press.

Jervis, Robert. 2017. *How Statesmen Think: The Psychology of International Politics*. Princeton, NJ: Princeton University Press.

Jiang, Shuguang, Qian Wei, and Luyao Zhang. 2020. 'Impacts of Cultural Difference on the Transmission of COVID-19: Individualism vs. Collectivism'. *SSRN*, 8 July. https://ssrn.com/abstract=3646229.

Johnson, Dominic D. P. 2004. *Overconfidence and War: The Havoc and Glory of Positive Illusions*. Cambridge, MA: Harvard University Press.

Johnson, Dominic D. P. 2020. *Strategic Instincts: The Adaptive Advantages of Psychological Biases in International Relations.* Princeton, NJ: Princeton University Press.

Johnson, Dominic D. P., and Elizabeth M. P. Madin. 2008. 'Paradigm Shifts in Security Strategy: Why Does It Take Disasters to Trigger Change?' In *Natural Security: A Darwinian Approach to a Dangerous World*, edited by R. D. Sagarin and T. Taylor, pp. 209–39. Berkeley, CA: University of California Press.

Johnson, Dominic D. P., and Dominic R. Tierney. 2019. 'Bad World: The Negativity Bias in International Relations'. *International Security 43* (3): pp. 96–140.

Johnson, Dominic D. P., Daniel T. Blumstein, James H. Fowler, and Martie G. Haselton. 2013. 'The Evolution of Error: Error Management, Cognitive Constraints, and Adaptive Decision-Making Biases'. *Trends in Ecology & Evolution 28* (8): pp. 474–81.

Jost, John T., Jack Glaser, Aarie W. Kruglanski, and Frank J. Sulloway. 2003. 'Political Conservatism as Motivated Social Cognition'. *Psychological Bulletin 129*: pp. 339–75.

Kahneman, Daniel. 2011. *Thinking, Fast and Slow*. London: Allen Lane.

Kenrick, Douglas T., and Vladas Griskevicius. 2013. *The Rational Animal: How Evolution Made Us Smarter Than We Think*. New York: Basic Books.

Korber, Bette, Will M. Fischer, Sandrasegaram Gnanakaran, et al. 2020. 'Tracking Changes in SARS-CoV-2 Spike: Evidence That D614G Increases Infectivity of the COVID-19 Virus'. *Cell 182* (4): pp. 812–27.

Lederberg. Joshua. 2000. 'Infectious History'. *Science 288* (5464): pp. 287–93.

Lieberman, Debra, John Tooby, and Leda Cosmides. 2007. 'The Architecture of Human Kin Detection'. *Nature 445*: pp. 727–31.

Ma-Kellams, Christine, Julie Spencer-Rodgers, and Kaiping Peng. 2011. 'I Am Against Us? Unpacking Cultural Differences in Ingroup Favoritism via Dialecticism'. *Personality and Social Psychology Bulletin 37* (1): pp. 15–27.

McCullough, Michael E. 2020. *The Kindness of Strangers: How a Selfish Ape Invented a New Moral Code*. New York: Basic Books.

Mesoudi, Alex 2011. *Cultural Evolution: How Darwinian Theory Can Explain Human Culture and Synthesize the Social Sciences*. Chicago, IL: University of Chicago Press.

Milne, Richard, and Clive Cookson. 2020. '"Ticking Bombs": Threat of Mink Coronavirus Mutation Sparks Anxiety'. *Financial Times*, 6 November.

Murdock, George. P. 1980. *Theories of Illness: A World Survey*. Pittsburg, PA: University of Pittsburgh Press.

Murdock, George P., and Suzanne Wilson. 1978. 'Cultural Theories of Illness'. *Ethnology 17*: pp. 449–70.

Nesse, Randolph M., Carl T. Bergstrom, Peter T. Ellison, et al. 2010. 'Making Evolutionary Biology a Basic Science for Medicine'. *Proceedings of the National Academy of Sciences (PNAS) 107*: pp. 1800–7.

Nesse, Randolph. M., and Stephen C. Stearns. 2008. 'The Great Opportunity: Evolutionary Applications to Medicine and Public Health'. *Evolutionary Applications 1*: pp. 28–48.

Nesse, Randolph M., and George C. Williams. 1995. *Why We Get Sick: The New Science of Darwinian Medicine*. New York: Times Books.

Nisbett, Richard E. 2003. *The Geography of Thought: How Asians and Westerners Think Differently—And Why*. London: Nicholas Brealey Publishing.

Olson, Mancur. 1965. *The Logic of Collective Action: Public Goods and the Theory of Groups*. Cambridge, MA: Harvard University Press.

Ostrom, Elinor. 1990. *Governing the Commons: The Evolution of Institutions for Collective Action*. Cambridge: Cambridge University Press.
Oyserman, Daphna, Heather Coon, and Markus Kemmelmeier. 2002. 'Rethinking Individualism and Collectivism: Evaluation of Theoretical Assumptions and Meta-Analyses'. *Psychological Bulletin 128* (1): pp. 3–72.
Pinker, Steven 2002. *The Blank Slate: The Modern Denial of Human Nature*. New York: Penguin Putnam.
Ridley, Matt. 1994. *The Red Queen: Sex and the Evolution of Human Nature*. London: Penguin.
Ridley, Matt. 1996. *The Origins of Virtue: Human Instincts and the Origins of Cooperation*. London: Penguin.
Roberts, Adam. 2020. 'Pandemics and Politics'. *Survival 62* (5): pp. 7–40.
Rozin, Paul, and Edward B. Royzman. 2001. 'Negativity Bias, Negativity Dominance, and Contagion'. *Personality and Social Psychology Review 5* (4): pp. 296–320.
Rozsa, Lajos 2000. 'Spite, Xenophobia, and Collaboration between Hosts and Parasites'. *Oikos 91* (2): pp. 396–400.
Ryan, Frank. 2009. *Virolution*. London: Collins.
Sagarin, Raphael D. 2012. *Learning from the Octopus: How Secrets from Nature Can Help Us Fight Terrorist Attacks, Natural Disasters, and Disease*. New York: Basic Books.
Sagarin, Raphael D., and Terence Taylor, eds. 2008. *Natural Security: A Darwinian Approach to a Dangerous World*. Berkeley, CA: University of California Press.
Sagarin, Raphael D., Candace Alcorta, Scott Atran, et al. 2010. 'Decentralize, Adapt and Cooperate'. *Nature 465*: pp. 292–3.
Sears, David. O., Leonie Huddy, and Robert Jervis. 2003. *Oxford Handbook of Political Psychology*. Oxford: Oxford University Press.
Sender, Ron. Yinon M. Bar-On, Avi Flamholz, et al. 2020. 'The Total Number and Mass of SARS-CoV-2 Virions in an Infected Person'. *medRxiv*. doi: 10.1101/2020.11.16.20232009.
Sharot, Tali 2011a. 'The Optimism Bias'. *Curent Biology 21* (23): R941–5.
Sharot, Tali 2011b. *The Optimism Bias: A Tour of The Irrationally Positive Brain*. New York: Pantheon.
Singelis, Theodore M., Harry C. Triandis, Dharm P. S. Bhawuk, and Michele J. Gelfand. 1995. 'Horizontal and Vertical Dimensions of Individualism and Collectivism: A Theoretical and Measurement Refinement'. *Cross-Cultural Research 29* (3): pp. 240–75.
Smith, Gavin J. D., Dhanasekaran Vijaykrishna, Justin Bahl, et al. 2009. 'Origins and Evolutionary Genomics of the 2009 Swine-Origin H1N1 Influenza A Epidemic'. *Nature 459*: pp. 1122–5.
Taras, Vas, Riikka Sarala, Paul Muchinsky, et al. 2014. 'Opposite Ends of the Same Stick? Multi-Method Test of the Dimensionality of Individualism and Collectivism'. *Journal of Cross-Cultural Psychology 45* (2): pp. 213–45.
Tetlock, Philip E. 1998. 'Social Psychology and World Politics'. In *Handbook of Social Psychology*, edited by D. Gilbert, S. Fiske, and G. Lindzey, pp. 868–912. New York: McGraw Hill.
Tetlock, Philip E. 2005. *Expert Political Judgment: How Good Is It? How Can We Know?* Princeton, NJ: Princeton University Press.
Thrall, A. Trevor, and Jane K. Cramer, eds. 2009. *American Foreign Policy and the Politics of Fear: Threat Inflation since 9/11*. New York: Routledge.

Tierney, John, and Roy F. Baumeister. 2019. *The Power of Bad: And How to Overcome It*. New York: Penguin.

Triandis, Harry. C. 1995. *Individualism and Collectivism*. Boulder, CO: Westview Press.

Van Egeren, Debra, Aalexander Novokhodko, Madison Stoddard, et al. 2020. 'Risk of Evolutionary Escape from Neutralizing Antibodies Targeting SARS-CoV-2 Spike Protein'. *medRxiv*. https://doi.org/10.1101/2020.11.17.20233726.

Villarreal, Luis P. 2005. *Viruses and the Evolution of Life*. Washington, DC: ASM Press.

Volz, Erik M., Verity Hill, John T. McCrone, et al. 2020. 'Evaluating the Effects of SARS-CoV-2 Spike Mutation D614G on Transmissibility and Pathogenicity'. *medRxiv*. https://doi.org/10.1101/2020.07.31.20166082.

Weissman, Drew, Mohamad-Gabriel Alameh, Tushan D. Silva, et al. 2020. 'D614G Spike Mutation Increases SARS CoV-2 Susceptibility to Neutralization'. *medRxiv*. https://doi.org/10.1101/2020.07.22.20159905.

Williams, George C., and Randolph M. Nesse. 1991. 'The Dawn of Darwinian Medicine'. *Quarterly Review of Biology 66* (1): pp. 1–22.

Wilson, Edward O. 1999. *Consilience: The Unity of Knowledge*. London: Abacus.

Wilson, Timothy D. 2004. *Strangers to Ourselves: Discovering the Adaptive Unconscious*. Cambridge, MA: Belknap Press.

Wright, Robert. 1994. *The Moral Animal: Why We Are, the Way We Are, The New Science of Evolutionary Psychology*. New York: Random House.

Wrotek, Sylwia, Edmund K. LeGrand, Artur Dzialuk, and Joe Alcock. 2020. 'Let Fever Do Its Job: The Meaning of Fever in the Pandemic Era'. *Evolution, Medicine, and Public Health*, eoaa044. https://doi.org/010.1093/emph/eoaa1044.

3

Will COVID-19 Bring Down Governments? Will It Bring Rebellions and Revolutions?

Jack A. Goldstone

There are two main paths by which pandemics create pressures for political change. The first is demographic; that is, if the impact on the population is so large as to substantially alter the level or trajectory of population growth, in a way that changes the balance of supply and demand for capital, land and labour, then changes in the leverage of governments and elites versus workers and peasants can arise that produce major shifts in wealth and political power (Scheidel 2018).

The Black Death, which in the early fourteenth century cut down roughly one-third of the population wherever it took hold, from Europe through the Middle East, Central Asia, and China, was one such pandemic catastrophe. Arising in central Asia, it was carried east to China and west to the Black Sea by Mongol armies, and thence to Europe by Italian traders from their base in Crimea (Kelly 2005). In Western Europe, the loss of labour to cultivate landed estates led to unsuccessful efforts by feudal lords to exert greater control over peasants. These efforts provoked uprisings such as the Peasant's Revolt of 1381 in England, which challenged the ability of princes to impose taxes and landlords to control peasants, thus helping to end serfdom (Jedwab et al. 2020). In the Near East, the Black Death undermined the Byzantine Empire and paved the way for the rise of the Ottomans (Ayalon 2014). In China and central Asia, the pandemic weakened the Mongol empires, including the Yuan dynasty in China, facilitating the rise of the Ming dynasty (Szczepanski 2019, Dennis 2020). In Egypt and other parts of the Middle East that depended on maintaining complex irrigation works, the major population losses led these systems to fall into decay, producing a long-term decline in their economies; this also contributed to the fall of the Mamluks in Egypt (Dols 1977; Borsch 2005). The impacts of these massive demographic losses, however, often took several decades after the onset of the pandemic to work through agricultural systems, the distribution of wealth, and the reigns of dynasties.

Nothing like that will result from the COVID-19 pandemic, which appears to have a fatality rate of somewhere between 1% and 2% of all those infected, and so far has killed just 0.2% to 0.5% of the population in the worst-affected states—for

Jack A. Goldstone, *Will COVID-19 Bring Down Governments? Will It Bring Rebellions and Revolutions?*.
In: *A Multidisciplinary Approach to Pandemics*. Edited by Philippe Bourbeau, Jean-Michel Marcoux, and Brooke A. Ackerly, Oxford University Press. © Oxford University Press (2022). DOI: 10.1093/oso/9780192897855.003.0004

example, 0.26% in the United States, 0.29% in Brazil, and 0.42% in Hungary. (Data on COVID-19 casualties throughout this chapter are from WorldOMeter 2022.) Even if this is a substantial undercount, COVID-19 is not severe enough to alter the size or trajectories of populations in any states. Unless its effects are much larger in the future, the disease will neither alter the tendency of rich countries to grow older nor that of fast-growing countries in Africa, the Middle East, and South Asia to grow much larger and younger. For example, even if COVID-19 killed one million people in the United States (the extreme high end of current estimates), and most of those were over the age of 60, that loss would hardly dent the expected increase in the United States of the 65 and older population, which the US Census has projected to grow by thirty million to 2050 (Vespa et al. 2018). Similarly, for fast-growing young countries, even a larger fraction of deaths, if they predominantly affect those over the age of 50, would have no effect on the growth trajectory of those countries, which is driven by the large numbers and high fertility of the cohorts of young women aged 15–30 (Guengant 2017).

Great pandemics such as the Justinian Plague or the Black Death, which kill one-quarter or more of the population are quite rare, occurring only once every few centuries (Harper 2021). Like most pandemics in history, which kill 5% or less of the population, and which typically are fatal mainly to the very old, or the very young, or the weak, it is likely that COVID-19 will be merely a blip in the ongoing trajectories of national populations, quickly made up by the normal pattern of births. We thus should not expect any political upheavals based simply on the mortality or demographic changes brought by this disease.

When the last novel, unexpected, and widespread epidemic disease struck (HIV/AIDS), concerns were raised by security experts and intelligence agencies that it might produce political instability, especially in relatively weak states in Africa, which also had the widest disease spread (National Intelligence Council 2000; Heinecken 2001; Elbe 2003; Garrett 2005; Feldbaum et al. 2006). Several pathways were suggested by which the epidemic might have such effects. First, in the absence of any treatments or early detection, it was feared that the disease might spread unchecked and lead to truly disruptive, 'great plague' levels of mortality (25% of the population or more) in some states. Second, HIV/AIDS had the unusual character, for epidemic disease, of primarily infecting and killing young adults, those aged 16–40, where most epidemics, like COVID-19, are fatal mainly to the very young or very old. Some analysts thus feared that the loss of workers in this age group could undermine the ability of governments to function, especially if critical professional groups—political leadership, military/police, engineers who maintain key infrastructure, medical personnel, transport workers—were particularly impacted (Garrett 2005: 10). Third, some observers were concerned that the deaths of so many young adults would leave a large cohort of orphans who would be poorly cared for and weakly socialized, and thus easy prey for recruitment to radical extremist groups.

In fact, HIV/AIDS treatments and testing were devised and distributed fairly rapidly, so that death rates stopped rising and then steadily declined. Global deaths per year from HIV/AIDS peaked in 2004 at 1.7 million, far less than the 3.48 million global deaths in the first 14 months of the COVID-19 pandemic. Even in the very worst-hit countries, such as South Africa, deaths attributed to HIV/AIDS over the entire period from 1997 to 2010 totalled only 5.5% of the 2010 population (Bradshaw et al. 2016). By 2019, global deaths attributable to HIV/AIDS had fallen by 60% from the 2004 peak; 'HIV is no longer on the World Health Organizations list of top 10 causes of deaths and has not been for several years' (Cichocki 2021). Treatments have now reached upwards of 90% of those with the disease, even in Africa (US State Department 2020: 15). Thus, the worst fears regarding major political consequences of HIV/AIDS were never realized.

Yet there is a second path by which pandemics cause political upheaval; that is by their economic effects. If the disease (or the effort taken to halt its spread) is so disruptive to commerce or production that it causes serious economic hardships, or significantly undermines or reshuffles state and elite revenues, that too can upset political relationships. If the government response is seen to be incompetent, corrupt, or ineffective, so that deaths and hardships are unnecessary, that can delegitimize a regime. What then becomes critical is how those hardships are viewed. If the epidemic appears to be an unavoidable natural disaster, and the government did all it reasonably could to limit and offset the impact of the disease, then the regime will likely find itself strongly supported. But if the epidemic appears to have been exacerbated by government policies or neglect, and the resulting hardships seem unequally and unfairly distributed, then the seeds of revolt may take root. As various social groups come to believe that state leaders are responsible for a weak, corrupt, or ineffective response to the crisis, then the legitimacy of the government can be undermined and the leverage of opponents can be increased.

This effect can occur either in authoritarian or democratic regimes. With regard to COVID-19, a number of both autocratic and democratic regimes have done well, and enjoyed a reinforcement of their authority and support. In democratic New Zealand, Japan, Australia, Canada, Taiwan, and South Korea, where governments acted quickly to limit contacts and trace and isolate the infected, and thus kept casualties low, the leaders have been rewarded with strong electoral mandates. In autocratic China, Cuba, and Vietnam, the governments also succeeded in keeping cases and deaths low, earning strong support for their ruling parties. All across Africa, regardless of regime, a relatively young population combined with a strong, continent-wide effort at infectious disease control headed off the worst-feared impacts (Chow 2020).

By contrast, in the democratic regimes of Western Europe and the United States, India, and across most of Latin America, governments have done poorly in controlling the spread of the pandemic. Not only did casualties initially reach high levels, but they have had multiple waves of infections, resulting in both initial lockdowns and succeeding further measures to limit the spread. These extended struggles to control the spread not only failed to limit casualties as much as in the success stories noted above, but they also produced deeper economic impacts in terms of negative growth and high unemployment. But some autocratic regimes have also failed to manage the pandemic well: Iran, Russia, Saudi Arabia, and Belarus are all in the top one-third of countries in deaths per million population. (Data on COVID-19 casualties throughout this chapter are from WorldOMeter 2022.)

In countries where governments have fared poorly in responding to the pandemic, a further consideration for political stability is how well the regime was able to offset the economic impacts, both in terms of overall gross domestic product (GDP) and distributional effects. Did the economy suffer major losses, and if so, were those losses distributed unequally? The latter situation is especially likely to bring political upheaval.

Such upheavals can take two forms. One is revolution, involving mass mobilization with the aim of overthrowing the existing regime. This is only likely in authoritarian regimes. The other is a major political party realignment and change of political direction brought about by opposition election victories. This is only likely in democracies and partial democracies. Thus, we need to consider the political effects of the pandemic separately for these different types of regimes.

COVID-19 and Political Change in Authoritarian Regimes

Globally, the regions that have managed the pandemic well are those that had prior experience with major epidemics and so were prepared to react swiftly to the appearance of the novel coronavirus (Penn 2020). In East Asia, which had experienced outbreaks of SARS-2 and avian influenza, governments were prepared to take decisive action and had populations that were motivated and aware of the need for compliance with public health measures. In Africa, which had experienced outbreaks of Ebola and HIV/AIDS, and had extensive ongoing programmes to deal with infectious diseases such as malaria, a similar willingness of governments to act quickly and decisively was widespread. Thus regimes as diverse as those of Thailand, China, Sri Lanka, Vietnam and Taiwan, or Tanzania, Burundi, Uganda, and Niger all have death rates per capita in the lowest one-sixth of all countries. By contrast, almost all the countries in the highest one-sixth of death rates per capita are in Europe or Latin America, plus the United States. In these regions, which had not experienced infectious disease pandemics for a century and did not expect them, the virus spread before they were prepared and caught them unawares. Then the policy response was constrained by the general population's unfamiliarity with, and distrust of, such public health measures as masking, distancing, lockdowns, and mass vaccination campaigns. As a result, their management of the disease has generally been disappointing.

If we ask whether the COVID-19 pandemic could give rise to revolutions, we have to focus on authoritarian regimes where the response to the pandemic went poorly. As there are not many regimes that are autocracies in Europe, Latin America, or the United States, the places where mishandling of the COVID-19 pandemic could give rise to a revolution are few. Instead, most of the world's autocracies have managed the disease well. The major exceptions–in the early stages of the pandemic in 2020–were Iran, Saudi Arabia, Russia, and Belarus.

For revolutions to occur, a conjunction of several factors is necessary: First, the government's financial resources and management must be under stress; that usually involves an accumulation of state debts and a decline in revenues or a major disruption to the economy. Otherwise, the government can usually pay off its enemies and generously reward its supporters, dividing and reducing the opposition. Second, influential elites must turn against the government, articulating a basis for a change in regime and supporting or rallying popular protest. If not, and key elites remain loyal, they can effectively wield the regime's coercive forces, defend the regime's legitimacy, and implement reforms to cope with current problems. Third, a broad coalition of popular groups must have the grievances, and the opportunity, to join up in mobilization for change. Uprisings by only some in urban areas, or only in some regions, can be isolated and effectively targeted for repression by the regime.

For smaller countries, a fourth condition is necessary: the international milieu must not produce intervention by more powerful countries to support the regime or undermine the opposition. Finally, for all countries a fifth condition is that a narrative takes hold that focuses grievances on the regime, and that unites diverse groups and classes into a broad anti-government coalition (Goldstone 2014).

In the case of COVID-19, given its modest demographic impact, it will be the health and economic effects of the policies chosen by governments that determine whether these factors arise. While these effects have been quite considerable, with lockdowns causing declines in economic output and government revenues almost everywhere, in most countries, the pandemic does not appear to be causing either sufficient elite divisions, nor widespread mobilization, to cause major unrest.

In Iran, despite the impact of international sanctions and declining oil prices, the government has managed to keep its military and officials loyal by rewarding them well, and has maintained popular support by relying on the fear of external enemies, including the United States, Israel and Saudi Arabia. While economic hardships and desires for a more open political regime have produced popular protests at regular intervals since the 1990s, most notably the failed 'Green Revolution' of 2009, none of these waves of protest have produced a broad, national anti-regime coalition. Instead, in different periods, different groups—students, or workers and professionals in the major metro centres, or residents of the smaller towns and the countryside—have acted separately, and been effectively repressed by the regime. So far, despite a lengthy battle with COVID-19, with five distinct waves of rising deaths between March 2020 and November 2021, the pandemic has not yet produced such a broad, national anti-regime coalition. Nor do the military and other elites show signs of defection from the regime. Thus, barring a new surge of disease that would discredit the regime, the risks of COVID-related revolution in Iran seem low.

Even the major surges of cases and deaths that occurred in Fall of 2020 and again in Fall of 2021, with daily new cases and deaths both quadrupling in weeks, have not shaken the regime. As of early 2022, Iran seems to have brought the effects of the pandemic under control, with cases and deaths per capita down to 40th among countries with one million or more population. Thus, another wave of popular anti-regime protests seems unlikely. Whether a democratizing 'colour' revolution will ever dislodge the Islamic regime will depend on the loyalty and unity of the Iranian Revolutionary Guard Corps (IRGC) and the Basij, its paramilitary militia. To date, in every crisis the IRGC and the Basij have held firm and defended the Supreme Leader. If that continues, so will the regime. Only if the pandemic toll reaches a level that undermines the cohesion and loyalty of these coercive forces will the regime be vulnerable to a new popular revolution.

In Saudi Arabia, Crown Prince Mohammed bin Salman has purged the country's leadership of anyone disloyal to the Prince, and increased public spending to retain popular support. Although Saudi Arabia's deaths per capita were in the top one-third of all countries by the summer of 2020, the number remained low—just over 7,200 deaths in a population of 35 million. Moreover, unlike most other countries, Saudi Arabia escaped further major waves of COVID-19 (although an Omicron wave is now beginning). Having sent home foreign workers, imposed curfews and lockdowns (including on mosques), and limited travellers for the Hajj to just 1,000 instead of the usual 2 million (Karadsheh and Qiblawi 2020), the Kingdom has kept the disease at bay. In addition, Saudi Arabia's regime is leveraging its relations with the United States to strengthen its position in the Middle East, helping to shore up its prestige, while highlighting the threat from Iran and Islamist extremists. Thus, it benefits from an international milieu that supports the regime. In this case, under current conditions, the risks of COVID-related revolution seem low.

In Russia, management of the epidemic has been quite poor: official figures give Russia the sixth largest number of cases of COVID-19 in the world, and the fourth largest number of deaths, at 320,600. This still gives Russia a death rate per 1,000 that is roughly the same as that of other European countries such as Italy, Spain, and France. Yet the official death totals are likely to be a substantial undercount: excess deaths in the summer of 2020 were three times higher than the reported number of COVID-19 fatalities (Tsvetkova 2020). And even the official death toll is now rising rapidly, doubled in summer of 2021 to over 5,000 per week, and then doubled again in November 2021 to 10,000 per week. It remains to be seen whether

Russia's vaccines can halt the epidemic, or if cases simply decline slightly and then return for a further wave in early 2022.

So far, President Putin has kept the elites loyal through economic rewards to his oligarch supporters and the persecution—even poisoning—of any serious political opponents (Seddon 2020). Nonetheless, the population seems restive. There have been major protests in the Far East (Higgins 2020), while the residents of Moscow, St Petersberg, and other major cities have come out in past protests against the regime. Yet, as in Iran, so far no nationwide coalition has formed to unite workers, professionals, and businessmen, or metropolitan and rural groups, against the regime. Moreover, President Putin is extremely anxious to halt any possibility of a 'color revolution', like those in Georgia or in Ukraine, that might seek to replace him with a democratic regime. This has led Putin to intervene in these countries and carve out sections of their territory to secure Russia's borders against any spread of such ideas. As this is being written in January 2022, Putin appears to be planning a military intervention in Ukraine, similar to past interventions in Moldova, Georgia and Crimea–perhaps in part to distract the population and short up support at home.

Nonetheless, Putin's position is not strong. Russia's financial reserves have been stressed by years of low oil and gas prices and years of military interventions in Georgia, Ukraine, and Syria. Such campaigns have won Putin nationalist and patriotic support, but at a significant financial cost. He is now facing the question of whether he can afford further military efforts to shore up allies in Libya and Nagorno-Karabakh against Turkish-supported military attacks. A decision to intervene will incur further financial pressures at a time when Putin is stretched to cover government salaries and public pensions at home; a failure to intervene may suggest weakness and an inability to play the role of the international strongman he has set for himself. Either course thus has risks. So far, Putin's tight rein on the oligarchs, government officials, media, and the military and intelligence services remains secure, and no widespread opposition seems viable. Yet if Putin remains bogged down in ever-expanding international wars, is unable to prevent the spread and increasing death toll from the coronavirus, and faces an economy that continues to stagnate, certainly not helped by the global economic downturn in the wake of the virus, his vulnerability to popular protests may grow.

Given the accumulation of pressures on the regime from its economic difficulties and military commitments, a further explosion of illness could tip the country into growing protests, as occurred in neighbouring Belarus. To be sure, compared to Belarus, Russia's government is stronger and the opposition currently weaker; but a similar trajectory is certainly possible in partial consequence of the COVID-19 pandemic, should the steady stream of deaths continue.

This brings us to Belarus. In 2020–2021, Belarus already has experienced an attempted colour revolution. Hundreds of thousands of protestors defied police to undertake public marches in the capital of Minsk for every weekend for months, demanding the resignation of President Alexander Lukashenka (Associated Press 2020). This became a truly national, cross-class protest, engaging everyone from workers and professionals to students and housewives, young and old, and in cities and towns across the country. People from all walks of life—from state television broadcasters and orchestra musicians to mothers, policemen, and factory workers—joined the protests.

COVID-19 was not the cause of the protests, but it did provide a push to help organize and trigger them. The root causes of the protests are the economic decline and the closure of political space in Belarus over the past decade. Up to 2014, Belarus fared reasonably well, refining cheap Russian oil to sell to Europe, and relying on state-owned enterprises to produce heavy trucks, logging/pulp and paper, and chemicals. But after oil prices and the Russian ruble collapsed in 2014, Russian subsidies were gradually withdrawn. State-owned enterprises did not adapt and the economy faltered. 'Belarusian GDP is the same today as it was in 2010, and real wages are 70 per cent of what they were a decade ago' according to Tadeusz Giczan, a researcher at University College London (Light 2020). Yet the government under Lukashenka made few efforts to cope with these changes. With no political parties and no real government except for Lukashenka and his appointees, Belarusians had no avenue to seek change.

When the COVID-19 epidemic came to Europe in March of 2020, particularly neighbouring Russia, Lukashenka downplayed the threat. He suggested a series of folk remedies, from saunas to drinking vodka, and refused to introduce any public health measures. When Belarus became the only country in Europe to continue to hold football matches and Victory Day parades, the people recognized that something was wrong. Sławomir Sierakowski wrote:

> Lukashenka's lack of an effective coronavirus response left him discredited. When he denied the threat and failed to intervene ... it seemed like a moral abdication. That was especially disappointing to the middle-aged, who feared for their parents. Belarusians had to deal with the threat of COVID-19 on their own and began banding together to buy masks and equipment, to help the sick, and to assist medical personnel. The regime lost ground, and civil society gained it. Bonds of solidarity were formed ... The regime lost legitimacy because it could no longer guarantee a basic level of security.
>
> (Sierakowski 2020: 10)

Lukashenka had scheduled an election for 9 August to confirm and extend his presidency. But by then, according to available statistics, Belarus had four times as many cases per capita as neighbouring Ukraine (Way 2020: 22). Opponents lined up to run against Lukashenka in the election, only to be arrested and jailed or forced into exile. Lukashenka eventually allowed Sviatlana Tsikhanouskaya, the wife of one of his jailed opponents, to run, but only because he thought she would embarrass herself. In fact, she proved to be a capable candidate and organizer, leading a growing opposition.

Popular support for Lukashenka was so low that there was a widespread certainty that the results were completely false when he announced his victory, claiming to have received 80% of the votes. The following day, protests that had been organized in advance emerged from the Metro stations in Minsk. The government responded with aggressive tactics by riot police, firing rubber bullets, conducting mass arrests, and beating people with truncheons. In the following days, thousands were arrested and hundreds told their families of torture in the detention facilities. Lukashenka had now gone to war against his people, but the protests briefly stopped.

Then on 13 August, thousands of women and girls, wearing white and holding flowers, took to the streets to demonstrate against the regime's violence. The next day, factory workers around the country went on strike, including the largest and most prestigious industrial centres. The regime had no answer to the spread of opposition; Lukashenka retreated to a policy of a barricading squares and trying to discourage mass protests, while playing for time.

In the meantime, the COVID-19 pandemic has, somewhat surprisingly, remained under control. Reported cases per capita have reached about the same level as in Germany and Denmark, but less than half as many as in France or, the UK, or the United States. Death rates per capita, at least officially, are even lower, only a fraction of that in Poland or Spain. This may be simply due to poor recording; but at least part is due to a conscientious effort by the population of Belarus, left to manage on their own, to safeguard the elderly by masking and distancing. In any event, the epidemic has not reached levels that would justify a severe lockdown, nor discourage the weekly public outdoor demonstrations involving hundreds of thousands across the country. Throughout 2021, new cases did not exceed 2,000 per day, and recorded COVID deaths remained under 125 per week, while most European countries were seeing over 100 deaths per day.

As of early 2022, the situation in Belarus remained an unstable stand-off between Lukashenka and the opposition. The government tried to arrest or exile the opposition's leaders, but they were replaced by others and the protests continued. Russia has contributed financial support and key workers for state television and police, but is very reluctant to intervene militarily to support Lukashenka. After all, Russia's interventions in Georgia and Ukraine only turned those countries away from Russia and towards the North Atlantic Treaty Organization (NATO), something it cannot afford with Belarus. Nor could it afford a prolonged occupation. So Russia seems willing to support Lukashenka as long as he can hold his resolve and that of his government. Lukashenka's popular support seems to be dwindling day by day, but strong Russian backing has helped him to keep the military and police loyal. In late May, Lukashenka seemed confident enough to have his military intercept a civilian airliner flying from Athens, Greece to Vilnius, Lithuania in order to remove and jail one of the passengers, a journalist who had been one of Lukashenka's chief critics. Lukashenka continued to jail journalists and opposition figures, and faces sanctions from Europe; but whether these will prove more dangerous to his continued rule than years of Western sanctions have been for his ally, Vladimir Putin, remains to be seen.

COVID-19 did not cause the ongoing revolution in Belarus. Yet it did provide a key tipping point in the growth of the opposition, the strengthening of civil society, and undercutting the legitimacy of Lukashenka's rule. So far, it remains the best, indeed the only, example of how mishandling the COVID-19 pandemic could contribute to revolution against an autocratic regime. Yet the revolution remains stymied, and both Putin and Lukashenka know that if autocracy falls in Belarus, Russia may not be far behind. Thus, Russia will seek to do all it can, albeit behind the scenes, to enable Lukashenka to wait out the opposition and prevail.

COVID-19 and Political Change in Democratic Regimes

The regimes that have done the most poorly in preventing the spread of COVID-19 have been the European democracies, the United States, India, and the countries of Latin America. Especially given the wealth and advanced medical systems of Europe and the United States, this has been a shock. As no effective medical preventive for infection by COVID-19 arrived until vaccines became available in the spring of 2021, stemming the spread during the first year of the epidemic had to rely on government public health measures. To be effective, these had to be early and decisive; yet in all of these countries they were neither.

The first wave spread from China to Europe, mutating there and spreading from winter ski resorts and port cities, quickly spreading all across Europe in February and March, and from there to the United States, and slightly later to Latin America. These first major outbreaks were concentrated in local 'hot zones' centred on major metropolitan areas; these were eventually beaten back with lockdowns and insistence on masking and distancing. In Western Europe, this succeeded in reducing cases and then fatalities to much lower levels, while Eastern Europe was largely spared the first wave altogether. Thus European governments, by and large, were spared any backlash, and began permitting summer travel and limited business openings. Unfortunately, however, their populations also seem to have become lax, and a new strain of coronavirus, the Delta strain, emerged in summer and was swiftly spread all across Europe by holidaymakers (Burger 2020).

This second wave spread rapidly in both Western and Eastern Europe; the spectre of overflowing hospitals and uncontrolled spread returned, leaving leaders with difficult choices. Politicians were extremely reluctant to bring back national lockdowns, as both the economic costs and the difficulty of getting compliance from populations already fatigued from the first wave made them unpopular. Nonetheless, Ireland, Iceland, Belgium, France, Italy, and the UK (and Israel) had to adopt national lockdowns. This wave also spread with new rapidity to previously more lightly affected areas. For example, Hungary had no significant spread before late August; but cases then grew from a few hundred per day in early September to a first peak of over 6.000 per day in December 2020, and then, after a short lull, reached a second peak of over 10,000 cases per day in March 2021, before suddenly dropping back to a few hundred cases per day in May. That sudden wave from autumn 2020 to spring 2021 produced almost 30,000 deaths, giving Hungary the fourth-highest rate of COVID-19 deaths per capita of any country in the world. Other European countries experienced similar surges of new cases and deaths from September 2020 to April 2021, although these waves ended with the onset of warmer weather and the arrival, but disappointingly slow distribution, of vaccines.

It is too early to tell whether there will be political fallout from this autumn 2020–spring 2021 wave. However, it is clear that there is growing impatience, criticism, and demonstrations against European leaders; increasingly violent anti-lockdown riots have occurred (Mitchell 2020). Could that herald a wave of regime changes at the polls? The most striking fact of European politics in the past decade has been the collapse or transformation of national parties and the wholesale replacement of the former establishment. In the UK, the once conservative Tory Party lost a referendum on Brexit, but then completely squashed the Labour Party and virtually drove the Liberal Democrats to extinction by allying with the upstart UK Independence Party and transforming itself into the party of Brexit. In France, the former establishment parties on both the right (UMP) and left (Socialistes) were thrashed at the polls by the upstart Emmanuel Macron, who won the presidency without a formal party, relying instead on a national movement, 'En marche'. Populist movements of the left (Podemos in Spain, the Five-Star party in Italy, Syriza in Greece) and of the right (Law and Justice in Poland, Fidesz in Hungary) came to power in several countries and continue to challenge traditional parties.

This new wave of populist parties with new nationalist leaders, who challenged both European unity and traditional democratic welfare policies, has now found itself with a new, continent-wide challenge. They may reinforce their prestige if they are successful in dealing with the pandemic; or they may get a strong backlash and be sent back to the political margins if they fail.

Thus far, however, no national leaders in Europe (excepting Lukashenka in Belarus, who has faced national protests, as noted in 'COVID-19 and Political Change in Authoritarian Regimes') have paid a price for a weak or ineffective reaction to COVID-19. Even Hungary, which suffered the worst of the autumn–spring wave, has seen no shift in the popularity of President Victor Orban, who has gathered support by being the only European leader to accept Chinese and Russian-made vaccines in response to the delayed distribution of European ones. In Sweden, where the ruling Social Democrats adopted a lax policy that resulted in 10 times as many deaths per capita as in neighbouring Norway, the ruling party still leads the national polls as of May 2021, with exactly the same percentage as it had in May 2019, before anyone had heard of the novel coronavirus; and as before, the main issue for the election will likely be immigration, not COVID-19 (Politico 2020d).

Other European leaders have also remained stable in the polls, despite anger over recent lockdowns and vaccine delays. In the UK, Prime Minister Boris Johnson's approval ratings had fallen for much of 2020, but recovered and were again very slightly net positive by May 2021 (YouGov 2021). In France, President Macron's approval, though still negative on balance, has improved significantly over the course of the epidemic (Politico 2020a). Only Spain, Italy, and Germany have seen a major shift between the left and right parties, with the conservatives in Spain winning a major victory in the 2021 regional elections, and the Italian ruling League Party and Germany's Christian Democrats losing much of their lead over their rivals (Politico 2020b, c, e); and the German results seem more tied to the coming departure of the popular Chancellor, Angela Merkel than to COVID-19 results. Overall, so far there is no sign that the COVID-19 pandemic is producing electoral upheavals.

The United States had a very muddled response to the pandemic. Public health professionals were not only late to develop testing and tracing, but then had to contend with a cavalier president, who worried that extreme public health measures would do irreparable harm to the economy. While many state governors took strenuous action, President Trump and leaders in his party remained opposed to testing, masking, business closures, and—much like Lukashenka in Belarus—refused to treat the virus as a serious threat. As a result, the United States became the world leader in both total cases and fatalities from COVID-19. Despite its world-leading wealth and sophisticated medical centres, the United States ranks seventh highest in deaths per capita among all countries with population greater than 10 million.

President Trump's approach was mirrored by other populist leaders in the Americas, such as Jair Bolsonaro in Brazil and Andres Manual López Obrador of Mexico, both of whom responded to rapidly rising infection and death counts by saying that the numbers were exaggerated and the problem was overblown. The result of a lack of strong response is that the United States and 4 Latin American countries (Brazil, Argentina, Colombia, and Mexico) comprise 5 of the 14 leading countries in the world in total COVID-19 cases. Worse yet, with Peru, these countries have had 6 of the 12 highest rates of COVID-19 deaths per capita in the world among countries with a population over 10 million.

Yet despite these high casualty rates, for most of these countries the political consequences have been slight. In northern South America, the bigger concern has been avoiding contagion from the disastrous collapse of Venezuela. In Brazil, the Bolsonaro regime has been so generous in providing emergency funds to the poor that it has actually gained in popularity (Sreeharsha 2020). In Mexico, López Obrador's approval has risen slightly since the start of the pandemic, from 59% in March 2020 to 61% in April 2021 (Zissis 2021). In the southern cone, Chile has voted overwhelmingly for a new constitution, to replace the restrictive one left over from the Pinochet government, but that followed massive protests in autumn 2020, over issues unrelated to COVID-19. Indeed, the lockdowns for COVID-19 temporarily ended those demonstrations. Only Argentina experienced widespread protests linked to COVID-19 in 2020 (BBC News 2020).

However, in 2021 and 2022, most of Latin America continues to experience exceptionally high rates of COVID-19 infections, driven by new variants of the virus that appear capable of infecting those who have already been ill from earlier strains. In Brazil, new cases started to rise in November 2020, reaching almost 100,000 per day in April 2021, and remaining nearly as high a month later, with deaths still over 2,500 per day in May. Argentina hit a new peak in new cases per day in May 2021, at over 35,000; daily deaths of 500–700 in May 2021 were also new records. In Paraguay, where there was no autumn/winter surge, new cases suddenly tripled from February to May 2021, and were still rising at the end of May; the sudden surge overwhelmed hospitals and daily deaths rose sixfold over this period. Colombia and Bolivia both experienced a fierce third wave of infections, with record numbers of new cases and deaths per day in April and May 2021. Peru had new peaks of daily cases and deaths in April, but these fell by about one-half over the course of May. In Chile, cases soared in March and April of 2021, but then levelled off, though deaths remained at levels not seen since July 2020. Uruguay, which had miraculously virtually escaped the pandemic until March 2021, had a sudden surge, with new cases going from a few hundred to over 5,000 per day in the 2 months from March to May; deaths per day followed suit, surging sixfold. Only Ecuador, which was hurt most severely in the early stages of the epidemic but only experienced a minor surge in early 2021, and Mexico, which had a fierce but brief surge in cases and deaths in January 2021 but then saw both fall by 70% by May, entered summer 2021 without raging epidemics.

It is hoped that vaccine distribution led by the World Health Organization will help Latin American countries follow the lead of Mexico, which rapidly brought its winter 2020/2021 record peak back down to levels not seen since the first months of the pandemic. Should that occur, it should remove the impact of COVID-19 on politics, just as López Obrador's popularity was unaffected by the massive but brief rise in deaths and cases in January 2021. However, if the wave of casualties that began in early 2021 continues, there is some possibility that it could roil politics in the region.

In the United States, it is remarkable that despite over 230,000 deaths, President Donald Trump is as popular as ever. To be sure, that means his popularity remains at no more than 45%, which was not enough to bring re-election against his favourably viewed competitor, Joe Biden (FiveThirtyEight 2020). But what is striking is that despite denying the severity of the epidemic, eschewing federal action, even (like Jair Bolsonaro and Boris Johnson), being hospitalized for COVID-19 and recovering, Trump lost none of his support. Although he lost his bid for re-election, he came within a few thousand votes of winning in Wisconsin, Arizona, and Georgia. His party, the Republican Party, which backed his COVID-19 policies, even gained seats in Congress. Moreover, Trump's loss appears mainly due to the strong vote against him by better-educated, suburban voters and African-Americans over issues of racial injustice. In regard to the pandemic, Trump actually gained votes in many states in the upper Midwest, where cases and deaths were rising fastest in the months before the election!

Though the economic impact of the pandemic on GDP and employment in the United States has been severe, this was offset for much of the population by a summer cash distribution and enhanced unemployment benefits, which were sufficient to fuel a strong economic recovery, and even increase household incomes. Thus, even as new cases surged to record levels in October 2020, Trump's polling remained steady. Trump's narrow defeat was because he was never able to raise his popularity ratings from the level of roughly 45% at which he started his term, not because the consequences of his COVID-19 policies lowered them.

One might expect that India, which is by far the largest democracy and the poorest country to suffer from a major epidemic of COVID-19, would see some political impact from the disease. Second in the world in total cases and third in total deaths (behind the United States and Brazil), although far lower in casualties per capita, India's response has not been good. Indeed, Prime Minister Modi's first policy response—a nationwide lockdown that was economically punishing to the poor, and which forced millions of impoverished Indians to trek to their home villages simply to obtain food, thus spreading the disease—was widely considered a disaster by epidemiologists.

After a first wave from May to December 2020, in which COVID-19 cases peaked near 100,000 per day and deaths at just over 1,000 per day, India experienced a lull from December 2020 to March 2021. However, as in Latin America, a surge driven by a new variant created a far more severe wave in March–May 2021, with new cases reaching 400,000 per day and deaths exceeding 4,500. Moreover, as hospitals across India reported running out of oxygen and crematoria reported being unable to keep up with the demand for firewood, a noted public health expert estimated the true number of deaths as closer to 25,000 per day (The Pioneer 2021). After the first COVID-19 wave receded, Prime Minister Modi's popularity soared (Sharma 2020), as Modi was given credit for his initial bold and sweeping action, regardless of the consequences. He never minimized the virus; instead, his early and total lockdown is given credit for showing that he took it seriously and would act to protect India. However, Modi acted differently in the second, far more severe wave, largely ignoring it, while promoting political rallies and religious festivals. This led his popularity to falter significantly for the first time since his election (Shivji 2021), falling from over 80% approval in May of 2020 to 64% a year later (Morning Consult 2021). To be sure, that does not put Modi in jeopardy. Moreover, even if India's total deaths should climb to 10 times their official level in May of 2021, they would still be only 0.2% of India's total population. Still, if any democratic leader may suffer from adopting an attitude of complete neglect in the middle of one of the most severe COVID-19 crises in the world, that could be Modi. However, the Spring 2021 wave faded as quickly as it appeared, virtually ending by July. Although a new, Omicron wave seems to have begun in December 2021, that too should quickly peak and fade, going by experience in other countries. If that holds, the epidemic may be a fading memory by the time Modi next faces a national election in 2024.

Conclusion

The COVID-19 pandemic has already been the deadliest and most sweeping single infectious disease outbreak since the 2018 Spanish flu, and it is far from over. Europe and the United States rolled out vaccines in spring 2021, in a race to immunize their population before more dangerous variants created new explosions of cases, as India and Latin America experienced.

Yet both the demographic and political impacts have, so far, been surprisingly slight. Thanks to improvements in treatment, the fatality rate per identified infection remains relatively low, at about 1–2%, and in even the worst-affected countries the overall death rates are no more than 3 or 4 per 1,000 of the total population. Of course, that is 900,000 deaths in a country of 330 million like the United States, which is a stunning tragedy (Rossen et al. 2020). Yet it is not enough to create a noticeable change in the size or trajectory of a population, and certainly not enough to create major labour shortages over a generation.

Sub-Saharan Africa, where HIV/AIDS was most severe, and where many feared the worst consequences of COVID-19 would arise, has been remarkably lightly affected. Excepting only South Africa, more or less all the countries of the region have had just one-fifth or less the rate of COVID-19 deaths per capita of major European countries. Perhaps that is because its population is overwhelmingly young, and young people seem far more resistant; perhaps it is because the heavy disease burden of Africa has provided some spill-over immunity. It is something of a mystery that will provide rich material for future research.

In most other regions, the lockdowns to combat the spread of the coronavirus have produced economic disruptions on the scale of a major recession (see Chapter 14 by Herrmann and Isabelle in this volume). Yet politicians have responded with massive financial interventions, justifying them as emergency responses to a natural disaster, and so providing more assistance than they have normally provided in economic downturns.

The overall result is that hardly any regimes—authoritarian or democratic—have faced major rebellions or revolutions, or even dramatic voting shifts, as a consequence of the disease. Almost all authoritarian regimes brought the pandemic quickly under control, as did the democracies in Asia and Oceana. Of the handful of authoritarian regimes that responded badly, so far only Belarus has faced a major challenge to its regime in which COVID-19 played a significant role, and that challenge so far has been unsuccessful. It is possible that Belarus, and eventually Russia, will face colour revolutions demanding more competent, less corrupt, and less closed governments, and that the history of those changes will be traced to the pandemic. But at present, that remains only a possibility.

In the democracies, no politicians have suffered a massive defeat as a consequence of their COVID-19 response. Indeed, most politicians are facing more backlash against lockdowns and other such measures than against the casualties that have occurred on their watch. Even in the United States, which had arguably the most spectacular government failure in dealing with the disease, given its advanced medical infrastructure and wealth, suffering by far the most cases and having one of the world's highest death rates per capita, the election contest between President Donald Trump and his challenger Joe Biden was polling in November 2020 almost exactly where it was in mid-March (FiveThirtyEight 2020), when there were 5,000 infections and 75 total deaths, as against 230,000 deaths by November. The expected punishing majority vote against Trump for his failure to stem the pandemic in the United States wholly failed to appear. In India, the other country that has suffered the most cases and one of the most disastrous policy actions, Prime Minister Modi's popularity has dimmed slightly, but he remains more popular than most other politicians could dream of.

In summary, despite its undoubted global health and economic impact, the political impact of COVID-19 appears, so far, to be negligible. While democratic leaders could yet be punished for a worse, coming wave of cases, the absence of any penalties for democratic leaders who have done little or nothing in the face of massive outbreaks suggests that other factors will be more important to their fate.

To be sure, this does not mean that we should be complacent about the future impact of global pandemics on political stability. The world was, despite the horrors and deaths brought by COVID-19, fairly lucky. This virus, at least in its original strain, was highly transmissible but had a case fatality rate of only 1–2% overall, and far less than that for people under age 65. By comparison, smallpox, when it was creating periodic pandemics, had a case fatality rate of 30%, and struck down the young as well as the old, and many in the prime of life. The bubonic plague, in its visitations in the sixth, fourteenth, and seventeenth centuries, may have had a case fatality rate of 50%. The interplay of animal viruses and human populations have repeatedly brought new diseases to the world; in recent years, the swine flu, avian flu, Ebola, SARS-1, MERS, and now SARS-2 (COVID-19). If COVID-19 had combined its current transmissibility with the case-fatality rate of

MERS, estimated at 25–50%, we would be dealing with a major plague event on the scale of those which brought down states and empires in the past.

The rapid development of a COVID-19 vaccine has been a major development that will further reduce the impact of the pandemic. Yet even this enormously rapid intervention took over a year to bring to mass production, and may take two years to reach global distribution. For a fast-acting pandemic which, like the plague or smallpox in the past, could kill upwards of 25% of an entire population in a year, even that is not sufficient to avert catastrophe.

The true lesson of the COVID-19 pandemic for political stability is best shown by the examples of Taiwan, Australia, New Zealand, and other countries that did extremely well in preventing even a modest death toll from the disease. That lesson is that swift, well-planned, and well-executed public health measures of a traditional kind—testing, tracing, masking, and distancing—can stop even an extremely contagious disease from causing widespread casualties. To ensure that the next major pandemic does not cause revolutions and rebellions, states would be wise to ensure their ability to execute these actions without delay and to train their citizens to comply. The next major pandemic may be far more deadly than COVID-19. If so, those citizens' lives, and the political stability of states around the world, will depend on it.

References

Associated Press. 2020. 'Nearly 3 Months after Vote, Belarus Protests Still Go Strong'. *US News*, 31 October.

Ayalon, Yaron. 2014. 'The Black Death and the Rise of the Ottomans'. In *Natural Disasters in the Ottoman Empire: Plague, Famine and Other Misfortunes*, edited by Yaron Ayalon, pp. 21–60. Cambridge: Cambridge University Press.

BBC News. 2020. 'Covid-19: Protests as Argentina's Cases Pass 900,000'. 13 October. https://www.bbc.com/news/world-latin-america-54522428.

Borsch, Stuart J. 2005. *The Black Death in Egypt and England: A Comparative Study*. Austin, TX: University of Texas Press.

Bradshaw, Debbie, William Msemburi, Rob Dorrington, Victoria Pillay-van Wyk, Ria Laubscher, and Pam Groenewald. 2016. 'HIV/AIDS in South Africa: How Many People Died from the Disease between 1997 and 2010?' *AIDS 30* (5): p. 771.

Burger, Ludwig. 2020. 'Scientists Identify Prolific Coronavirus Strain which Started in Spain and Spread across Europe'. *Reuters*, 29 October. https://in.reuters.com/article/health-coronavirus-spain-variant/scientists-identify-prolific-coronavirus-strain-which-started-in-spain-and-spread-across-europe-idINKBN27E2RS.

Cichocki, Mark. 2021. 'How Many People Die from HIV Each Year?' *VeryWell-Health*, 15 February. https://www.verywellhealth.com/how-many-people-die-from-aids-each-year-49053.

Chow, Denise. 2020. 'Africa Has Held off the Worst of the Coronavirus. Researchers are Working to Figure out How. *NBC NEWS*. 25 September. https://www.nbcnews.com/science/science-news/africa-has-held-worst-coronavirus-researchers-are-working-figure-out-n1241026.

Dennis, Laurie. 2020. 'The Impact of the Black Death on 1300s China: No Plague = No Ming'. *LaurieDennis.com*. https://lauriedennis.com/2020/05/02/the-impact-of-the-black-death-on-1300s-china-no-plague-no-ming.
Dols, Michael W. 1977. *The Black Death in the Middle East*. Princeton, NJ: Princeton University Press.
Elbe, Stefan. 2003. *Strategic Implications of HIV/AIDS*. Oxford: Oxford University Press.
Feldbaum, Harley, Kelley Lee, and Preeti Patel. 2006. 'The National Security Implications of HIV/AIDS'. *PLoS Med 3* (6): e171. https://doi.org/10.1371/journal.pmed.0030171.
FiveThirtyEight. 2020. 'Who's Ahead in the National Polls?' Updated 31 October. https://projects.fivethirtyeight.com/polls/president-general/national.
Garrett, Laurie. 2005. *HIV and National Security: Where Are the Links?* New York: Council on Foreign Relations.
Goldstone, Jack A. 2014. *Revolutions: A Very Short Introduction*. New York: Oxford University Press.
Guengant, Jean-Pierre. 2017. 'Africa's Population: History, Current Status, and Projections'. In *Africa's Population: In Search of a Demographic Dividend*, edited by Hans Groth and John F. May, pp. 11–31. New York: Springer.
Harper, Kyle. 2021. *Plagues upon the Earth: Disease and the Course of Human History*. Princeton, NJ: Princeton University Press.
Heinecken, Lindy. 2001. 'HIV/AIDS, the Military and the Impact on National and International Security'. *Society in Transition 32* (1): p. 120.
Higgins, Andrew. 2020. 'Defying Kremlin, Protesters Stage Biggest Rally Yet in Russian Far East.' *New York Times*, 18 July. https://www.nytimes.com/2020/07/18/world/russian-protests.html.
Jedwab, Remi, Noel D. Johnson, and Mark Koyama. 2020. 'The Economic Impact of the Black Death'. *Journal of Economic Literature* (forthcoming).
Karadsheh, Jomana, and Tamara Qiblawi. 2020. '"Unprecedented" Hajj Begins—with 1,000 Pilgrims, Rather than the Usual 2 Million'. *CNN Travel*, 29 July. https://www.cnn.com/travel/article/hajj-2020-coronavirus-intl/index.html.
Kelly, John. 2005. *The Great Mortality: An Intimate History of the Black Death, the Most Devastating Plague of All Time*. New York: Harper Collins.
Light, Felix. 2020. 'How Poor Handling of Covid-19 Has Caused Uproar in Belarus'. *NewStatesman.com*, 24 June. https://www.newstatesman.com/world/europe/2020/06/how-poor-handling-covid-19-has-caused-uproar-belarus.
Mitchell, Charlotte. 2020. 'Another Weekend of Violent Anti-Lockdown Protests in Europe: Clashes in Italy and Spain as Belgium Becomes the Latest to Lock Down and Restrictions Tighten across Continent'. *Daily Mail*, 30 October. https://www.dailymail.co.uk/news/article-8898657/Anti-lockdown-protesters-throw-bricks-Barcelona-police-clash-Spains-new-Covid-19-rules.html.
Morning Consult. 2021. 'Global Leader Approval Rating Tracker'. Updated 11 November. https://morningconsult.com/form/global-leader-approval/#section–70.
National Intelligence Council. 2000. 'National Intelligence Estimate: The Global Infectious Disease Threat and Its Implications for the United States'. *Environmental Change and Security Project Report 6*: p. 33.
Penn, Michael. 2020. 'How Some Asian Countries Beat Back COVID-19: Experience Matters When Confronting a Novel Infectious Disease, DGHI Policy Expert Says'. Duke Global Health Institute, 12 August. https://globalhealth.duke.edu/news/how-some-asian-countries-beat-back-covid-19.

Pioneer, The. 2021. 'Daily Covid Deaths Must Be 25,000 in India, Says Expert'. 11 May. https://www.dailypioneer.com/2021/page1/daily-covid-deaths-must-be-25-000-in-india—says-expert.html.

Politico. 2020a. 'France—President Emanuel Macron's Approval Rating'. https://www.politico.eu/europe-poll-of-polls/france.

Politico. 2020b. 'Italy—National Parliament Voting Intention'. https://www.politico.eu/europe-poll-of-polls/italy.

Politico. 2020c. 'Spain—National Party Voting Intention'. https://www.politico.eu/europe-poll-of-polls/spain.

Politico. 2020d. 'Sweden—National Parliament Voting Intention'. https://www.politico.eu/europe-poll-of-polls/sweden/.

Politico. 2020e. 'Germany—2021 General Election'. https://www.politico.eu/europe-poll-of-polls/germany/.

Rossen, Lauren M., Amy M. Branum, Farida B. Ahmad, Paul Sutton, and Robert N. Anderson. 2020. 'Excess Deaths Associated with COVID-19, by Age, Race and Ethnicity—United States, January 26–October 3, 2020'. *Centers for Disease Control and Prevention, Morbidity and Mortality Weekly Report 69* (42): p. 1522.

Scheidel, Walter. 2018. *The Great Leveler: Violence and the History of Inequality from the Stone Age to the Twenty-First Century*. Princeton, NJ: Princeton University Press.

Seddon, Max. 2020. 'Putin Opponent Alexei Navalny in a Coma after Suspected Poisoning'. *Financial Times*, 20 August. https://www.ft.com/content/ee2ab4b2-ddb3-4d01-81a3-db2318ea8e71.

Sharma, Mihir. 2020. 'View: Despite All Problems, Why Is Modi Still the Most Popular Leader?' *Economic Times*, 11 September. https://economictimes.indiatimes.com/news/politics-and-nation/view-despite-all-problems-why-modi-is-still-the-most-popular-leader/articleshow/78052453.cms?utm_source=contentofinterest&utm_medium=text&utm_campaign=cppst.

Shivji, Salimah. 2021. 'Popularity Crumbles for Indian PM Modi as Devastating COVID-19 Surge Continues'. *CBC News*. 15 May. https://www.cbc.ca/news/world/modi-india-coronavirus-1.6027346.

Sierakowski, Sławomir. 2020. 'The Making of a Revolution'. *Journal of Democracy 31* (4): p. 5.

Sreeharsha, Vinod. 2020. 'COVID-19 Batters Brazil, but Its Leader Is More Popular Than Ever'. *Wall Street Journal*, 13 September. https://www.wsj.com/articles/covid-19-batters-brazil-but-its-leader-is-more-popular-than-ever-11599998401.

Szczepanski, Kallie. 2019. 'How the Black Death Started in Asia and Subsequently Spread across the Middle East and Europe'. *ThoughtCo*. https://www.thoughtco.com/black-death-in-asia-bubonic-plague-195144.

Tsvetkova, Maria. 2020. 'Russian Excess Deaths over Summer Outstrip COVID Toll by More Than 3 to 1'. *Reuters*, 14 September. https://www.reuters.com/article/us-health-coronavirus-russia-mortality/russian-excess-deaths-over-summer-outstrip-covid-toll-by-more-than-3-to-1-idUSKBN2652CO.

US State Department. 2020. 'Office of the U.S. Global AIDS Coordinator and Health Diplomacy. PEPFAR: 2020 Annual Report to Congress'. September. https://www.state.gov/wp-content/uploads/2020/09/PEPFAR2020ARC.pdf.

Vespa, Jonathan, David M. Armstrong, and Lauren Medina. 2018. 'Demographic Turning Points for the United States: Population Projections for 2020 to 2060'. US Census Bureau, March P25–1144.

Way, Lucan A. 2020. 'How a Dictator Became Vulnerable'. *Journal of Democracy 31* (4): p. 17.

WorldOMeter. 2022. 'COVID-19 Coronavirus Pandemic'. https://www.worldometers.info/coronavirus.

YouGov. 2021. 'Boris Johnson Approval Rating'. https://yougov.co.uk/topics/politics/trackers/boris-johnson-approval-rating.

Zissis, Carin. 2021. 'Approval Tracker: Mexico's President AMLO'. Americas Society Council of the Americas, 13 October. https://www.as-coa.org/articles/approval-tracker-mexicos-president-amlo.

4
Bioterrorism and Pandemics

Matthieu J. Guitton

From inequalities to public health systems limits, the COVID-19 pandemic has highlighted a lot of weaknesses in our modern societies. From a security perspective, one of the main lessons the pandemic has taught us is about our vulnerability, as individuals and as societies, to biological threats (see the Introduction to this volume by Ackerly et al. and Chapter 2 by Johnson). Obviously, we were not ready when the pandemic struck us, despite all our knowledge on microbiology, virology, infectious diseases, and epidemiology on the one hand, and despite the existence of centralized structures aimed at preventing the spread of diseases, such as the World Health Organization (WHO) on the other hand. The worldwide COVID-19 pandemic was the first of its kind. However, it is unlikely to be unique, as chances are very good that similar events will occur in the near future, whether because of new waves of COVID-19 or pandemics triggered by other emerging pathogens. Indeed, because of the magnitude of international exchanges and of travel among the global population, pathogens can get propagated from one country to another, increasing the odds for any outbreak to become a pandemic. This interconnection of people and systems forces us to question our vision of international dynamics in the light of the possibility of biological threats.

The tremendous advances in science, and specifically in the field of biotechnologies, are bringing new challenges for nations. Some of them are economic (e.g. pharmaceutical companies and biotech start-ups being particularly targeted by industrial espionage), some are related to public health (such as issues related to access to health care and medicine), and some are geopolitical (notably with questions related to food security, especially in a climate change context) (see Chapter 13 in this volume by Bergeron and Darveau and Chapter 15 by Parent). In addition, some of these challenges are related to security (see Chapter 10 in this volume by Muggah). In a globalized context of democratization of biotechnologies, one of these security challenges is represented by bioterrorism.

Defining bioterrorism is not necessarily an easy task, as the definition of terrorism itself can vary across countries and among scholars. Furthermore, bioterrorism encompasses not only the conventional notions of political

Matthieu J. Guitton, *Bioterrorism and Pandemics*. In: *A Multidisciplinary Approach to Pandemics*.
Edited by Philippe Bourbeau, Jean-Michel Marcoux, and Brooke A. Ackerly, Oxford University Press.
 DOI: 10.1093/oso/9780192897855.003.0005

terrorism, but also dimensions of biosecurity and biosafety (Nestle 2003). However, a conservative definition of bioterrorism is the use of biotechnologies (particularly of natural or human-made pathogen agents) to conduct terrorist actions (Henderson 1999). Militarization of biological agents is not purely a scholarly view. Indeed, this possibility already exists in the eyes of the population, as evidenced by the numerous movies, games, and other popular culture artefacts using biological weapons as a trope. The COVID-19 pandemic provides clear examples of how people can attribute a malevolent origin to an outbreak. Indeed, in the early weeks of the pandemic, Donald Trump, the president of the United States, openly accused China of having engineered the virus in its military laboratories, despite being contradicted both internally by US security agencies and externally by the WHO (Singh et al. 2020).

Whether of natural origin or genetically engineered for military purposes, pandemics share the same determinants and are likely to elicit similar responses from governments and populations alike. Yet bioterrorism adds a layer of fear and psychological warfare that could potentiate the tensions among the population, making the challenges to control a pandemic much more complex. Furthermore, bioterrorism can target not only humans, but also crops or cattle, and bioterrorist actions can enter into deadly synergies with natural pathogens.

By analysing the potential synergy between pandemics and bioterrorism, this chapter aims to identify the main threats related to bioterrorism in a context of global pandemics, and to discuss strategies to mitigate these threats. Of note, there has not been, as of yet, a co-occurrence of bioterrorism and a pandemic, or a bioterrorism event leading to a pandemic. One of the reasons for this is that the technology that would allow engineering a pathogenic agent strong enough to lead to an uncontrolled pandemic is still recent. Thus, there have not been case histories documented so far. In addition, despite a growing focus on bioterrorism over the past 20 years, a quick reality check demonstrates that this focus did not make us more attuned to identify and respond to a pandemic, despite these two phenomena sharing numerous determinants and risks. Therefore, this chapter will take a mostly prospective perspective regarding these questions. We will first describe how bioterrorism and pandemics can enter into a synergy, and what the risks and threats are of such synergies for modern societies. We will then analyse how the convergence of technology between biotechnologies and cybertechnologies can potentiate the combined negative impacts of bioterrorism and pandemics. From a security perspective, we will explore some of the challenges related to the responses of security services and propose elements to optimize the action of counter-intelligence services in the context of bioterrorism. Finally, we will emphasize the importance of educating the population and the necessity of preparedness on the part of decision leaders and governments.

Synergy of Risks and Threats

In the first half of the 1990s, the various terrorist attacks perpetrated by the Aum Shinrikyo movement, including several attempts to use various strains of *Bacillus anthracis* to cause anthrax infections (Takahashi et al. 2004), culminating with the Tokyo subway sarin attack, elicited noticeable alarm. It is easy to foresee that even a single attack with an agent such as anthrax in the context of a pandemic would trigger far greater panic. Yet the interactions between bioterrorism and pandemics can be much more complex than a single event and can take place on a considerably larger scale, thus leading to a marked degradation of health-care systems' capacity to manage the health of the population, and, ultimately, to a sizable increase in potential casualties. Weaponized biological agents can be designed to target the population or resources (crops and cattle). Of note, if artificial pathogens can touch the population as a whole without discrimination, they could also be engineered to target only some segments of the population, by targeting only individuals carrying some specific biomarkers (Bossi et al. 2006).

Bioterrorism and pandemics can interact in various ways. In a minimalistic scenario, isolated bioterrorism events could occur during a pandemic. On the contrary, a human-made pandemic could occur at the same time as a natural-borne pandemic. Between these two extremes, all the configurations are possible. Whether their origin would be natural or artificial, a situation of synergistic pandemics would clearly put a considerable stress on health-care systems. The early months of the COVID-19 pandemic demonstrated the limits in terms of capacity of public health-care systems—and these limits were seen in almost all the countries of the world. Furthermore, not only was the maximal capacity of health-care systems reached, but it was reached incredibly quickly—in less than a week in some cases. The direct and predictable result of a saturation of health-care systems' capacities in a situation of synergistic pandemics or other biological events would be an increase in human deaths.

Several factors are increasing the vulnerability of our societies to bioterrorist attacks. The first of these factors is without doubt the increased accessibility of technologies (Guitton 2020). Once confined to just a few laboratories in a limited number of major public or industrial research centres, biotechnologies are now widespread. From a theoretical perspective, biotechnology is taught worldwide as an academic field. From a practical perspective, the equipment and components related to the biosciences are now highly accessible and readily available (at least, outside of an immediate pandemic context). Even technologies such as genome editing, thought of as cutting edge just a few years ago, are now available in laboratories all over the world. Despite a clear international consensus not to do so, editing human genome has even been accomplished by a Chinese team (Normile 2018, 2019). If a public university laboratory can perform this type of experiment despite the regulations of its own country, it is difficult to see what would stop non-state laboratories from doing the same. Developing or modifying an existing pathogen is not as resource-consuming as it used to be. A lot of the intermediate steps can be outsourced (e.g. ordering DNA sequences can be done without real control). Therefore, an individual with sufficient knowledge in molecular biology (knowledge that is easily obtained from any legitimate graduate programme in molecular biology or associated disciplines at any university worldwide) and with limited resources could potentially generate harmful biological agents.

The second factor of vulnerability is the escalation of global risk. There is probably no need to elaborate on the fact that international tensions have been growing over the past few years. A quick look at the daily news provides numerous examples of this. Yet this has consequences for the management of potential biological risks, both at the national and the international levels. Indeed, the deterioration of international relations leads to a decrease of trust among traditional partners and allies, resulting in a decrease of data-sharing and a lack of transparency between countries. The beginning of the COVID-19 crisis provided a dramatic example of this phenomenon, when China did not fully disclose the information it had on the outbreak. Another example of this lack of communication regarding biotechnology-related information that might have global significance is provided by the case we mentioned earlier regarding the use of genome-editing technology in humans by Chinese scientists. While these experiments were not officially sanctioned, nor were they endorsed by Chinese authorities, the authorities were nonetheless able to recover the data related to the experiment during the investigations—yet these data were not shared with the international research community. If information related to public health is not being shared freely, it is reasonable to think that information regarding weaponized biological agents will not be readily shared either.

The third factor is related to changes in the distribution of the population, specifically the increase in the urban–rural population ratio and the density of population. This progressive displacement of populations from rural to urban areas is now global (Young 2013). Indeed, it has taken place in European countries for at least a century and a half, and has been observed with an accelerated pace in Asia and Africa over the past few decades. This increased inter-individual proximity clearly potentiates the risks of human-to-human transmission of pathogens, as well as animal-to-human transmission (zoonosis), thus favouring the propagation of diseases and the emergence of multiple pandemic clusters.

Finally, but not least, the diminution of food self-sufficiency observed in a lot of countries is a major factor of vulnerability. In our globalized world, supply chains are international, and countries heavily rely on international trade to obtain basic food products (D'Odorico et al. 2014). This dependency on supply chains was seen during the COVID-19 pandemic, when disruption of international trade led to major disturbances in the supply of basic products. Of note, all countries were affected to some extent, including those with the strongest pre-COVID-19 economies. This last factor is extremely important when considering potential synergies between bioterrorism and pandemics. Indeed, while public attention is currently focusing on human diseases, pathogens can be designed to contaminate agricultural targets, whether crops or cattle, compromising the population's access to food even more profoundly. In the context of a pandemic—especially if the country has been targeted by bioterrorism—tensions could escalate into resource conflicts. It is easy to understand that these resource conflicts could quickly move into international wars, especially if some specific areas are associated with the origin of terrorists.

As for biological war, bioterrorism relies on a form of weaponized biological agents. Yet, although weaponized biological agents for biological war and for bioterrorism share the same determinants, they do not share the same constraints. In the case of biological war, the country militarizing the agent has to keep in mind its own population. In other words, a country could not use a pathogen as a weapon without already having the cure—for instance, a vaccine in the case of a virus. As we well know thanks to the COVID-19 pandemic, engineering a vaccine for an uncommon virus is time-consuming and resource-consuming, and can be complex—maybe even more complex than it would be to bioengineer a new virus. This seriously hinders the capacity of nations to use biological agents for large-scale military purposes. On the contrary, bioterrorists are not restrained by this issue. Indeed, bioterrorists can use pathogen agents without caring about whether they have a potential cure for it.

An opposite set of constraints exist in the case of bioterrorism arising from state actors compared to biological wars. If a country aims to use bioterrorism (for instance, as a means to destabilize another country), it would be important to make sure that the biological agents could not be tracked back to their source. In other words, a state actor would not want to be identified as the source of the pathogen. Indeed, if the targeted country could identify the aggressor with certainty, this would lead to a de facto (biological) war situation. In such a case, it is unlikely that the country that engineered and militarized the pathogen would receive any kind of support from the international community. These two sets of different constraints for non-state and state actors nonetheless have something in common: they make bioterrorism menaces more difficult to predict, to detect in their early stages, to counter, and to contain.

Convergence of Technologies

Although terrorist actions are often associated with dramatic events causing numerous deaths, terrorism is not by definition associated with mass murders. Instead, as suggested by the name itself, terrorism aims to use 'fear' as a weapon to push a specific political agenda. In this view, a pandemic is a perfect moment to launch a terror attack because the population is already experiencing fear—or at the very least, they are primed to experience it. Since fear is the very material on which terrorism is based, it is important to analyse the processes of ontogeny of fear when exploring modern forms of terrorism—particularly bioterrorism. In an age of ubiquitous technology, social media, and continuous and global communication, it is impossible to understand the ontogeny of fear or to analyse the mechanisms of its propagation among the different segments of the population without considering new technologies of information in the equation. Indeed, although fear is an emotion, it can easily be created by social engineering through digital spaces.

When it comes to fear, the perception of facts is more important than the facts themselves. This perception is constantly moving alongside a continuum ranging from reality (rational) to fantasy (irrational). The further this perception is from the rational end of the spectrum, the more fear can anchor itself. By pushing perceptions in the irrational direction, disinformation nurtures fear. From fake news to propaganda, disinformation is powered up in digital spaces (Shin et al. 2018; Colliander 2019). This echo-chamber effect gets even more pronounced as people spend more time on social networks—which is typically the case during the massive lockdowns associated with pandemic peaks, as seen during the COVID-19 crisis (Beaunoyer et al. 2020). However, the possibility of manipulating the perception of fear through digital spaces goes way beyond an echo chamber. Indeed, digital spaces offer several ways to manipulate human behaviour (Colliander 2019; Guitton 2019; Frissen 2021; Luqiu et al. 2019). In this aspect, it is important to remember something obvious that we nonetheless tend to forget. Communication technologies are exactly that: technological means to support and enhance communication between individuals. This means that terrorist groups can use them to communicate as well. Using encrypted messaging applications has become a favoured way for terrorists to communicate with each other, to coordinate their actions, and to recruit new members (Frissen 2021). The numerous websites and forums such groups can sustain also provide a powerful vector to convey their messages without leaving the security of their hideout, even from foreign countries.

Whether in a context of a pandemic, bioterrorism, or a combination of the two, fear powered in digital spaces may lead to two types of divisions in the population. The first division is a dichotomist separation of the population between two major factions. A first group is made up of those who will 'follow' the official voices—people who will trust their governments, who will follow the recommendations of health authorities, who won't systematically question every piece of information released by officials. In opposition to this group, a second part of the population gathers those who would believe—or want to believe—in alternate interpretations of the facts. This second category includes, for instance, conspiracy theorists, people who deny the version of the authorities regarding the magnitude of the threat, or those who don't in general want to obey government orders. Prior to the rise of the internet, this second group would typically represent a small minority. Indeed, conspiracy theorists have been around for decades, if not centuries. But before the internet, it was difficult for them to share their ideas, and they tended to remain at the margin of the information market. The internet has been a game-changer because it provided them with a platform to push their ideas. Conspiracy theories nowadays have a wide exposure and gather large audiences—so much so, in fact, that the president of the United States did not hesitate to endorse some of these theories through platforms such as Twitter.

The second type of division in a society that can be observed during biological threat events is related to the stigmatization of some groups, leading to a segmentation of the population. First, social media can increase the risk for some populations to be labelled as scapegoats. For instance, an increase in anti-Asian racism was observed at the beginning of the COVID-19 outbreak in several countries, including the United States (Pomfret 2020), the UK (Campbell 2020), France (d'Adhémar 2020), and Canada (Aguilera 2020). Second, the dependency on the internet puts aside those who are excluded from the digital market, either because of socio-economic conditions or low levels of digital literacy (Beaunoyer et al. 2020). Third, social media discourses can create a final category made up of populations who perceive themselves as being excluded by the system. For instance, a lot of Afro-American people have perceived the decisions made by President Trump's administration regarding the management of the pandemic as being disadvantageous to them. The main risk, then, is for three groups of stigmatized people (scapegoats, those who are excluded from the digital world, and those who perceive themselves as excluded by the system) to be perceived as opposed to the majority of 'good citizens'. Therefore, in addition to the already-existing issues, governments (and security services) will have to deal with unwanted mob behaviour, such as various forms of lynching. These two types of divisions in society (official version versus alternate version followers; stigmatized people versus good citizens) that appear during a pandemic can be potentiated by terrorist events.

As demonstrated here, there is a convergence of technologies between biotechnology and cybertechnology. This convergence needs to be taken into account not only from a theoretical perspective, but also for its practical implications. From a state perspective, the authorities might have to deal not only with the combined impacts of a pandemic and bioterrorist event on the public health front, but also might have to deal with large-scale fear-induced troubles among the population. Therefore, in a bioterrorism/pandemic synergy context, governments and other public services would have to simultaneously fight on two fronts. First, the sanitary or 'biological' front would deal with managing health-care systems to keep patient numbers and health status under control, while also ensuring that the food supply remains secure (or at the very least wasn't overwhelmingly impacted). Second, the ideological or 'informational' front would focus on efforts to disseminate government-validated messages on the one hand, and to control the propagation of unwanted messages and other fake news on the other hand. In the context of bioterrorist events occurring during a pandemic, the control of the messages (and consequently of the perceptions of the population) is as important as the control of the pathogen(s). More than for any other form of biological-based threat, fighting bioterrorism would not primarily be about fighting a biological conflict, but would foremost be about fighting a communication war. Preparedness is key when dealing with biological threats. Yet preparedness should not solely focus on health-care systems. Active and optimal communication between governmental services, on the one hand, and between the authorities and the population, on the other hand, would be a cornerstone of an efficient response.

Security Perspective

The vulnerability of Western societies to bioterrorism finds some of its explanation in the absence of an appropriate frame of reference. Indeed, bioterrorism is not fully equivalent to the other more conventional forms of terrorism. Furthermore, some of the notions at the basis of current anti-terror security responses, such as that of an asymmetrical war, are not necessarily adapted to conceptualize and reflect the threats that biological agents may represent. Indeed, biological war—of which bioterrorism is a specific form—takes place in the context of a double rupture, both sociotechnical and cultural, between Western societies, on the one hand, and other state and non-state entities, on the other hand. The sociotechnical rupture occurs because, since the second half of the twentieth century, Western countries have built their defence strategies upon their technical advances. They thus favoured technological weapons (from nuclear warheads to drones) over chemical weapons (whose massive use by Western armies almost disappeared after the Vietnam War) and biological weapons. The cultural rupture results from the fact that the ethics of research, human rights, and animal rights have become extremely important in Western societies. Although there is absolutely no question that such standards are required to guide the path of progress, these ethical and legal frameworks nonetheless impose constraints on Western research that are not imposed in some other parts of the world. This overwhelming cultural perspective conditions the way biological risks are conceived of and approached.

As a direct consequence of this lack of operational frame of reference, the degree of preparedness of Western societies is not as high as it should be. The centrality of the adaptation of public health systems as a cornerstone to respond to pandemics should not be questioned. Yet, and independently of the responses that need to be found and implemented at the level of public health systems, other state structures need to be adapted to optimally answer biological threats. This is notably the case for security services. Schematically, the missions of security services can be divided into two main lines: preventing trouble (this is typically the mission of intelligence and counter-intelligence services) and, if the threats cannot be countered at an early stage, managing the trouble (which is the mission of police forces).

Intelligence and counter-intelligence inherently deal with information gathering. Thus, the link between intelligence and cybertechnology is easy to understand. Quite naturally, intelligence and counter-intelligence professionals have embraced the emerging information technologies in their practice. Most intelligence academic curricula these days include strong elements of cybersecurity (although the emphasis is often on technical aspects, rather than cyberbehaviour), technology-based information-gathering methods, and data analysis. The situation is, however, utterly different when it comes to biotechnologies. Indeed, primarily because of the disciplinary distance between the fields of security and biology, it is extremely difficult to include in-depth knowledge of biotechnology in an intelligence formation curriculum while keeping enough internal coherence (Guitton 2020). Several pedagogical formats can be used to provide security specialists with functional knowledge of biology, ranging from short academic formations to intensive internships or online courses (Guitton 2020).

Whatever the solution—or the combination of solutions—that is selected, it is critical to increase the literacy of intelligence and counter-intelligence experts in biotechnology for an appropriate defence against bioterrorism to emerge. In any case, given the pace of evolution of technologies and the geostrategic context, the initial formation of intelligence and counter-intelligence professionals cannot be considered as sufficient—even if it were to include a base level of biology. Instead, initial formation has to be completed by continuous, lifelong learning. Strictly mono-disciplinary approaches are fated to fail to produce the experts we need to deal with the threats related to bioterrorism. Therefore, implementation of counter-intelligence-targeted continuous education should avoid focusing solely on specific (often technical) issues, but rather embrace a much wider perspective.

During a pandemic, the role of police forces is extremely important. Indeed, in addition to all their regular tasks and missions, police forces will have to deal with an overly worried population. In such a context, public gatherings may be prone to degenerating into riots. At the same time, police forces will have to enforce the decisions made by the authorities. In addition, they might have to protect vulnerable populations and potentially defend stigmatized segments of the populations (see 'Convergence of Technologies' above). The way the management of biohazards by security forces is conceptualized typically relies on the principles of chemical, biological, radiological, and nuclear (CBRN) defence. The central element of this frame of reference is the notion of confinement. The COVID-19 pandemic, however, demonstrated the limits of the confinement of the population. The confinement of officers is typically done using heavy protective suits, referred to as CBRN suits. However, these strategies have some important limits. While CBRN suits are perfectly adapted to a laboratory setting, they are much less so in an open space. CBRN suits offer some measure of protection to the officers, but not to the populations. They do not prevent the diffusion of the pathogen in the environment. CBRN measures are extremely difficult to operationalize (and almost impossible in an urban landscape at a large scale). Finally, from the population perspective, CBRN approaches do not take into account the human factor. The vision of a group of fully equipped technicians wearing CBRN suits ordering people to stand aside in decontaminated plastic-clad modules might be enough to create more panic among the victims than the actual menace warrants.

All in all, the use of such suits is not feasible in a context of crowd management, either in the case of legitimate gatherings or in the case of riots. At this point, it is interesting to look at the current equipment of anti-riot units. There has been an overall reduction in the length of the primary melee weapons used by law enforcement forces over the past few decades. Long anti-riot sticks (such as the 'jo', a long stick still used by some Japanese anti-riot police units as part of their standard equipment) have been progressively replaced by side-handle batons (derived from the Okinawa tonfa, with a typical length of 61 centimetres or 24 inches) and, more recently, by shorter telescopic batons (also known as tactical batons). As the length of the melee weapons decreases, the distance of contact between officers and civilians gets shorter, leading, in the context of biological risk, to an increase in contamination risk for officers. This might lead to law enforcement forces feeling a lack of safety that might lead them to favour the use of distance weapons instead of melee weapons—which comes with increased risk of accidents for civilians. Within a pandemic context, governments might be prompted to take measures of force majeure that would, for instance, soften the use of firearms by anti-riot units.

Providing a 'right to shoot' to police forces during a pandemic is a good example of how a lack of appropriate preparedness could endanger social cohesion. From the reduction of freedom of movement to issues with medical privacy, a pandemic could easily erode fundamental rights and enter into conflict with national and international legal obligations. This was exemplified by the early weeks of the COVID-19 pandemic. Whether we are discussing counter-intelligence forces or police forces, the responses that will be adopted by security services bear risks for social cohesion and for individual liberties, including (but not limited to) rights to privacy, civil rights, and public rights. In the case of a synergy between a pandemic and bioterrorism, the predictable increased security response should not be used by nations as an excuse to increase state power. Since the declaration of the War on Terror by the United States in the early 2000s, the evolution of counterterrorism has elicited numerous controversies related to fundamental rights. As a consequence, the scrutiny of security policies by the population has increased. The support of the population for the government is more fragile than it was a few decades ago. Therefore, social acceptability is central if one wants to adjust security strategies without impairing social cohesion. This social acceptability will heavily depend on the transparency of the decisions made by the governments and on the accountability of security services. The mission of intelligence and counter-intelligence—which counterterrorism is but a specific form of—is to protect society, and this mission is shared with police forces. Undertaking this mission might have a cost, and this cost is likely to translate to a (hopefully transient) reduction of some of our liberties. How much we, as individuals and as societies, are ready to sacrifice to ensure the safety of the population is the core question of the security debate in a pandemic/bioterrorist context. The line is thin, especially in a context of biological threats, where the health of the population—and thus the lives of tens of thousands of people—is directly threatened.

Conclusion

As the world becomes more globalized, the implications of technological advances on national, economic, health, or food security cannot be neglected. The interconnection of these implications is obvious when it comes to biological threats, whether that threat comes from a pandemic or from bioterrorism. However, the vulnerability of our societies to biological threats, which was revealed starkly by the COVID-19 pandemic, is not inescapable. As the situation is likely to happen again, we must get ready to answer future crises. Biology is not just a way to better human health anymore—it is now also a potential source of tactical and geostrategic weapons. This new reality emphasizes the strategic importance of research. Therefore, and to summarize what we have discussed in this chapter, governments will need to re-evaluate the risks and threats, their international alliances, the preparedness of the population, the formation of security and counter-intelligence services, and the strategic importance of research to be ready for future bioterrorist events.

Whether to better human health or to fight against climate change, the convergence of technologies is bringing major hope for humankind. However, this convergence can also, as we demonstrated in this chapter, bring its share of threats. The response of governments will have to take into account this evolving reality in a world characterized by unstable equilibriums. Answering these challenges properly, while still maintaining a socially acceptable level of individual liberties, will not be an easy task. A significant part of the solution will come from education: education of health-care professionals, education of security services agents, and education of the general population as a whole. Yet besides education, in-depth debates among governmental agencies, between decision-makers and the population, and among the population as a whole will be required to ensure that the strategies adopted to cope with potential future military-grade pandemics are being implemented in such a way that will be satisfying from a societal perspective.

To close this chapter on the interactions between bioterrorism and pandemics, we will make a final note on sovereignty. The COVID-19 pandemic has shown the importance of social media in the management of large-scale, long-lasting crises, both as an ally and a valuable tool for communicating official messages or instructions and as a foe and danger when it comes to propagation of erroneous—or even malevolent—information. The widespread mastery many people have over biotechnologies leads to the possibility of a bioterrorism event occurring during a pandemic context, and this blurs the boundaries between state and non-state actors and their respective control over population health—a domain so far under the sole control of state actors. Post-COVID-19, international relations and dynamics will necessarily be different than those that were taking place prior to the pandemic. Therefore, the COVID-19 pandemic might contribute to redefining the importance of multidisciplinary in counterterrorism and counter-intelligence approaches, rethinking the potential evolution of global warfare, and, ultimately, questioning some of the norms and limits of state sovereignty.

References

Aguilera, Jasmine. 2020. 'Xenophobia "Is a Pre-Existing Condition." How Harmful Stereotypes and Racism Are Spreading around the Coronavirus'. *Time*, 1 February, updated 3 February. https://time.com/5775716/xenophobia-racism-stereotypes-coronavirus.

Beaunoyer, Elisabeth, Sophie Dupéré, and Matthieu J. Guitton. 2020. 'COVID-19 and Digital Inequalities: Reciprocal Impacts and Mitigation Strategies'. *Computers in Human Behavior 111*: 106424.

Bossi, Philippe, Daniel Garin, Amélie Guihot, et al. 2006. 'Bioterrorism: Management of Major Biological Agents'. *Cellular and Molecular Life Sciences 63*: p. 2196.

Campbell, Lucy. 2020. 'Chinese in the UK Report "Shocking" Levels of Racism after Coronavirus Outbreak'. *The Guardian*, 9 February, updated 10 February. https://www.theguardian.com/uk-news/2020/feb/09/chinese-in-uk-report-shocking-levels-of-racism-after-coronavirus-outbreak.

Colliander, Jonas. 2019. '"This Is Fake News": Investigating the Role of Conformity to Other Users' Views When Commenting on and Spreading Disinformation in Social Media'. *Computers in Human Behavior 97*: p. 202.

d'Adhémar, Margaux. 2020. 'Rentre chez toi, garde ta maladie! Quand le coronavirus sert d'excuse au racisme antiasiatique'. *Le Figaro*, 30 January. https://www.lefigaro.fr/actualite-france/rentre-chez-toi-garde-ta-maladie-quand-le-coronavirus-sert-d-excuse-au-racisme-antiasiatique-20200130.

D'Odorico, Paolo, Joel A. Carr, Francesco Laio, Luca Ridolfi, and Stefano Vandoni. 2014. 'Feeding Humanity through Global Food Trade'. *Earth's Future 2* (9): p. 458.

Frissen, Thomas. 2021. 'Internet, the Great Radicalizer? Exploring Relationships between Seeking for Online Extremist Materials and Cognitive Radicalization in Young Adults'. *Computers in Human Behavior 114*: 106549.

Guitton, Matthieu J. 2019. 'Manipulation through Online Sexual Behavior: Exemplifying the Importance of Human Factor in Intelligence and Counterintelligence in the

Big Data Era'. *International Journal of Intelligence, Security, and Public Affairs 21* (2): p. 117.

Guitton, Matthieu J. 2020. 'Using Biotechnology to Build a Workforce for Intelligence and Counterintelligence'. *International Journal of Intelligence and CounterIntelligence 33* (1): p. 119.

Henderson, Donald A. 1999. 'The Looming Threat of Bioterrorism'. *Science 283* (5406): p. 1279.

Luqiu, Luwei Rose, Michael Schmierbach, and Yu-Leung Ng. 2019. 'Willingness to Follow Opinion Leaders: A Case Study of Chinese Weibo'. *Computers in Human Behavior 101*: p. 42.

Nestle, Marion. 2003. *Safe Food: Bacteria, Biotechnology, and Bioterrorism*. Berkeley, CA: University of California Press.

Normile, Dennis. 2018. 'Shock Greets Claim of CRISPR-Edited Babies'. *Science 362* (6418): p. 978.

Normile, Dennis. 2019. 'Government Report Blasts Creator of CRISPR Twins'. *Science 363* (6425): p. 328.

Pomfret, John. 2020. 'The Coronavirus Reawakens Old Racist Tropes against Chinese'. *Washington Post*, 5 February. https://www.washingtonpost.com/opinions/2020/02/05/coronavirus-reawakens-old-racist-tropes-against-chinese-people.

Shin, Jieun, Lian Jian, Kevin Driscoll, and François Bar. 2018. 'The Diffusion of Misinformation on Social Media: Temporal Pattern, Message, and Source'. *Computers in Human Behavior 83*: p. 278.

Singh, Maanvi, Helen Davidson, and Julian Borger. 2020. 'Trump Claims to Have Evidence Coronavirus Started in Chinese Lab but Offers no Details'. *The Guardian*, 1 May. https://www.theguardian.com/us-news/2020/apr/30/donald-trump-coronavirus-chinese-lab-claim.

Takahashi, Hiroshi, Paul Keim, Arnold F. Kaufmann, et al. 2004. 'Bacillus anthracis Bioterrorism Incident, Kameido, Tokyo, 1993'. *Emerging Infectious Diseases 10* (1): p. 117.

Young, Alwyn. 2013. 'Inequality, the Urban–Rural Gap, and Migration'. *Quarterly Journal of Economics 128* (4): p. 1727.

5

Europe and the Pandemic

Christopher Bickerton

There is no such thing as a single 'European experience' of the ongoing COVID-19 pandemic. This is curious. We would expect a public health emergency of this kind to present the European Union (EU) with all the cross-border externality challenges best managed when national states 'pool' their sovereignty in a regional union. We would expect a region so thoroughly integrated in its laws and policymaking to stand out from countries far less connected with one another. And yet, prima facie evidence suggests that this was not the case. Events move fast, of course, especially those driven by the spread of disease, and EU member states are still operating under lockdowns and feeling the full effects of the pandemic that started in early 2020. So far, it would seem that other factors—such as a prior experience of similar pandemics and the impact of this on individual behaviour—have been far more decisive in shaping the spread, effects, and government responses to COVID-19.[1]

As emphasized by Greer and de Ruijter (2020: 623), '[p]ublic health is a strange place to rein in European integration, for everything we know about the movement of diseases, animals and people show that there already is European public health'. What emerges from this chapter is something similar to the Eurozone crisis of the 2010s and the challenge it posed to the future of the EU. On the one hand, the crisis was a reflection of the high level of financial interdependence that characterized the national economies of the EU and of the Eurozone in particular. On the other hand, the crisis exposed a deficit in transnational solidarity, manifest in an unwillingness to make cross-border fiscal transfers that could have balanced out the effects of the crisis. This sort of integration without solidarity continues to be a feature of the EU. At the same time, the coronavirus crisis has transformed the EU in important ways. One way is through the fiscal stimulus promised to

[1] This chapter focuses on the 2020 COVID-19 pandemic. Existing EU policies and national experiences have also been shaped by previous virus-related crises, in particular Severe Acute Respiratory Syndrome (SARS) in 2003 and AH1N1 (swine flu) in 2009. 2020 has unsurprisingly been the occasion for revisiting earlier European experiences, for instance of Spanish flu (1918–1919). On the historical lessons of pandemics, see Jones (2020).

Christopher Bickerton, *Europe and the Pandemic.* In: *A Multidisciplinary Approach to Pandemics.*
Edited by Philippe Bourbeau, Jean-Michel Marcoux, and Brooke A. Ackerly, Oxford University Press.
 DOI: 10.1093/oso/9780192897855.003.0006

member states as part of the 'NextGenerationEU' fund.[2] Another way is through the institutional experimentation undertaken around collective vaccine procurement, which was rolled out in the course of 2021. This chapter reflects on why national experiences have differed so much within a regional union characterized by high levels of political and economic integration. Some of the explanation must lie in the balance of competences over health policy, with power skewered heavily towards the member states. But policy-specific explanations have their limits. The role of regional integration in the experience of the pandemic also tells something more fundamental about the nature of the EU and its place in the lives of Europe's citizens.

Effects, Responses, Styles: A Chronicle of European Diversity

The first wave of the coronavirus crisis in the late winter/early spring of 2020 hit countries such as Italy, Spain, and the UK with devastating effect. Much of Eastern Europe was spared, relatively speaking, with countries such as the Czech Republic fêted for its exemplary response. Czech citizens even held a large party celebrating the 'defeat' of the virus at the beginning of the summer (Cameron 2020). Germany stood out as an instance of early action in testing and tracing working to bring infections and hospitalizations down (Chazan 2020). The second wave that came after the summer hit much of Eastern Europe very hard, including the Czech Republic, drawing these countries into a continent-wide second lockdown. On 21 October, the German health minister, a figure often touted as a possible successor to Angela Merkel, Jens Spahn, self-isolated after testing positive for COVID-19. Doubts raised about Germany's status as pandemic success story (e.g. Robinet-Borgomano 2020) deepened in the first months of 2021 as complaints flared up about the slow pace of the country's vaccine campaign. Differences in experience in 2021 were shaped by a combination of different exposures to variant strains of coronavirus and the highly variable roll out of vaccines across Europe.

All countries in Europe have been marked by the spread of the pandemic. According to Tooze (2020), '[t]he crisis is being fought nation by nation, with whatever resources are available'. However, in some countries, the sense of national crisis and catastrophe was so acute that it will live on in the minds and habits of its citizens. The experience of the need to triage treatment given to patients according to age, which hit Northern Italy in early 2020, added to a sense of urgency and profound crisis. The lack of protective equipment and medical devices in some Italian

[2] The impact of this fund is at present unknown, since the money allocated to countries has not yet been distributed, let alone spent. This chapter focuses on the practical and symbolic effects associated with its creation.

hospitals during this period created an apocalyptic sense of facing a threat without adequate resources. In Spain, the PSOE–Podemos government pushed through coronavirus measures by decree, encapsulating a form of what Jonathan White has called 'governing by emergency' (White 2020). Elsewhere, the spread was slower and the bottlenecks within public health services were fewer than expected. In the UK, a coronavirus-dedicated hospital—the Florence Nightingale, in the London docklands area, a stone's throw from London City Airport—remained largely empty in spite of the very high levels of COVID-19-related deaths, second only to Italy.[3]

As well as the different *effects* of the pandemic, government *responses* have varied considerably. In France, its lockdown arrangements have included the requirement that anyone moving outside of their home must carry an official document stating the reason for their movements. Only a small number of justifications were accepted. Inhabitants of sparsely inhabited zones—such as in the far North West of Brittany—were unable to take their customary coastal walks in spite of it being unlikely that one would meet anyone at all for the whole duration of the outing. Across the Channel in the UK, lockdown measures never involved the same degree of state coercion. Fines by the police were rare and rules regarding quarantining after international travel were thinly policed until well into 2021. Studies in the UK suggest that only a small proportion of people have followed many of the COVID-19-related rules, such as the need to self-isolate when given a notification to do so via the official NHS app. Elsewhere, such as in much of Italy, compliance rates have been very high.

An extreme outlier was Sweden, where the government introduced stricter quarantine rules very late on, after a sustained effort at achieving 'herd immunity'.[4] For much of the first six months of Europe's coronavirus crisis, Swedish schools remained open and people moved around within many restrictions. In Spain, whole families lived in small, inner-city apartments for months on end, with trips outside restricted to essential shopping and some daily exercise. When Denmark and Norway imposed travel restrictions on Swedish citizens because of the higher infection rates in Sweden, these differences in approach were brought into stark relief. A region characterized by high-frequency cross-border travel was transformed into one with carefully monitored national borders.

As well as effects and responses, European experiences differed in terms of *political styles* and the internal politics surrounding COVID-19. Angela Merkel's cautious and methodical approach in Germany contrasted with the bluster and hubris of Boris Johnson. Italy's Giuseppe Conte found that his ratings rose sharply over the course of the first wave and the ensuing health crisis in Italy, reflecting his

[3] At the time of writing, that is, end of November 2020.

[4] Even these stricter rules were light by comparison to other countries. Notwithstanding very high infections and death rates in the second wave, Sweden does not quarantine the close contacts of infected people and does not require the wearing of masks.

standing as a non-partisan figure (Lazar 2020). The later arrival of Mario Draghi at the helm of the Italian government in February 2021 brought a new political style, one that combined Draghi's unquestioned commitment to pan-Europeanism with firm commitment to pursuing Italy's interests within the EU. The pandemic also sharpened territorial conflicts in Europe. Consensual forms of decentralized power—in Germany, for instance—performed well by devolving responsibilities for key tasks such as testing and tracing contacts to the local level (Chazan 2020). Territorial conflicts in Spain and the UK got in the way of government responses, creating divisions between cities or regions and national authorities.

One obvious explanation for the variety of European experiences of the pandemic is the absence of supranational European public health policy (Greer and de Ruijter 2020). European member states have been careful to limit the EU's powers in this area, with the result that enormous diversity continues to characterize health provision and policy across member states. As single market integration has progressed, a tense stand-off has developed between the imperatives of free movement (of goods and services) and the restrictions associated with sustaining a functioning national health-care system (De Ruijter et al. 2020). Such health systems are shielded from the usual single market rules of free competition: patients do not shop around for their doctor or their hospital in the way that they would when seeking a mortgage or booking a holiday. Fears about the survival of public services as single market integration deepens have been strong enough to push member states to seek legal guarantees protecting their national health-care sectors from the involvement of the EU.

This limitation in juridical competence certainly goes some way to explaining why—hitherto—European integration seems to have played a limited role in shaping the experience of the pandemic in Europe for the continent's citizens. There was some evidence of policy learning over the course of 2020 and 2021, and this is likely to continue. When EU member states began to plan their strategy for vaccine procurement, it was decided that the efforts would be centralized via an EU Commission-led collective procurement arrangement. Small member states were particularly concerned at the prospect of being cut out of deals with pharmaceutical companies struck with the larger member states. In Germany, there was a strong desire to avoid the scramble for scarce virus-related supplies that had featured in the early months of 2020. For the French government, a Commission-led strategy would be a means to bring down the costs of vaccination whilst also demonstrating the value of the regional union over the national strategies pursued by the UK and the United States. Even here, however, we can see how collective agreements harbour a multiplicity of aims, in ways that can make it difficult to achieve the stated policy goal (Majone 2015; Bickerton 2021).

Sangiovanni (2013) is quite right to caution against applying to Europe the solidaristic standards of an integrated global community of cosmopolitans. But even according to his more limited 'internationalist' standard, the EU's record since the beginning of the pandemic has been mixed. It thus makes some sense to distinguish between solidarity at the national level and solidarity at the EU level. Since the beginning of the COVID-19 pandemic, solidarity has been at the very heart of national responses. It has been the principle justification used when asking people to observe lockdown rules, and the level of acceptance of this kind of solidarity has been exceptionally high. In terms of health risks, the coronavirus of 2020 was much more threatening for older generations; in terms of economic costs of containment measures, those of working age and younger were hit the hardest in terms of lost income, unemployment, and deteriorating future economic prospects. National governments have urged citizens to accept this uneven intergenerational burden—in effect, a wealth transfer from the young to the old—in the name of solidarity. Another sort of solidarity has been evident in the support given to doctors and nurses: national publics demonstrably recognized the way in which these professions exposed themselves to high levels of risk in order to treat sick patients and control the effects of the pandemic (Jones 2020: 1682). Solidarity has been at the centre of how national public health regimes function and how pandemic-related responses have been legitimized. But its place within health-related policy coordination at the EU level is, as one might expect, a more complex matter (de Ruijter et al. 2020: 8).

The EU's Role in Fighting COVID-19

'European solidarity is in high demand but in short supply' (Genschel and Hemerik 2018: 1). This section of the chapter looks at the EU's role in tackling the COVID-19 pandemic. It distinguishes between the EU's role during the first wave of the pandemic (February–May 2020) and during the second wave (September 2020—present).[5] The chapter also differentiates between economic and health-related EU interventions. This section provides a narrative of EU actions and then provides a simple classificatory framework in terms of policy instruments and the relevant actors involved. Whereas the EU's role in sustaining the European economy throughout 2020 was significant and extensive, its involvement in the public health dimension of the fight against the pandemic was—with the exception of vaccine procurement—more limited.

Fighting the 'First Wave'

News of a new coronavirus in China reached Europe in early January 2020. China embarked on a radical lockdown in the city of Wuhan on 23 January. A month

[5] The chapter does not discuss what has come to be known as the 'third wave', referring to the levels of infections and transmission within an established and ongoing vaccination campaign.

later, there were over 2,000 infections in Europe and already 35 deaths in Italy. Northern Italy emerged as the first epicentre of the outbreak. The virus hit hardest in the regions of Piedmont, Lombardy, and Veneto. Officials cordoned off a cluster of small villages in Lombardy and subjected them to a strict lockdown. Whilst most other European countries were registering only a handful of cases, Italy had reached 500. With the number of new cases per day increasing exponentially, Italy was in 'the eye of the storm' (Majoli 2020). Other outbreaks were occurring at the same time, such as the one in the Tyrolian ski resort of Ischgl, where cases were reported in late February. The Austrian outbreak became an important 'super-spreader' moment: even after cases of the virus had been reported, foreign tourists were allowed to return home. This had the effect of spreading the virus to places as far afield as Singapore and Israel, leading to subsequent outbreaks in these countries (Chazan and Jones 2020).

By the end of the first week of March, national governments across Europe began to respond in earnest. On 3 March, French President Emanuel Macron requisitioned all the existing French stock of masks. On 4 March, Germany banned the export of all personal protective equipment (PPE). A week later, Germany unilaterally closed its borders, leading to 50-km traffic hold-ups on the Polish border. At this time, the European Commission launched a Joint Procurement Agreement (JCA) for PPE. This made use of a voluntary procurement scheme that was introduced in the wake of the EU's experience of the April 2009 swine flu epidemic.[6] On 19 March, the European Commission announced the creation of a stockpile of medical equipment, known as RescEU. Member states could propose themselves as the host for the stockpile and the Commission would finance the purchases of equipment. The stockpile arrangement was coordinated through the EU Civil Protection Mechanism (EUCPM). The EUCPM had already been mobilized for the repatriation of citizens from EU member states who were stranded in various parts of the country as pandemic-related travel restrictions were introduced. The European Response Coordination Centre, set up as part of the EUCPM, was responsible for coordinating the distribution of emergency supplies. The first action of RescEU was to deliver masks to Italy, but this came long after the critical shortages in March. In mid-April, the Commission issued a communication regarding the coordination of restrictions on non-essential travel, but this came over a month after member states had imposed these measures themselves, without any systematic coordination between them (Deruelle 2020).

The health-related responses to the 'first wave' of the virus were national in character. Whilst much of health policy in the EU remains a competence of national governments, there is an EU solidarity clause (Article 222 of the Treaty on the Functioning of the European Union (TFEU)) which states that in case of a terrorist

[6] During the swine flu crisis, national antiviral procurement had created important imbalances between member states that failed to correspond with immediate need.

attack, man-made or natural disasters, member states should provide emergency assistance to one another and coordinate their efforts. No such efforts featured in the course of the first wave of the coronavirus. At the end of February, the Italian government issued a call for help to the European Commission, which uploaded Italy's request to the EU's Common Emergency Communication and Information System (CECIS). No member state responded to the call (Boffey et al. 2020). In effect, Italy had triggered the solidary clause to no effect (Atlantic Council 2020).[7] Instead of pooling resources through the RescEU stockpile to a meaningful degree, national governments built up their own national supplies, irrespective of the immediate demands they were facing.

There were echoes here of the way European Economic Community (EEC) member states responded to the Organization of the Petroleum Exporting Countries (OPEC) oil crisis of 1973. Because of their different standing in the Arab world, some of the European countries were able to secure more oil supplies than others. France, for instance, with a foreign minister dubbed 'Jobert of Arabia' fared much better than the Netherlands.[8] A plea to pool oil supplies within the EEC was met only with disagreement and delay.[9] It is easy, of course, with hindsight to observe that in late Feburary/early March, the need for PPE and medical devices (especially ventilators) was most acute in some parts of Italy, whereas it was much less urgent in other parts of Europe. At the time, governments were looking forwards, seeking to protect their citizens against the coming of the virus. By the end of March, aid packages from China were alleviating some of the equipment shortages. As aid arrived to Italy from China, the country's foreign minister, Luigi di Maio, declared that 'we are not alone, there are people in the world who want to help Italy' (Atlantic Council 2020). De Maio's words captured a sentiment that was prevalent in Italy at the time: that in a moment of great national emergency, the country had not been able to rely on help from immediate European neighbours or from the EU. On 16 April, the President of the European Commission acknowledged the limits of the EU's action in the first wave. Addressing the European Parliament, Ursula Von de Leyen apologized to Italy 'on behalf of the European Union as a whole'.

Coordination in macro-economic policymaking was more successful during the first wave, though initially it deepened the asymmetry between monetary and fiscal policy. The European Central Bank (ECB) reacted quickly. The collapse in the oil price in March triggered a global sell-off in stocks. In response, the

[7] In Besch's words, '[t]he EU and its member states fell short in their initial response to the outbreak. When the Italian government first activated the EU's solidarity mechanism, not one country came to its aid. Instead some, including Germany and France, initiated export bans on medical equipment.' Besch notes that the EU performed better during later stages of the crisis (see Atlantic Council 2020).

[8] Michel Jobert was foreign minister under George Pompidou, during 1973–1974. Born in Morocco, he enjoyed good relations with many leaders and politicians in the Middle East.

[9] For an extended account of the OPEC oil crisis and its impact on Europe, see Möckli 2008.

ECB launched the Pandemic Emergency Purchase Programme, an asset-buying programme totalling 750 billion Euros. This set the stage for ECB intervention that took the central bank far beyond what it had done since 2008. Adam Tooze (2020) noted the marked contrast between the speed of the ECB's actions in 2020 and those during the Eurocrisis. In his words, '[i]n 2012 Mario Draghi's admission that the ECB would do "whatever it takes" to save the Euro was the climax of more than two years of political and economic struggle. This time around it was the first principle of central bank intervention.' The swift and very significant action by the ECB contrasts with a much more modest EU-level response in fiscal and supply-side policies. On the fiscal side, consistent with the EU's limited powers, national government decisions reflected the different positions of member states. Germany's COVID-19 fiscal stimulus package was far greater than Italy's, due to the latter's far higher levels of sovereign debt. The EU's principal interventions in this area were to support flexible interpretations of state aid rules in support of national assistance programmes. The European Commission made targeted interventions through regulatory changes to support specific sectors. The European Investment Bank provided some support to pharmaceutical research, channelling 100 million Euros of investment into BioNTech, a German pharmaceutical company that was the first to produce—in conjunction with Pfizer—a working vaccine using novel mRNA technology.

Fighting the Later Waves

In the course of the summer of 2020, rates of infection fell considerably across Europe. Some sense of normality returned, albeit in a patchy manner and in the context of many discussions about a return of the virus during the winter months. Across the continent, 'staycations' became the norm as travel bans and quarantine restrictions hit international travel hard. Nevertheless, governments phased out national lockdowns. Primary and secondary schools began to open, partially or in a staggered fashion, making an enormous difference to those expected to 'work from home' and 'home school' simultaneously. City centres began to fill up as non-essential shops reopened. New restrictions led to very different environments for shoppers (closed changing rooms and an interdiction to touch some items) but consumption picked up and began, once again, to drive economies reliant upon services and high consumer demand. Fears about a 'second wave' were moderated by government promises to develop an effective test-and-trace infrastructure.

September 2020 signalled a turn for the worse. The re-opening of schools proceeded almost everywhere, reflecting a commitment by national politicians not to impose restrictions that would do permanent damage to children's education. This came with a rise in infections, especially in secondary schools. The start of the academic year for universities was another important factor in driving infections: many students arrived at university and very soon found themselves sick with COVID-19, obliged to isolate in their own student rooms: 'locked down and locked in', as one journalist put it. Various systems were put in place to manage the onset of a 'second wave' of infections. The French government had introduced a 'traffic light' system, intended to pin point epidemic trouble spots, whilst protecting areas without much infection from the socio-economic costs of another lockdown. In Spain, different rates of infection across cities and regions were managed through a variety of different rules, with city mayors often complaining about the severity of the restrictions placed on their own cities. In the UK, resistance to a second lockdown persisted throughout the autumn. The government introduced a system of tiers, with those living in tiers 2 or 3 subjected to more restrictions than those in tier 1.

The 'second wave' in Europe was different from the first in many ways, not least in terms of mortality and hospitalizations. For a number of reasons, but in particular because of greater awareness about the need to swiftly close down clusters of infections, mortality rates rose but at a much slower pace than in March or April. In March, foreign tourists returned from Austrian ski resorts, spreading the virus to all corners of the continent. In the UK, hospitals discharged sick elderly patients into care homes in order to keep hospital beds free for COVID-19 cases. The effect was to bring infections into the elderly care sector, with devastating effects. Learning from these mistakes brought death rates down. Eventually, however, lockdowns returned. Even countries with effective test-and-trace systems—such as Germany—found themselves overwhelmed with new cases. Efficient contract tracers were no match for a rapid increase in infections: the spread meant that there were simply too many contacts for tracers to call. Ireland was the first to bring in a second lockdown (on 22 October), followed swiftly by the Czech Republic. In Belgium, infection rates rose to the highest in Europe in per capita terms. Since the end of the summer, the Belgian government had introduced a variety of restrictions, including a midnight to 5 a.m. curfew (Looi 2020). There was some homogenization in government responses to the 'second wave' but only because the wave itself was less discriminating and more comprehensive in its reach. The principal difference between the first wave and the later waves was the arrival of variant strains of COVID-19. Whilst medical treatment had improved, and governments were more willing to deploy stringent social distancing measures, transmissibility rates increased as more virulent variants of the virus took hold.

The action at the EU level differed considerably from the first wave, but principally with respect to EU-level fiscal stimulus, not in relation to direct pandemic-related measures. Risk management (see 'The EU's Actions during the Pandemic—a Summary and Assessment' below) remained the preserve of governments, with great differences between member states. On 27 May 2020, the Commission presented its 'Recovery Plan' for Europe. Based on close consultation with member states, the idea was to create a new recovery instrument ('Next Generation EU') that would sit alongside the 2021–2027 budget. Totalling 750 billion Euros, the Recovery Fund consists of one half in loans, the other half in grants. How to finance the fund was an issue of considerable conflict. Many EU member states did not want to sign up to a financial package that could leave them more indebted than ever. Moreover, loans carried with them the negative connection to intrusive forms of conditionality.[10] This sentiment was strongest in countries that had been on—or almost been on—the receiving end of EU loans in the past, particularly at the time of the Troika-managed bail-outs. At the same time, member states committed to fiscal rectitude—the so-called 'frugal four'—resisted any idea that financial assistance could come in the form of direct transfers to the hardest-hit member states.

Franco–German agreement on the Recovery Fund was a crucial factor in unblocking disagreement, as was a compromise where the package would include grants and loans. On the French side, the plan reflected a longstanding desire to have some form of debt mutualization for the Eurozone and it was consistent with Emmanuel Macron's call for more 'European sovereignty' made in his September 2017 Sorbonne speech. German support was more difficult to fathom, given longstanding opposition within Germany to any sort of Euro-bond initiative. The German government found itself pulled in different directions. On the one side were the fears about debt mutualization, familiar since the Eurozone crisis debates. On the other side was the growing opposition to the expanding activities and powers of the ECB. This opposition was political, institutional (via the concerns of the Bundesbank) and juridical (as articulated by Germany's own constitutional court). The great advantage of taking such an important forward step on the fiscal side for Germany was that it would take some pressure off the ECB and its emerging legitimacy deficit.

In the third week of July 2021, heads of state and government struck an agreement on the 2021–2027 budget and the Recovery Fund. This signalled an important shift towards fiscal redistribution within the EU. It gave the EU significant capacity to borrow on international markets for the purpose of supporting member states hardest hit by COVID-19. Moreover, by locating this financial instrument within the European Commission, the Recovery Fund is likely to empower the Commission. The Commission will have new oversight powers and will have the power over the regulation of member state requests for EU funds, similar to, but also in a more permanent fashion with, what was observed in the formation of the Troika. The effect of these oversight powers have already been felt: the collapse of the second Conte government in Italy in early 2021 was prompted by doubts expressed by other politicians (notably Matteo Renzi) about the strength

[10] The stigma was also attached to the European Supervisory Mechanism (ESM). 'No ESM' was the position taken by many member states when negotiating the fiscal package.

of Italy's plan for spending the 'NextGenEU' money. For financial markets, the Recovery Fund constitutes an important event—in terms of the size of the new tranche of triple A-rated bonds that will come with it, along with the effect of creating a new safe asset for international investors.

Member states reached an agreement on the EU-level COVID-19 fiscal strategy during the summer of 2021, but it has taken time for the NextGenerationEU fund to become operational. After agreeing the fiscal stimulus as part of the negotiations around the multi-annual budget, the German presidency and the European Parliament agreed on linking access to EU funds to conditionality surrounding the rule of law. This provoked very negative reactions in Hungary and Poland, the two countries targeted by the European Commission for violation in the area of the rule of law, and led to a stand-off between the Polish and Hungarian governments and the rest of the EU. Even after the budget was passed, ratification at the national level has been slowed down because of political disputes within some member states.

A significant new element in EU public health policy has emerged over the course of 2021, namely, the pan-European vaccine procurement initiative and its delivery of vaccines. Originally, this began as an alliance between four EU member states—Germany, Italy, France, and the Netherlands. Governments in these countries were anxious that whereas the United States, the UK, and some other countries were already in advanced negotiations with pharmaceutical companies, including extensive upfront financing, EU member states had agreed nothing by the beginning of June 2020. A 'pre-agreement' with Astra Zeneca for 300 million doses struck by this alliance of four member states prompted the rest of the EU to act, out of fear that they would find themselves cut out of the first tranche of vaccine deliveries. Later in June, the European Commission announced a collective procurement arrangement, made up of 2.1 billion Euros for advanced vaccine contracts (via the Emergency Support Instrument) and 750 million Euros from member states themselves. The responsibility for negotiating with vaccine producers was passed on to the Commission. A contract with Astra Zeneca was finally agreed in August 2021. One with Sanofi was signed in September, with Johnson and Johnson in October, with Pfizer–BioNTech, Curevac, and Moderna in November. One of the goals of the Commission was to secure doses at the best price possible. It was successful in doing so: for a population of 448 million, the EU spent well under 3 billion Euros on vaccines. For a population of only just over 66 million, the UK spend well over 4 billion Euros. The result, however, was a slower delivery of vaccines than those countries that had spent a premium on doses and had provided pharmaceutical companies with more assurances and more investment up front. One of the reasons the EU was so affected by the supply difficulties faced by Astra Zeneca was that its negotiators had refused a larger order from Pfizer–BioNTech, making them dependent on a small number of vaccine producers. Moreover, one of the EU's earliest contracts was with the Sanofi–GSK vaccine, which was at a relatively early stage of development. This product, not yet available, has been beset by a number of problems at the trial stage (Barnéoud 2021).

The EU's Actions during the Pandemic—a Summary and Assessment

Looking back at the narrative concerning member states and EU-level responses to COVID-19 across the first and subsequent waves, we can see that the EU's involvement spanned both public health and economic measures. Given the varying levels of integration across these areas, the economic (monetary and fiscal) measures were significantly greater in scale compared with the public health measures. Writing about the EU's role in public health, Deruelle (2020) describes this asymmetry between economic and health policies. Regarding the latter, he distinguishes between risk assessment and risk management (2020: 4). At the beginning of the pandemic, the EU had some role in the former but very little in the latter. This has evolved to an extent, but the imbalance remains.

Risk assessment refers to 'the identification of risks through the evaluation of the magnitude, mechanisms and gravity of threats to public health' (Deruelle 2020: 4). This involves work by scientists in terms of analysis and forecasting. The relevant bodies at the EU level are the DG Santé within the Commission and the European Centre for Disease Prevention and Control (ECDC).[11] The ECDC collects data from national health authorities and facilitates the exchange of information between member states. National health authorities also meet in the Health Security Committee (HSC). Originally an informal body, it was given a more formal status as a committee in a joint decision of the European Parliament and the European Council in 2013. In contrast, risk management refers to the multiple actions taken by governments in dealing with a health emergency such as COVID-19—from treatment responses such as vaccines to measures relating to mobility (i.e. the lockdown decisions and all restrictions falling short of a full lockdown, such as the introduction of a tiered system). As Deruelle (2020) notes, within member states there is no real separation between risk assessment and risk management. The executive fuses the two together, as evidenced by the role scientific advisors have played in national politics. Up-to-date epidemiological information is fed into decision-making at the very top of the state. The only instance of such fusion at the EU level is in joint procurement. The legal basis for Joint Procurement Agreements (JCAs) goes back to 2013. These are voluntary procurement initiatives that aim to boost the purchasing power of governments in the field of medical equipment and supplies, as well to achieve a better allocation of such supplies across

[11] The ECDC was established in 2005, after the 2003 SARS outbreak. It is based in Solna, Sweden, a suburb north of Stockholm. It hosts the EU's early warning and response system. It has a staff of fewer than 300 and an annual budget of 60 million Euros.

member states, based on need. The most dramatic use of this initiative—with mixed results—was the joint purchase of coronavirus vaccines.

Tables 5.1 and 5.2 provide a more schematic account of the policy domains in which the EU has intervened during the pandemic and the various instruments deployed. Table 5.1 refers to health-related policy interventions. Table 5.2 focuses on the macro-economic policy measures.

It is too early to judge with any certainty what effect the pandemic will have on health policy at the EU level. In some ways, the pandemic may even have reinforced the gap between the transnational dimensions of a virus of this kind and the resolutely national capacities of member states to tackle it. It has certainly been common to observe that over the course of the pandemic, we have seen a 'return of the state' across Europe—in the form of intrusive national regulation of individual behaviour as well as the imposition of restrictions on travel. In those countries that were hardest hit at the beginning of the pandemic, such as Italy, the sentiment of having been abandoned by other member states will take time to dissipate. The NextGenerationEU Fund comes with a particular infrastructure that will require member states to succumb to extensive EU-level oversight. As during the Eurocrisis, this may lead to new conflicts between member states and the Commission.

On the fiscal side, we should not underestimate the significance of the Recovery Fund, both practically and symbolically. Eurozone macroeconomic policy has

Table 5.1 Health measures

Action	Relevant body	Example
Joint procurement of medical equipment and supplies	RescEU stockpiling initiative; EU vaccines strategy	Joint Procurement Agreement (JPA) for PPE signed on 28 February; JPA for ventilators (17 March); EU vaccines strategy launched on 17 June, including pooled effort at securing vaccines (via Advanced Purchase Agreements with pharmaceutical companies and via changes to EU regulatory environment)
Monitoring role	ECDC, DG Santé (Health and Food Safety)	Active since early January reporting on the spread of the virus
Member state coordination	European Council, European Commission, Health Security Committee	European Council meeting on 10 March devoted to the COVID-19 emergency; the Commission issues a communication on how to coordinate restrictions on non-essential travel (16 April)

Sources: Deruelle 2020; Boffey et al. 2020

Table 5.2 Economic measures

Action	Relevant body	Example
Interventionist monetary policy	European Central Bank	Pandemic Emergency Purchase Programme (18 March): 750 billion Euros (increased to 1.3 trillion Euros on 4 June)
Fiscal stimulus	European Commission	Recovery Plan for Europe (launched 27 May; agreed by EU leaders 21 July; completing national ratifications)
State aid rules	European Commission	Adoption of temporary framework (19 March) on state aid to maximize room for manoeuvre for member states introducing national measures to assist companies/sectors
Sector-specific assistance via regulatory changes	European Commission	Actions to assist agri-food sector and to assist banking sector by adopting new or changed regulations (e.g. to ensure continued lending in banking sector); Capital Markets Recovery Package (24 July)
Investment in vaccine research by pharmaceutical industry	European Investment Bank	100 million Euros financing for BioNTech vaccine research

Sources: Deruelle 2020; Tooze 2020

long been characterized by the asymmetry between supranationalized monetary policy and nationalized fiscal policy. This fund is a step towards greater symmetry. Moreover, as noted above, it empowers the Commission in a variety of ways. It remains to be seen whether or not the fund will lead to some levelling out across member states. The size of the transfers are fairly limited, especially for the larger member states such as Italy and Spain. It is unlikely that the Recovery Fund will be able to eliminate those structural divergences which have become a feature of life within the Eurozone.

Conclusion

In seeking to generalize about government responses to the pandemic, observers have stressed the difference between successful containment in much of Asia and Australasia and the failures in both Europe and the United States, along with a number of countries in South America. What seems to have been decisive is the behaviour and habits of citizens. In those countries most exposed to prior pandemics, such as severe acute respiratory syndrome (SARS), compliance with pandemic-related measures was swift and uncontested. In countries that had been close to these earlier outbreaks, such as New Zealand, governments were more accustomed to taking costly decisions up front in order to minimize the spread of the virus.

In this assessment of the EU's role in the pandemic, we find that the greatest changes so far have been in fiscal policy rather than in health policy. This is not just a reflection of a pre-existing and treaty-determined delineation of competences, as these sorts of constraints have not stopped policymakers from creating new fiscal powers for the EU. It suggests a deeper tension between European integration and the integration of national health policies. As noted above, national welfare states stand out as exceptions to the logic of European economic integration. This is because they institutionalize a set of limits to the logic of market exchange and market competition. The pandemic in Europe has wrought many changes at the individual and collective level, but the 'outsiderness' of national welfare states to the process of European integration is—thus far—not one of them.

References

Atlantic Council. 2020. 'Is China Winning the Coronavirus Response Narrative in the EU?'. *Atlantic Council*, 25 March. https://www.atlanticcouncil.org/blogs/new-atlanticist/is-china-winning-the-coronavirus-response-narrative-in-the-eu/.

Barnéoud, Lise. 2021. 'Vaccins contre la COVID-19: Dans les coulisses des contrats entre l'UE et les groupes pharmaceutiques'. *Le Monde*, 3 février. https://www.lemonde.fr/planete/article/2021/02/03/vaccins-contre-le-covid-19-dans-les-coulisses-des-contrats-europeens_6068574_3244.html.

Bickerton, Christopher. 2021. 'Europe Failed with Vaccines. Of Course It Did'. *New York Times*, Guest Essay, 19 May 2021.

Boffey, Daniel, Celine Schoen, Ben Stockton, and Laura Margottini. 2020. 'Italy's Call for Urgent Help Was Ignored as Coronavirus Swept through Italy'. *The Guardian*, 15 July. https://www.theguardian.com/world/2020/jul/15/revealed-the-inside-story-of-europes-divided-coronavirus-response.

Cameron, Rob. 2020. 'A Sense of Optimism'. *BBC News*, 1 July 2020. https://www.bbc.co.uk/news/world-europe-53244688.

Chazan, Guy. 2020. 'How Germany Got Coronavirus Right'. *Financial Times Magazine*, 4 June. https://www.ft.com/content/cc1f650a-91c0-4e1f-b990-ee8ceb5339ea.

Chazan, Guy and Sam Jones. 2020. 'Merkel Calls for Ski Resorts across EU to Close'. *Financial Times*, 27 November. https://www.ft.com/content/7b734ba3-8248-4cfd-9bdd-2752f02bc130.

De Ruijter, Anniek, Roed Beetsma, Brian Burgoon, Francesco Niccoli, and Frank Vendenbroucke. 2020. 'EU Solidarity and Policy in Fighting Infectious Diseases: State of Play, Obstacles, Citizen Preferences and Ways Forward'. Amsterdam Centre for European Studies Research Paper No. 2020/6.

Deruelle, Thibaud. 2020. 'Beyond Health: Looking for Europe's Strategy vis-à-vis the COVID-19 Crisis'. *Aljazeera Centre for Studies*, 28 May. https://studies.aljazeera.net/en/reports/beyond-health-looking-europe's-strategy-vis-à-vis-covid-19-crisis.

Genschel, Philippe and Anton Hemerijck. 2018. 'Solidarity in Europe'. School of Transnational Governance EUI, Policy Brief 2018/1.

Greer, Scott and Anniek de Ruijter. 2020. 'EU Health Law and Policy In and After the COVID-19 Crisis'. *European Journal of Public Health 30* (4): pp. 623–4.

Jones, David S. 2020. 'History In a Crisis—Lessons for COVID-19'. *New England Journal of Medicine 381*: pp. 1681–3.

Lazar, Marc. 2020. 'Leaders Revealed by Covid-19: The Curious Case of Giuseppe Conte', Institut Montaigne, 1 September. https://www.institutmontaigne.org/en/blog/leaders-revealed-covid-19-curious-giuseppe-conte.

Looi, Mun-Keat. 2020. 'Covid-19: Is a Second Wave Hitting Europe?' *British Medical Journal 371*: m4113, 28 October. https://www.bmj.com/content/371/bmj.m4113.

Majoli, Alex. 2020. 'The Eye of the Storm'. *Vanity Fair*, 26 March. https://www.vanityfair.com/news/2020/03/coronavirus-in-italy-scenes-from-the-eye-of-the-storm.

Majone, Giandomenico. 2015. 'The Deeper Euro-Crisis: or the Collapse of the EU Political Culture of Total Optimism'. European University Institute Working Paper, EUI LAW 2015/10.

Möckli, Daniel. 2008. *European Foreign Policy during the Cold War: Heath, Brandt, Pomidou and the Dream of Political Unity*. London: Bloomsbury.

Robinet-Borgomano, Alexandre. 2020. 'Coronavirus 2.0: How Germany Could Lose Control', Institut Montaigne, 27 October. https://www.institutmontaigne.org/en/blog/coronavirus-20-how-germany-could-lose-control.

Sangiovanni, Andrea. 2013. 'Solidarity in the European Union', *Oxford Journal of Legal Studies 33* (2): pp. 213–241.

Tooze, Adam. 2020. 'Shockwave'. *London Review of Books 42* (8): 16 April.

White, Jonathan. 2020. *Politics of Last Resort: Governing by Emergency in the European Union*. Oxford: Oxford University Press.

6

Pandemics and Environmental Crises

Similar Problems; Different Governance Systems

Jean-Frédéric Morin, Sikina Jinnah, and Amandine Orsini

Pandemics and environmental degradation are both deadly global crises, which often disproportionately impact the world's most vulnerable populations (see the Introduction to this volume by Ackerly et al.). The 2014 Ebola outbreak, for example, killed more than 11,000 people across several of the world's poorest countries in Africa. Many environmental crises, such as climate change-related weather events, have similar distributional impacts. The 2003 heat wave in Europe, for example, affected at least 16 countries and caused more than 70,000 excess deaths, disproportionately impacting the elderly. Hurricane Mitch, the second deadliest hurricane on record, killed 10,000 people in Honduras and Nicaragua in 1998.

The scale of devastation for both pandemics and environmental problems can be immense. At its peak in the mid-2000s, for example, the HIV/AIDS pandemic was responsible for the death of almost 2 million people per year. Similarly, according to the World Health Organization (WHO), known avoidable environmental risks, such as air pollution, cause 13 million deaths each year (WHO 2019a: 2).

This chapter compares pandemics and environmental crises on two dimensions: their underlying problem structures and governance systems. Several political scientists assume that policymakers design governance systems to fit with the characteristics of the specific problems they try to address (Koremenos et al. 2001, Koremenos 2016). For example, studies have found that states favoured the WHO's high-level design because it simultaneously protected global health and did not interfere too deeply in states' sovereign control of health policy and decision-making (Ip 2020; Benvenisti 2020). Other studies have shown that the nature of the problems raised by environmental degradation influences the design of international environmental agreements (Mitchell 2006; Mitchell and Keibach 2001). One conjecture resulting from this line of thinking is that states will prefer similar governance systems for different issue areas if they have similar problem structures, and different governance systems for problems with different problem stuctures (Mitchell 2006).

Jean-Frédéric Morin, Sikina Jinnah, and Amandine Orsini, *Pandemics and Environmental Crises.* In: *A Multidisciplinary Approach to Pandemics.* Edited by Philippe Bourbeau, Jean-Michel Marcoux, and Brooke A. Ackerly, Oxford University Press. © Oxford University Press (2022). DOI: 10.1093/oso/9780192897855.003.0007

This chapter highlights how pandemics and environmental degradation present similar problem structures. Yet they have triggered very different policy responses, and their governance systems are also different. Moreover, even if pandemics and environmental degradation are similar types of problems, there is little attempt to coordinate policies that tackle the interrelated aspects of these issues. We explain these incongruities by power differentials and perception biases that lead to an underinvestment in environmental degradation compared to pandemics.

The chapter is divided into two parts. The first part illuminates the problem structures of pandemics and environmental degradation, including their similarities and interactions. The second part compares the existing approaches governing each of these issues and explains this variation. We conclude by discussing policy solutions to create positive synergies between the two issue areas.

Pandemics and Environmental Crises

Similar Problem Structures

Pandemics and environmental degradation have similar problem structures, which might suggest similarities in governance responses. This section focuses on five key similarities: global interdependence, exponential dynamics, disproportionate impacts, scientific uncertainty, and their relationship to economic liberalization. These characteristics are not exclusive to pandemics and environmental crises; the problem structures of several other global issues share one or two of these features, but few share all five.

First, both problems are characterized by a high degree of global interdependence. The health of a population and the quality of its environment are both dependent on the health and environmental conditions of other populations. This is because governments cannot stop viruses and pollution from crossing borders. In this context of interdependence, government actions to protect a population in one country may benefit other countries. Conversely, a government's failure to address health or environmental problems may be detrimental to other countries. Implementing health and environmental measures can be expensive, which means that governments may be tempted to 'free ride', letting other states foot the bill. Governments rarely have to pay for the consequences that their policies have on foreign countries. The full costs of an infectious disease outbreak or deforestation of the Amazon, for example, are not borne by the responsible parties. Rather, these costs are distributed globally through, for example, loss of human and non-human life. Individualistic state behaviour can exacerbate these impacts and occurs particularly when there is a shortage of scarce resources—for example, when a government restricts exports of valuable pharmaceutical products during a pandemic to safeguard its own stock or when a state siphons excess water from a transboundary river for its own use. This type of behaviour may serve individual states in the short term, but it leads to suboptimal outcomes at the global level: it results in unfair and inefficient resource distribution (Morin et al. 2020).[1]

A second key feature of pandemics and environmental degradation is their exponential dynamics. They are both non-linear problems, which amplify at an increasing rate over time. For example, if each infected person transmits a virus to two individuals every day, the infected population goes from 1 to 81 individuals in just 5 days and then jumps to 19,683 individuals five days later. Similarly, the biosphere is characterized by various feedback loops that accelerate the speed of climate change. For example, if the temperature were to rise sufficiently to melt the permafrost, this would release huge quantities of methane, a powerful greenhouse gas, into the atmosphere, and it would amplify climate change significantly. As a result, epidemiologists and earth scientists alike are trying to identify the thresholds beyond which a crisis spirals out of control. For a pandemic, this tipping point is based on the capacity of the health-care infrastructure to treat infected patients. For climate change, it is estimated that an increase of 2 degrees Celsius would create large-scale environmental discontinuities (Intergovernmental Panel on Climate Change (IPCC) 2018). Therefore, the governance challenge for both issues is to implement measures to flatten the exponential curve (of infected people or carbon dioxide in the atmosphere). The idea of an exponential curve putting human populations at risk has been well understood since Thomas Malthus's work in the eighteenth century. However, studies have found that the human mind has difficulty grasping its explosive nature. Exponential dynamics are consistently underestimated as a result (Wagenaar and Sagaria 1975; Kunreuther and Slovic 2020).

Another common feature of pandemics and environmental problems is that historically marginalized populations are disproportionally impacted (Venkatapuram 2011; Anand 2017; Mascarenhas 2020). When a crisis occurs, the most vulnerable groups often include lower socio-economic classes, ethnic minorities, and women. This occurs both within and between countries. Within countries, for example, Indigenous groups and black communities in the United States have borne disproportionate impacts of ill health, pandemics, climate change, oil exploration, and toxic exposure (Bullard 2020; Clark et al. 2020; Pellow 2018; Quinn et al. 2011; Watt-Cloutier 2018; Whyte 2020; Yancy 2020). At the international level, least-developed countries and developing countries often lack the necessary resources to protect their populations or adapt to changing circumstances. The poorest people in the poorest countries in the world, for example, are expected to bear the brunt of climate impacts, such as fisheries depletion

[1] Like that of the environment, the preservation of public health is a public good. Chapter 14 in this volume by Herrmann and Isabelle also discusses how, even at the micro level, individuals may opt for suboptimal behaviours for a societal point of view in the context of a pandemic if they adopt them based only on calculations involving their private benefit.

(Blasiak et al. 2017; Byers et al. 2018), and developing countries who are least responsible for global emissions are the most vulnerable to climate impacts (Althor et al. 2016). Similarly, global health research is increasingly illuminating the social determinants of (ill) health, such as lower socio-economic status and the impacts of pandemics (Donkin et al. 2018; Singu et al. 2020).[2] Redistributive measures, in addition to mitigation and adaptation policies, are required to tackle the regressive effects of health and environmental crises. Yet redistributive measures are often politically contested, both domestically and internationally.

The problem structure of pandemics and environmental degradation is also characterized by a degree of scientific uncertainty. When a new crisis arises, scientists are often unsure about the causes, the consequences, and the most effective responses; we saw such a dynamic with the initial HIV/AIDS outbreak and the discovery of the ozone hole in the 1980s. Scientists work with incomplete information, contested assumptions, and unstable models during the initial stages of a crisis. They make progress incrementally. In this context, some groups advocate action to protect human health and the environment, as the precautionary principle suggests (Vogel 2012), despite limited scientific evidence. Political opponents of the precautionary principle typically start by denying that the problem exists and then minimize its importance. As scientific knowledge advances and the magnitude of the crisis can no longer be credibly denied, opposition groups typically argue that there is no effective solution or seek to place blame on others to avoid responsibility for (in)action. As diverse political actors make scientific claims, the boundary between science and politics becomes increasingly unstable and blurred. Ultimately, difficult policy decisions, such as imposing a three-month shelter-in-place order to avoid disease transmission, or cutting CO_2 emissions by 20% by 2020 (a European Union target), are not simply based on science, they are also deeply political. They involve various ethical considerations that science alone cannot arbitrate (see the Introduction to this volume by Ackerly et al.).

One last similarity that health and environmental problems have is their tense and ambiguous relationship with economic liberalization. Globalization has created conditions that facilitate the diffusion of pandemics and accentuate environmental degradation. For this reason, several health and environmental groups are calling for policies, such as local supply chains, that run against the principles of economic liberalism. In contrast, certain industrial groups claim that health and environmental regulations are unnecessary and expensive job-killing measures (Tienhaara 2014). At the international level, some of the most controversial trade disputes concern health or environmental measures. The disputes are arbitrated by the World Trade Organization (WTO) and include issues such

[2] See Chapter 14 in this volume by Herrmann and Isabelle for a discussion on the distribution of the health and economic impacts of the COVID-19 pandemic across groups with different pre-existing vulnerabilities.

as asbestos, genetically modified organisms, beef hormones, and fisheries (such as the tuna/dolphin and shrimp/turtle controversies). Interestingly, several health and environmental measures are covered under WTO law by the same exception, which refers to measures that are 'necessary to protect human, animal or plant life or health' (GATT Article XX para. b). At the same time, globalization supports scientific innovation, essential for tackling both environmental and health crises. It also helps to reduce the cost of key technologies, such as pharmaceutical products or solar panels (Lafond et al. 2018).

Given the five key similarities in their problem structure, one might expect that similar global governance systems would govern pandemics and environmental degradation (Onzivu 2016; Koremenos et al. 2001). However, as the next section discusses, pandemics and environmental degradation also interact, which further suggests that a shared governance response might be appropriate (Thomas 2001).

The Health Consequences of Environmental Degradation

Although health and environmental crises are often treated as separate problems, they are intricately linked in multiple and complex ways. Environmental health is the field of study that analyses the health-related impacts of environmental problems (Negri 2019). It shows that environmental degradation increases the risks and consequences of disease, including pandemics.

In particular, biodiversity loss increases the likelihood of zoonotic diseases—diseases caused by pathogens that 'jump' from wildlife to humans. An estimated 75% of new human pathogens originate from non-human animals (Jones et al. 2008; UNEP and International Livestock Research Institute 2020). Examples of zoonotic diseases include HIV/AIDS, SARS, Ebola, and COVID-19. They are increasingly frequent, which is largely because of the destruction of natural habitats (through urbanization or deforestation), which brings wildlife and humans into closer contact. Wildlife trade also contributes to the greater interaction between wildlife and humans (UNEP 2020b).

Climate change can exacerbate the development of vector-borne infectious diseases. With rising temperatures or higher rainfall, certain vector-borne diseases may spread to higher altitudes and different latitudes (IPCC 2018: 9). This can prolong transmission seasons in some endemic regions. Malaria, Zika virus, Lyme disease, and dengue fever are all zoonotic diseases that are on the rise in several areas. Climate hazards and reduced agricultural production because of climate change can also force people to live in crowded, unsanitary conditions or to migrate, thus increasing the risks of contagion. Extreme weather events, such as flooding, heat waves, and tornadoes, put exceptional pressure on hospitals and emergency services, limiting their capacity to respond to a pandemic (Phillips et al. 2020).

Air pollution is another risk multiplier. The WHO estimates that air pollution causes around 7 million preventable deaths per year (WHO 2019a). The emission of ground-level ozone, dioxins, mercury, benzene, particulate matter, and other pollutants can exacerbate respiratory diseases. During the SARS and COVID-19 outbreaks, for example, air pollution was linked to the higher rates of mortality among infected people (Cui et al. 2003; Fattorini and Regoli 2020). Although pollution may be temporarily reduced during a pandemic, a lifetime of breathing polluted air, both indoors and outdoors, can make people more susceptible to respiratory infections.

The lack of sufficient safe water can also exacerbate health risks during infectious disease outbreaks. Frequent handwashing, which requires a continuous supply of clean water, is one of the most important public health indications to limit contagion. Yet, according to the WHO, 'more than half the world's population is still exposed to unsafely managed water, inadequate sanitation and poor hygiene' (WHO 2019a: 2). Pollution of water sources and destruction of natural habitats around river basins are partly responsible for these poor sanitary conditions. The WHO estimates that 'more than 800,000 preventable deaths each year' result from the lack of sufficient safe water (WHO 2019a: 2). This figure may increase significantly in the event of a pandemic in populations where people do not have access to clean water to wash their hands and where sanitary facilities are shared by a large number of people.

Polluted cities with few green spaces and little access to nature can worsen mental health problems when new pandemics occur. New health risks generate uncertainty, social isolation, and financial losses, which are stressors that can contribute to distress and mental illness. During the spring of 2020, a higher proportion of the population suffered from anxiety and depressive disorders compared to the previous year (Centers for Disease Control and Prevention (CDC) 2020). In short, environmental degradation can create and exacerbate health hazards, which get worse during times of pandemics.

The Environmental Impacts of Pandemics

Pandemics also have adverse consequences on the environment. In the early stages, their environmental impact might appear to be positive; for example, the economic slowdown they induce might reduce air and water pollution. In the first months of 2020, daily CO_2 emissions dropped significantly compared to the previous year. In some countries, emissions decreased by more than 25% (Le Quéré et al. 2020). Newspapers reported that blue skies were visible once more in cities usually smothered by heavy smog, and wildlife was increasingly visible in areas suddenly devoid of economic activities (Rutz et al. 2020). Yet, as with other types of economic downturn, pandemics are followed by economic recovery and increased pollution levels (Kuzemko et al. 2020). Temporary reductions in pollution, even when they are significant, as in the case of the COVID-19 pandemic, are too short-lived to have a meaningful long-term environmental impact (Forster et al. 2020). The planet needs more than a few months to get its breath back.

Pandemics can exacerbate environmental degradation in many different ways. One of their immediate environmental consequences is linked to greater waste production, including medical products and protective equipment (masks, gloves, gowns, etc.). The United Nations Conference on Trade and Development estimates that global sales of disposable masks alone jumped from $800 million in 2019 to $166 billion in 2020 (UN 2020). A pandemic also leads to a resurgence of disposable, single-use plastic products to reduce contagion, including bags, cups, and plates. Some waste is burned in the open, releasing toxins into the environment, and some ends up in the sea. Greater quantities of active pharmaceutical ingredients may be released into the environment via saturated sewage systems, further polluting ecosystems. This pollution reveals and exacerbates a host of environmental justice-related impacts associated with, for example, adequate protection for workers who manage such waste.

Pandemics can also have adverse effects on biodiversity. During the COVID-19 pandemic, several developing countries saw a major reduction in safari tourism and ecotourism, depriving parks and reserves of an important source of income for anti-poaching surveillance (UNEP 2020a). At the same time, the economic recession induced by COVID-19 may increase the incentives to hunt wild animals, thereby paradoxically also increasing exposure risk to zoonotic diseases. In some communities, hunting can provide necessary food or a source of income. Likewise, when tourism no longer provides income for local communities, farmers may be tempted to kill wild animals to protect their crops and livestock (Buckley 2020; Lindsey et al. 2020). Governments may see the overexploitation of natural resources, including forests and fish stocks, as a short-term solution to the major economic downturn created by a pandemic.

More broadly, a pandemic and the associated economic downturn can create political conditions that are favourable to more lax environmental regulations. Public opinion tends to be less enthusiastic about environmental measures in times of economic recession (Ratter et al. 2012). Short-term economic sacrifices for long-term environmental gains are difficult to accept when the economy is hit by a pandemic. As unemployment soars, more people are likely to perceive environmental regulations as an extravagant inhibitor of economic growth (Kenny 2018). During the Great Recession of 2007–2009, surveys reported a decline in the level of concern for climate change (Kenny 2019; Brulle et al. 2012; Kahn and Kotchen 2011; Scruggs and Benegal 2012; Shum 2012). There is not a strong correlation between the magnitude of the economic downturn and the disinterest in environmental protection (Bakaki and Bernauer 2018; Andreas et al. 2017; Skovgaard 2014). However, recessions create favourable conditions so that political leaders opposed to environmental measures can make their voices heard and gain influence (Mildenberger and Leiserowitz 2017). As such, during the first months of the COVID-19 pandemic, several governments suspended the enforcement of their pollution regulations, relaxed environmental impact assessments for infrastructure projects, and postponed their investment in renewable energy. The need to create jobs fast, combined with a greater concentration of executive power (often a feature of public health emergencies) paves the way for those who profit from environmental degradation (Russel and Benson 2014).

In short, environmental crises and pandemics interact in ways that make both problems worse. Importantly, historically marginalized populations are disproportionately impacted by these crises because of a lack of capacity and resources to protect their communities (see the Introduction to this volume by Ackerly et al.). As much as pandemics and environmental crises exacerbate one another, social inequalities become further entrenched and more difficult to correct. That said, since health and environmental systems are closely interrelated, there is an opportunity for governments to design policy measures that have positive effects on both. For example, reducing air pollution, designing transportation systems that encourage active transport, providing access to family planning services, and encouraging people to eat less red meat can improve health and have a positive environmental impact (IPCC 2014; Quam et al. 2017; Schucht et al. 2015). Yet, as the next section discusses, few governments are striving to achieve these co-benefits.

Health and Environmental Governance

Contrasting Reactions to Health and Environmental Crises

Despite similar problem structures, the global governance systems for health and environmental issues are remarkably different. They both have strengths, weaknesses, room for improvement, and more alignment to maximize synergies (see Chapter 12 in this volume by Davies for the challenge of global health governance). Of the two, the global health governance system appears better equipped to face global crises.

Very few governance initiatives have succeeded in solving global environmental problems. In most cases, actions are geared to limiting the pace of degradation, instead of stopping it or restoring the environment. Overall, public policies related to climate change and biodiversity loss are inadequate to tackle these crises of such immense magnitude. In contrast, some health responses to viral epidemics have been effective. While deaths are not always avoided, efficient treatments and preventative measures have been developed. Notably, smallpox was eradicated in 1980, and polio has almost been eradicated worldwide. These are two of the most remarkable achievements of global health governance.

A key asset of the global health governance system in addressing global crises is its higher degree of centralization, relative to the global environmental governance system (Fazal 2020). Centralization is a key asset when it comes to dealing with global crises. Health governance coalesces around the WHO, in Geneva, whereas environmental governance is notoriously fragmented into myriad institutions around the world (Biermann et al. 2009). The United Nations Environment Programme (UNEP) in Nairobi does not enjoy the same degree of political clout and autonomy as the WHO, as evidenced most basically by its designation as a 'programme', not an organization within the UN system. It also faces intense competition from several other intergovernmental organizations and programmes under the UN umbrella. While fragmentation and competition can make a governance system more innovative and adaptive in the long run, centralization and autonomy can facilitate effective decision-making in times of crisis (Biermann and Kim 2020).

Related to the issue of centralization, the most active global health organizations have more resources than their environmental counterparts. For example, the WHO's annual budget is around US$2.5 billion per year (WHO 2019c). In contrast, the UNEP has an annual budget of less than one-fifth of that amount (UNEP 2018). This disparity is also manifest in the resources available to key foundations and non-governmental organizations (NGOs) in both fields. The Bill & Melinda Gates Foundation, a leading actor in global health, spends around US$5 billion every year (Gates Foundation 2020). In contrast, Greenpeace International, a major environmental NGO, has a budget of less than one-twentieth of that amount (Greenpeace 2019).

The COVID-19 pandemic revealed that public health policies can be implemented promptly, even when they are expensive. Governments around the world (with some notable exceptions) implemented emergency measures to protect public health. This disrupted economic activities and limited individual freedom. No government has ever implemented such drastic measures to reduce greenhouse gas emissions or curb environmental pollution. Yet environmental crises will ultimately be responsible for far more deaths than COVID-19 (WHO 2019a: 2).

Political systems across the globe were much more responsive to COVID-19 than they ever have been for an environmental crisis. Journalists reported daily statistics for COVID-19 infections and victims, while the death toll associated with environmental degradation rarely hits the headlines. Some government leaders, who previously questioned the validity of climate science to avoid action or claimed that economic development should come before environmental protection, gave press conferences during COVID-19 announcing major restrictions on economic activities in the name of health imperatives. Even government leaders who initially underestimated the gravity of the pandemic gradually became more supportive of basic public health measures. Several political leaders wanting to be seen as public health champions used the opportunity to boost their popular support. In some countries, opposing health measures became politically toxic. Even industries severely hit by COVID-19, such as airline companies, did not organize opposition to public health measures, unlike the oil and gas industries, which have opposed measures to tackle climate change for decades. COVID-19 demonstrated that governments can act decisively, with little political opposition and strong public support, when confronted with a major crisis. We saw similar trends with the 2003 outbreak of SARS and the 2014 outbreak of Ebola. Yet these same governments have failed to act decisively on the same scale for climate change, biodiversity loss, or ocean pollution.

Clearly, global health responses have not always been as reactive as they were during the COVID-19 crisis. HIV/AIDS responses were initially slow (Sell and Prakash 2004), and Ebola has long remained a neglected disease (Nunes 2016). Further, as the COVID-19 case demonstrates, when some states fail to act, the crisis can be prolonged unnecessarily. The governance of pandemics also suffers, like global environmental governance does, from an imbalance between prevention and treatment (Dauvergne 2005). Governments tend to favour short-term solutions to health and environmental crises, despite the fact that investment in prevention pays off in the long run. Nevertheless, the governance responses to health crises appear to be more decisive than the response to environmental crises.

Explaining Variations in Policy Responses

At least three factors can explain this discrepancy in policy responses to environmental and health crises: income distribution and political influence, perceived urgency, and the presence of identifiable victims.

The first relates to income distribution and the political influence of the people impacted. Pandemics and environmental degradation disproportionally affect the most vulnerable populations. However, pandemics such as COVID-19 and HIV/AIDS are more directly life-threatening to rich and powerful individuals than are climate change or biodiversity loss. In the first few months of 2020, the COVID-19 pandemic was particularly prevalent in high-income countries, at least according to official records. The contagion was acute in highly connected global cities, such as New York and London, which are home to many of the transnational elite. Even government leaders and royalty were diagnosed with COVID-19 during the spring of 2020, including the British prime minister and the Prince of Wales. In contrast, rich and powerful individuals may have the impression that environmental degradation does not directly threaten their lives. When leaders (mis)perceive a crisis as a problem that affects foreign countries, they are unlikely to implement expensive preventative measures. In several high-income countries, the response of policymakers to climate change is biased by a spatial overoptimism (Gifford et al. 2009). This type of optimism bias only lasted a few weeks during the COVID-19 pandemic, when it was limited to Asia in January 2020. However, climate change is still perceived as a problem that affects geographically or socio-economically distant populations.

Another key factor is the degree of perceived urgency related to a public policy problem. Environmental degradation is often (mis)perceived as a crisis to come that will affect future generations, not an immediate crisis. The sudden SARS and COVID-19 crises called for immediate short-term reactions. For COVID-19, in February and March of 2020 several political leaders actually announced that public health measures would probably only last for a few weeks. In contrast, climate action advocates have been calling for reduced greenhouse gas emissions for decades. Moreover, the effects of climate change will slowly unfold over decades, even after drastic cuts in greenhouse gas emissions. This reduces the perceived urgency to act. It allows for psychological adjustments to a new normal and suggests that we might have time to find solutions before it is too late. The climate crisis requires immediate and drastic action if we are to avoid catastrophic scenarios, but it is rarely perceived as an urgent crisis. Mark Carney, the head of the Bank of England, describes this short-term bias as the 'tragedy of the horizon' (BBC 2019).

Finally, a crucial variable that explains differences in policy response is the presence of identifiable victims. In a pandemic, viral infections can be connected to specific contagious contacts. Many people diagnosed with COVID-19 know when, where, and by whom they were infected. There are 'identifiable victims' in the sense that their disease can be causally linked to the pandemic. On the contrary, it is not possible to identify the victims that will fall prey to a specific source of greenhouse gas emissions. Viral infections have direct and traceable effects, whereas the consequences of greenhouse gas emissions are diffuse. It is not even possible to assert with certainty that a specific weather event was caused by a high level of greenhouse gases in the atmosphere. Climate change has probabilistic effects and only causes so-called 'statistical victims'. The WHO estimates that climate change will cause 250,000 additional deaths per year on average between 2030 and 2050 (WHO 2018). However, none of these victims will have 'climate change' listed as the cause of death on their death certificate. The diffuse effect of climate change reduces the collective motivation to take decisive action (Marx et al. 2007). On the contrary, the direct consequences of a pandemic like COVID-19 trigger an immediate response.

Strengthening the Health–Environment Linkage

Several international institutions have already linked human health and environmental protection. The vast majority of global environmental governance is fundamentally anthropocentric—that is, the primary motivations for protecting the environment are explicitly related to the well-being of humans, including human health. The 1992 Rio Declaration on Environment and Development, one of the pillars of global environmental governance, was revealing. Its first principle states that 'Human beings … are entitled to a *healthy* and productive life in harmony with nature' (UN 1992, emphasis added).

Human health has motivated the conclusion of several environmental agreements, including the following: the 1987 Montreal Protocol on the ozone layer, the 1992 Basel Convention on hazardous wastes, the 2004 Stockholm Convention on Persistent Organic Pollutants, and the 2013 Minamata Convention on Mercury. The Paris Agreement on climate change argues that greenhouse gas reductions are justified on human health grounds. It also includes a provision stipulating that when states act to address climate change, they should 'respect, promote and consider their respective obligations on the right to health' (UN 2015 preamble). Morin and Blouin (2019) have identified a total of 338 environmental treaties that refer explicitly to human health.

Intergovernmental organizations devoted to environmental protection and human health are already cooperating. As early as 2002, the WHO and UNEP launched the Health and Environment Linkages Initiative to support actions in developing countries to reduce environmental threats to health. Since 2000, the WHO has partnered with UNEP and the World Meteorological Organization to raise awareness about the health impacts of climate change. In 2010, the secretariat of the Convention on Biological Diversity reinforced its cooperation with the WHO in the framework of a joint work programme to produce and diffuse scientific knowledge on health and biodiversity. The WHO, the World Organization for Animal Health, and the UN Food and Agriculture Organization created an early warning system for animal diseases and zoonoses. These are just a few of the existing institutional linkages between intergovernmental organizations that create synergies between human health and environmental protection.

Some transnational civil society organizations are also actively promoting synergies between health and the environment, for example, the EcoHealth Alliance and the Healthy Environments for Children Alliance. Several of these groups meet annually at the Global Climate and Health Summits, which are organized in parallel to the Conference of the Parties to the UN Framework Convention on Climate Change. These groups combine public health and environmental concerns to form broad coalitions to coordinate convincing advocacy narratives for policy action (Mayer 2009).

Several international institutions and actors are promoting new paradigms to reinforce the synergies between health and environmental policies. In recent decades, the concepts of 'sustainable development' and 'green growth' have brought together broad coalitions that have developed global policy actions geared towards the joint objectives of economic development and environmental protection (Morin et al. 2020). After COVID-19, concepts that connect human health to environmental protection are likely to gain prominence in global debates. Possible candidates include 'one health' and 'planetary health'. These two concepts are already being promoted by organizations such as the Wildlife Conservation Society, the Rockefeller Foundation, and the International Development Research Centre. While the two concepts differ, they stress the interdependence between human health, the health of other animals, and healthy ecosystems. They also call for a holistic and interdisciplinary understanding of health.

Despite this, the governance of human health and environmental protection is not fully integrated and several potential synergies are not exploited. According to the WHO, in 2019 half of its member-states did not have a strategy to tackle the twin issues of public health and climate change, and several countries that did have a strategy failed to implement it (WHO 2019b). This suggests that environmental and health policymaking remains largely siloed.

The social and economic disruption caused by the COVID-19 pandemic provides an opportunity to engage in recovery plans that address environmental protection like never before. Public measures could have a multiplier effect on the economy, by providing jobs and income to economic victims of COVID-19, while at the same time accelerating the transition towards a greener economy. For example, public money could be invested in renewable energy infrastructure, public transportation systems, modernizing the electric grid, or renovating buildings for energy efficiency. These investments would create jobs and significantly reduce greenhouse gas emissions (Hepburn et al. 2020; IRENA 2020). In addition, public support to industries that were heavily impacted by COVID-19 could be conditional on new environmental requirements. The significant reduction in oil prices makes 2020 a good time to introduce carbon taxes and eliminate consumption subsidies for fossil fuels. Although COVID-19 has had tragic consequences, it has also pushed governments to design recovery plans, which open up new opportunities for environmental protection (Kuzemko et al. 2020; McNamara and Newman 2020; OECD 2020).

Nonetheless, governments around the world might be more inclined to focus their recovery plans solely on economic growth because of pressure to boost the economy. The 2008 economic crisis revealed that not all political leaders are interested in creating synergies between economic development and environmental transition. It also suggested that the window of opportunity for large-scale initiatives is short-lived. After the 2008 economic crisis, new equilibriums emerged, and political groups jointly opposed reforms (Geels 2013). Post-COVID-19 recovery plans might provide a rare opportunity to boost the environmental transition.

Conclusion

Despite similarities and interactions between health and environmental crises, very different policy responses have emerged to tackle them. Governments have adopted drastic policy changes and agreed to massive public investments to address pandemics such as COVID-19, while similar measures appear out of reach for environmental problems like climate change. Moreover, few synergies exist between policy responses to health and environmental issues.

The relative success of global health governance, as indicated by, for example, the swift government response to COVID-19 in many countries, offers lessons for global environmental governance. In particular, environmental governance could be more effective if it (1) framed environmental impacts more explicitly in human health and economic terms; (2) made victims more visible and proximate; and (3) communicated the short-term consequences for all, across geographies and classes. Some of this could be done via 'bandwagoning', or more generously put, by creating 'strategic linkages' between global environmental and health governance (Jinnah 2011). Rather than creating new institutions, strategic linkages capitalize on existing untapped capacities within international institutions to identify overlaps that can maximize synergistic cooperation and even open up new sources of funding by identifying previously opaque connections (Jinnah 2014).

The COVID-19 crisis has also drawn into sharp relief some of the shortcomings of global health governance. There is a need for greater international coordination on things like medical supply production and distribution, public messaging, and coordinated responses. Further, the COVID-19 crisis illuminated the social determinants of health, such as ethnicity, class, and gender, which have deep implications not only for health vulnerability, but also for environmental vulnerability. In order for countries to make equitable progress in either domain, redistributive support is imperative, and a failure to address these systemic problems head on will only further entrench and exacerbate existing inequalities.

Global challenges require systemic changes as related to both formal institutions and norms of what is right and what is possible. Strong government action is needed not only to respond to the crises as they emerge, but to prevent them from emerging in the first place. Investment in prevention, such as by ensuring health-care access for all and transitioning away from fossil fuels, is necessary to prepare not just for the next pandemic or environmental crisis, but also to create long-term, healthy living conditions for all. Prevention is a cheaper, safer, and more equitable option.

References

Althor, Glenn, James E. M. Watson, and Richard A. Fuller. 2016. 'Global Mismatch between Greenhouse Gas Emissions and the Burden of Climate Change'. *Scientific Reports* 6: 20281. https://doi.org/10.1038/srep20281.

Anand, Ruchi. 2017. *International Environmental Justice: A North–South Dimension*. Abingdon: Routledge.

Andreas, Jan-Justus, Charlotte Burns, and Julia Touza-Montero. 2017. 'Renewable Energy as a Luxury? A Qualitative Comparative Analysis of the Role of the Economy in the EU's Renewable Energy Transitions during the "Double Crisis"'. *Ecological Economics 142*: pp. 81–90.

Bakaki, Zorzeta, and Thomas Bernauer. 2018. 'Do Economic Conditions Affect Public Support for Environmental Policy?' *Journal of Cleaner Production 195*: pp. 66–78.

BBC. 2019. 'Bank of England Chief Mark Carney Issues Climate Change Warning'. 30 December. https://www.bbc.com/news/business-50868717.

Benvenisti, Eyal. 2020. 'The WHO—Destined to Fail? Political Cooperation and the COVID-19 Pandemic'. University of Cambridge Faculty of Law Research Paper No. 24, 30 June.

Biermann, Frank, and Rakhyun E. Kim, eds. 2020. *Architectures of Earth System Governance: Institutional Complexity and Structural Transformation*. Cambridge: Cambridge University Press.

Biermann, Frank, Philipp Pattberg, Harro Van Asselt, and Fariborz Zelli. 2009. 'The Fragmentation of Global Governance Architectures: A Framework for Analysis'. *Global Environmental Politics 9* (4): pp. 14–40.

Blasiak Robert, Jessica Spijkers, Kanae Tokunaga, Jeremy Pittman, Nobuyuki Yagi, and Henrik Österblom. 2017. 'Climate Change and Marine Fisheries: Least Developed Countries Top Global Index of Vulnerability'. *PLoS One 12* (6): e0179632. https://doi.org/10.1371/journal.pone.0179632.

Brulle, Robert J., Jason Carmichael, and J. Craig Jenkins. 2012. 'Shifting Public Opinion on Climate Change: An Empirical Assessment of Factors Influencing Concern over Climate Change in the U.S., 2002–2010'. *Climatic Change 114* (2): pp. 169–88.

Buckley, Ralf. 2020. 'Conservation Implications of COVID-19: Effects via Tourism and Extractive Industries'. *Biological Conservation 247*: 108640.

Bullard, Robert D. 2020. 'From Civil Rights to Black Lives Matter'. In *Lessons in Environmental Justice: From Civil Rights, to Black Lives Matter, to Idle No More*, edited by Michael Mascarenhas, pp. 2–18. Thousand Oaks, CA: Sage Press.

Byers, Edward, Matthew Gidden, David Leclère, et al. 2018. 'Global Exposure and Vulnerability to Multi-Sector Development and Climate Change Hotspots'. *Environmental Research Letters 13*: 055012. https://doi.org/10.1088/1748-9326/aabf45.

Centers for Disease Control and Prevention (CDC). 2020. 'Anxiety and Depression: Household Pulse Survey'. https://www.cdc.gov/nchs/covid19/pulse/mental-health.htm.

Clark Eva, Karla Fredricks, Laila Woc-Colburn, Maria Elena Bottazzi, and Jill Weatherhead. 2020. 'Disproportionate Impact of the COVID-19 Pandemic on Immigrant Communities in the United States'. *PLOS Neglected Tropical Diseases 14* (7): e0008484. https://doi.org/10.1371/journal.pntd.0008484.

Cui, Yan, Zuo-Feng Zhang, John Froines, et al. 2003. 'Air Pollution and Case Fatality of SARS in the People's Republic of China: An Ecologic Study'. *Environmental Health 2* (15).

Dauvergne, Peter. 2005. 'Cancer and Global Environmental Politics: Proposing a New Research Agenda'. *Global Environmental Politics 5* (3): pp. 6–13.

Donkin Aangela, Peter Goldblatt, Jessica Allen, Vivienne Nathanson, and Michael Marmot. 2018. 'Global Action on the Social Determinants of Health'. *BMJ Global Health 3*: e000603.

Fattorini, Daniele, and Francesco Regoli. 2020. 'Role of the Chronic Air Pollution Levels in the COVID-19 Outbreak Risk in Italy'. *Environmental Pollution 264*: 114732.

Fazal, Tanisha. 2020. 'Health Diplomacy in Pandemical Times'. *International Organization 74* (supp): pp. E79–E97.

Forster, Piers M., Harriet I. Forster, Mat J. Evans, et al. 2020. 'Current and Future Global Climate Impacts Resulting from COVID-19'. *Nature Climate Change 10*: pp. 913–19. https://doi.org/10.1038/s41558-020-0883-0.

Gates Foundation. 2020. 'Who We Are: Financials'. https://www.gatesfoundation.org/Who-We-Are/General-Information/Financials.

Geels, Frank W. 2013. 'The Impact of the Financial–Economic Crisis on Sustainability Transitions: Financial Investment, Governance and Public Discourse'. *Environmental Innovation and Societal Transitions 6*: pp. 67–95.

Gifford, Robert., Leila Scannell, Christine Kormos, et al. 2009. 'Temporal Pessimism and Spatial Optimism in Environmental Assessments: An 18-Nation Study'. *Journal of Environmental Psychology 29* (1): pp. 1–12.

Greenpeace. 2019. 'International Combined Financial Statement'. https://storage.googleapis.com/planet4-international-stateless/2020/06/a3d5435f-greenpeace-international-combined-financial-statement-2019.pdf.

Hepburn, Cameron, Brian O'Callaghan, Nicholas Stern, Joseph Stiglitz, and Dimitri Zenghelis. 2020. 'Will COVID-19 Fiscal Recovery Packages Accelerate or Retard Progress on Climate Change?' *Oxford Review of Economic Policy 36* (S1): pp. S359–S381.

Ip, Eric C. 2020. 'The Constitutional Economics of the World Health Organization'. *Health Economics, Policy and Law 16* (3): pp. 1–15.

Intergovernmental Panel on Climate Change (IPCC). 2014. 'Climate Change 2014: Synthesis Report. Contribution of Working Groups I, II and III to the Fifth Assessment Report of the Intergovernmental Panel on Climate Change'. Geneva: IPCC.

IPCC. 2018. 'Global Warming of 1.5°C'. https://www.ipcc.ch/sr15.

International Renewable Energy Agency. 2020. *The Post-COVID Recovery: An Agenda for Resilience, Development and Equality*. Abu Dhabi: IRENA.

Jinnah, Sikina. 2011. 'Climate Change Bandwagoning: The Impacts of Strategic Linkages on Regime Design, Maintenance, and Death'. *Global Environmental Politics 11* (3): pp. 1–9.

Jinnah, Sikina. 2014. *Post-Treaty Politics: Secretariat Influence in Global Environmental Governance*. Cambridge, MA: MIT Press.

Jones, Kate E., Nikkita G. Patel, Marc A. Levy, et al. 2008. 'Global Trends in Emerging Infectious Diseases'. *Nature 451*: pp. 990–4.

Kahn, Matthew E., and Matthew J. Kotchen. 2011. 'Business Cycle Effects on Concern about Climate Change: The Chilling Effect of Recession'. *Climate Change Economics 2* (3): pp. 257–73.

Kenny, John, 2018. 'The Role of Economic Perceptions in Influencing Views on Climate Change: An Experimental Analysis with British Respondents'. *Climate Policy 18* (5): pp. 581–92.

Kenny, John. 2019. 'Economic Conditions and Support for the Prioritisation of Environmental Protection during the Great Recession'. *Environmental Politics 29* (6): pp. 937–58.

Koremenos, Barbara. 2016. *The Continent of International Law: Explaining Agreement Design*. Cambridge: Cambridge University Press.

Koremenos, Barbara, Charles Lipson, and Duncan Snidal. 2001. 'The Rational Design of International Institutions'. *International Organization 55* (4): pp. 761–99.

Kunreuther, Howard, and Paul Slovic. 2020. 'Learning from the COVID-19 Pandemic to Address Climate Change'. 29 May 2020. https://riskcenter.wharton.upenn.

edu/wp-content/uploads/2020/06/Learning-from-the-COVID-19-Pandemic-to-Address-Climate-Change_wp.pdf.

Kuzemko, Caroline, Michael Bradshaw, Gavin Bridge, et al. 2020. 'COVID-19 and the Politics of Sustainable Energy Transitions'. *Energy Research & Social Science 68*: 101685.

Lafond, François, Aimee Gotway Bailey, Jan David Bakker, et al. 2018. 'How Well Do Experience Curves Predict Technological Progress? A Method for Making Distributional Forecasts'. *Technological Forecasting and Social Change 128*: pp. 104–17.

Le Quéré, Corinne., Robert B. Jackson, Matthew W. Jones, et al. 2020. 'Temporary Reduction in Daily Global CO_2 Emissions during the COVID-19 Forced Confinement'. *Nature Climate Change 10*: pp. 647–53.

Lindsey, Peter, James Allan, Peadar Brehony, et al. 2020. 'Conserving Africa's Wildlife and Wildlands through the COVID-19 Crisis and Beyond'. *Nature, Ecology & Evolution 4*: pp. 1300–10.

Marx, Sabine M., Elke U. Weber, Benjamin S. Orlove, et al. 2007. 'Communication and Mental Processes: Experiential and Analytic Processing of Uncertain Climate Information'. *Global Environmental Change 17* (1): pp. 47–58.

Mascarenhas, Michael. 2020. *Lessons in Environmental Justice: From Civil Rights, to Black Lives Matter, to Idle No More*. Thousand Oaks, CA: Sage Press.

Mayer, Brian. 2009. *Blue-Green Coalitions: Fighting for Safe Workplaces and Healthy Communities*. Ithaca, NY: Cornell University Press.

McNamara, Kathleen R., and AAbraham L. Newman. 2020. 'The Big Reveal: COVID-19 and Globalization's Great Transformations'. *International Organization 74* (supp): pp. E59–E77.

Mildenberger Matto, and Anthony Leiserowitz. 2017. 'Public Opinion on Climate Change: Is There an Economy–Environment Tradeoff?' *Environmental Politics 26* (5): pp. 801–24.

Mitchell, Ronald B. 2006 'Problem Structure, Institutional Design, and the Relative Effectiveness of International Environmental Agreements'. *Global Environmental Politics 6* (3): pp. 72–89.

Mitchell, Ronald B., and Patricia M. Keilbach. 2001. 'Situation Structure and Institutional Design: Reciprocity, Coercion, and Exchange'. *International Organization 55* (4): pp. 891–917.

Morin, Jean-Fréféric, and Chantal Blouin. 2019. 'How Environmental Treaties Contribute to Global Health Governance'. *Globalization and Health 15* (1): p. 47.

Morin, Jean-Frédéric., Amandine Orsini, and Sikina Jinnah. 2020. *Global Environmental Politics. Understanding the Governance of the Earth*. Oxford: Oxford University Press.

Negri, Stefania, ed. 2019. *Environmental Health in International and European Law*. Abingdon: Routledge.

Nunes, João. 2016. 'Ebola and the Production of Neglect in Global Health'. *Third World Quarterly 37* (3): pp. 542–56.

Onzivu William. 2016. 'Rethinking Transnational Environmental Health Governance in Africa: Can Adaptive Governance Help?' *Review of European, Comparative & International Environmental Law 25* (1): pp. 107–22.

Organisation for Economic Co-operation and Development (OECD). 2020. *Making the Green Recovery Work for Jobs, Income and Growth*. Paris: OECD.

Pellow, David Naguib. 2018. *What Is Critical Environmental Justice?* Cambridge: Polity Press.

Phillips, Carly A., Astrid Caldas, Rachel Cleetus, et al. 2020. 'Compound Climate Risks in the COVID-19 Pandemic'. *Nature Climate Change 10*: pp. 586–8.

Quam, Vivian G. M., Joacim Rocklöv, Mikkel B. M. Quam, and Rebekah A. I. Lucas. 2017. 'Assessing Greenhouse Gas Emissions and Health Co-Benefits: A Structured Review of Lifestyle-Related Climate Change Mitigation Strategies'. *International Journal of Environmental Research and Public Health 14* (5): p. 468.

Quinn, Sandra Crouse, Vicki S. Supriya Kumar, Donald Musa Freimuth, Nestor Casteneda-Angarita, and Kelley Kidwell. 2011. 'Racial Disparities in Exposure, Susceptibility, and Access to Health Care in the US H1N1 Influenza Pandemic'. *American Journal of Public Health 101*: pp. 285–93.

Ratter, Beate M. W., Katharina H. I. Philipp, and Hans von Storch. 2012. 'Between Hype and Decline: Recent Trends in Public Perception of Climate Change'. *Environmental Science & Policy 18*: pp. 3–8.

Russel Duncan, and David Benson. 2014. 'Green Budgeting in an Age of Austerity: A Transatlantic Comparative Perspective'. *Environmental Politics 23* (2): pp. 243–62.

Rutz, Christian, Matthias-Claudio Loretto, Amanda E. Bates, et al. 2020. 'COVID-19 Lockdown Allows Researchers to Quantify the Effects of Human Activity on Wildlife'. *Nature Ecology & Evolution 22*: pp. 1–4.

Schucht, Simon, Aaugustine Colette, Shilpa Rao, and Mike Holland. 2015. 'Moving towards Ambitious Climate Policies: Monetised Health Benefits from Improved Air Quality Could Offset Mitigation Costs in Europe'. *Environmental Science & Policy 50*: pp. 252–69.

Scruggs, Lyle, and Salil Benegal. 2012. 'Declining Public Concern about Climate Change: Can We Blame the Great Recession?' *Global Environmental Change 22* (2): pp. 505–15.

Sell, Susan, and Aseem Prakash. 2004. 'Using Ideas Strategically: The Contest between Business and NGO Networks in Intellectual Property Rights'. *International Studies Quarterly 48*: pp. 143–75.

Shum, Robert Y. 2012. 'Effects of Economic Recession and Local Weather on Climate Change Attitudes'. *Climate Policy 12* (1): pp. 38–49.

Singu, Sravani, Arpan Acharya, Kishore Challagundla, and Siddappa N. Byrareddy. 2020. 'Impact of Social Determinants of Health on the Emerging COVID-19 Pandemic in the United States'. *Frontiers in Public Health 8*: p. 406.

Skovgaard, Jakob. 2014. 'EU Climate Policy after the Crisis'. *Environmental Politics 23* (1): pp. 1–17.

Thomas, Caroline. 2001. 'Environmental and Health Research: Overlapping Agendas'. *Global Environmental Politics 1* (4): pp. 10–7.

Tienhaara, Kyla. 2014. 'Varieties of Green Capitalism: Economy and Environment in the Wake of the Global Financial Crisis'. *Environmental Politics 23* (2): pp. 187–204.

United Nations (UN). 1992. 'Report of the United Nations Conference on Environment and Development'. 3–14 June 1992. https://www.un.org/en/development/desa/population/migration/generalassembly/docs/globalcompact/A_CONF.151_26_Vol.I_Declaration.pdf.

UN. 2015. 'Paris Agreement'. https://unfccc.int/sites/default/files/english_paris_agreement.pdf.

UN. 2020. 'Five Things You Should Know about Disposable Masks and Plastic Pollution'. 30 July. https://news.un.org/en/story/2020/07/1069151.

UN Environment Programme (UNEP). 2018. 'UNEP Annual Report 2018'. https://wedocs.unep.org/bitstream/handle/20.500.11822/27689/AR2018_EN.pdf?sequence=1&isAllowed=y.

UNEP. 2020a. 'Virus which Causes COVID-19 Threatens Great Ape Conservation'. Interview with Johannes Refisch, United Nations Great Apes Survival Partnership Programme, Manager and Coordinator.

UNEP. 2020b. 'Three Ways the United Nations Environment Programme Works to Address Illegal Trade in Wildlife'. 17 February.

UNEP and International Livestock Research Institute. 2020. *Preventing the Next Pandemic: Zoonotic Diseases and How to Break the Chain of Transmission*. Nairobi: UNEP.

Venkatapuram, Sridhar. 2011. *Health Justice: An Argument from the Capabilities Approach*. Cambridge: Polity Press.

Vogel, David. 2012. *The Politics of Precaution: Regulating Health, Safety, and Environmental Risks in Europe and the United States*. Princeton, NJ: Princeton University Press.

Wagenaar, William A. and Sabato D. Sagaria. 1975. 'Misperception of Exponential Growth'. *Perception & Psychophysics 18* (6): pp. 416–22.

Watt-Cloutier, Sheila. 2018. *The Right to Be Cold: One Woman's Fight to Save the Arctic and Save the Planet from Climate Change*. Minneapolis, MN: University of Minnesota Press.

Whyte, Kyle Powys. 2020. 'Environmental Justice, Indigenous Peoples and Consent'. In *Lessons in Environmental Justice: From Civil Rights, to Black Lives Matter, to Idle No More*, edited by Michael Mascarenhas, p. 35. Thousand Oaks, CA: Sage Press.

World Health Organization (WHO). 2018. 'Climate Change and Health, Key Facts'. Updated 30 October 2021. https://www.who.int/news-room/fact-sheets/detail/climate-change-and-health.

WHO. 2019a. 'Health, Environment and Climate Change'. A72/15, 18 April.

WHO. 2019b. 'Health and Climate Change Survey Report'. WHO/CED/PHE/EPE/19.11.

WHO. 2019c. '2018–2019 Annual Report'. https://www.who.int/about/finances-accountability/reports/results_report_18-19_final1.pdf?ua=1.

World Trade Organization (WTO). n.d. 'GATT Article XX: General Exceptions'. https://www.wto.org/english/res_e/publications_e/ai17_e/gatt1994_art20_gatt47.pdf.

Yancy Clyde W. 2020. 'COVID-19 and African Americans'. *Journal of the American Medical Association 323* (19): pp. 1891–2.

7

Pandemics and the City

COVID-19 and the Future of Urban Density and Densification

Michael Hooper

Pandemics have long affected the public's perceptions of, and officials' responses to, urban risk. As in past pandemics, the COVID-19 pandemic has raised urgent questions for urban planners and policymakers. Many of these questions concern density, a topic that has come to occupy an increasingly prominent position in urban politics, policy, and planning. Urban density refers to the number of people and the built floor area of an urban area. As the COVID-19 pandemic emerged, many people argued that it, and the threat of other pandemics, calls into question the future of dense cities and of densification efforts. These claims have been particularly prominent in the news and popular media. They are important because many planners and city officials have seen promoting density and densification as among their most important tasks over the past decades. Densification, they have claimed, brings environmental, social, and economic benefits. As I will argue, while many observers have likely overstated the case made by pandemics against density, the current crisis does raise vital and enduring questions about the way in which densification efforts are undertaken and the manner in which the costs and benefits of urban density are distributed. Importantly, the current pandemic offers learning opportunities for planners and policymakers that can help ensure future efforts to build dense urban neighbourhoods do not exacerbate existing inequalities or increase the vulnerability of residents to future pandemics and other forms of risk (relatedly, see the Introduction to this volume by Ackerly et al., and Chapter 9 by Smith).

A Brief History of Densification

For the past several decades, planners have sought to densify cities and neighbourhoods for a variety of environmental, social, and economic reasons. Indeed,

Michael Hooper, *Pandemics and the City*. In: *A Multidisciplinary Approach to Pandemics*.
Edited by Philippe Bourbeau, Jean-Michel Marcoux, and Brooke A. Ackerly, Oxford University Press.
 DOI: 10.1093/oso/9780192897855.003.0008

densification has become a key component in planners' toolkits and has been taught to urban planning students as a pillar of sustainable urbanization. Densification efforts, which seek to increase the density of cities and neighbourhoods, have fallen under a number of closely related labels and are part of a variety of planning strategies, including 'compact cities', 'green urbanism', 'smart growth', and 'sustainable urbanism' (Lehmann 2019). These efforts share a vision of relatively dense urban areas focused on compact forms of development.

The push for urban densification stems in large part from its perceived environmental benefits and it has been argued that urban planning is increasingly focused on 'sustainability-as-density' (Quastel et al. 2012). Studies have shown that such environmental benefits are considerable and serve as a powerful justification for advancing both dense development and densification efforts. Summarizing these claims, the United Kingdom (UK)'s Urban Task Force argues that the compact city is the most sustainable urban form (Urban Task Force 1999). As described by Lehmann (2019), there is extensive evidence that compact cities with higher densities encourage public transportation use, walking and cycling, are more efficient in terms of land-use, allow for preservation of peripheral open-space and agricultural land, and allow more efficient siting and provision of infrastructure and services, including water and electricity. There are also social and economic benefits from densification, including potential reductions in social segregation and improved access to services, amenities, and employment (Burton 2000; Dempsey et al. 2011). From an economic standpoint, it has been argued that dense cities are better able to efficiently provide key forms of infrastructure and services (Alvarez et al. 2014).

Building on the growing evidence that density has environmental, social, and economic benefits, densification strategies have been increasingly adopted in both the Global North and the Global South (Dave 2010; Organisation for Economic Co-operation and Development (OECD) 2012; UN Habitat 2016). The proliferation of densification plans has particularly increased as the implications of climate change have become apparent and cities are forced to address the energy and environmental costs associated with diffuse development and sprawl. Densification plans have been proposed in cities as diverse as Ulaanbaatar, Mongolia (Anderson and Hooper 2017), and Christchurch, New Zealand (Vallance et al. 2005). Planners have also pursued densification in diverse spatial contexts, including in urban and peri-urban settings such as in Toronto, Canada (Charmes and Keil 2015) and Lyon, France (Rousseau 2015), as well as in more suburban environments, including in Phoenix, Arizona (Atkinson-Palombo 2010), and Charlotte, North Carolina (Delmelle et al. 2014).

While planners and policymakers have voiced growing support for densification, these strategies have often been contested, as neighbourhoods have resisted such change. Where densification is undertaken, it is often unsuccessful or results in conflict (Cook et al. 2013; Filion 2003; Peirce 2002; Vallance et al. 2005).

Researchers have shown that efforts to increase density in cities are often met by anti-densification activism of resident groups (Peters 2016). The Urban Land Institute has argued that, due to local backlash, there is a long history of failed densification efforts around the globe (Scott 2015). Strong resistance to densification has been reported in such diverse locations as Berkeley, California (Dougherty 2017), and Ulaanbaatar, Mongolia (Anderson et al. 2017).

Despite the challenges that many densification efforts encounter, there have been some notable recent successes in planners' efforts to both increase the public acceptance of density and to advance densification plans (Manville et al. 2020). Perhaps most well documented are relatively recent moves by several cities to transition away from the single-family house as the default zoning type. In 2019, Minneapolis, Minnesota, adopted a new comprehensive plan that allows up to three units on residential lots as the citywide minimum (Wegmann 2020). Also passed in 2019, Oregon's Bill 2001 permits, in cities with more than 10,000 residents, duplex housing in areas that currently allow single-family houses and higher levels of density in cities with more than 25,000 residents (Miller 2019). Similar efforts have been discussed at the city level in California, including by the mayors of Oakland, Sacramento, and San Jose (Dillon 2019).

In addition to the zoning changes mentioned above, related successes have made it easier to construct accessory dwelling units (ADUs) in many cities. ADUs are small, second dwellings on the same lot as, or sometimes attached to, a single-family house. In California, legislation has enabled the construction of many new ADUs and has allowed some of those already built to be retroactively brought within the law (Mukhija 2014). Lane-way houses, which are similar to ADUs, but are built with access to the lanes between streets have also seen an increase in public and legal acceptability, including in Canada. For example, Vancouver's zoning and development bylaw allows lane-way houses in all single-family residential zones (City of Vancouver 2020).

Beyond the specific policy changes mentioned above, there has also been a broader acceptance among planners and the public of increased density as an appropriate mode of urban development. The urban models that receive normative and rhetorical support among planners increasingly focus on higher densities. For example, it has been argued that the widely discussed 'Vancouver model' of density is the 'true New Urbanism ... shaping the way more people live than any variation on early-twentieth century American suburbia' and is 'the portal through which the twenty-first-century is being conceived' (Boddy 2004: 19). The growing acceptance of density and densification can also be seen in the rise of new pro-densification groups, such as the YIMBY (Yes in My Backyard) movement. This movement promotes denser development to address the global housing affordability crisis. YIMBY groups have arisen in many cities across North America and Europe, they host an annual conference, and have achieved notable successes. For example, in Cambridge, Massachusetts, YIMBY activists gained approval for a multi-unit housing project and in Boulder, Colorado, they stopped a growth-restricting ballot initiative (Stahl 2018).

Pandemics and Density: A History

The debate around urban density sparked by the COVID-19 pandemic has been heated and complex and has implications for how we think about cities, density, and risk more broadly. The many critiques offered have ranged from arguing that high urban densities are dangerous to forecasting the demise of large cities as centres of economic growth and prosperity. The negative focus on density is perhaps not surprising, as it was pinpointed as a key element in many COVID-19 responses adopted by cities and institutions. For example, when Harvard University closed its campus in March 2020, it called this an explicit 'de-densification' effort (Hassan and Ries 2020). Similarly, many workplaces initiated efforts to 'de-densify', using this language specifically (Wells 2020). City officials also began relatively early to adopt the language of de-densification. For example, in South Africa, officials announced 'urgent plans to de-densify' informal settlements (Luckhoff 2020). Given that so many institutions adopted de-densification as a strategy for addressing the pandemic, it should perhaps be no surprise that broader questions about the acceptability and safety of urban density quickly gained ground. New York governor Andrew Cuomo captured the sentiments of many regarding urban density and pandemics when he tweeted in March 2020 that, 'There is a density level in NYC that is destructive' (Wiener and Iton 2020).

In addition to the adoption of campus, workplace, and institutional de-densification strategies, reports also emerged of urban residents voluntarily fleeing cities for the countryside, including to holiday and second homes (Holpuch 2020). The many stories documenting the movement of people to the countryside were accompanied by startling headlines—such as 'Land of the Flee' in the *New York Post*—and evocative photographs showing, for example, movers and moving vans crowding city streets (Delves-Broughton 2020). Reflecting the apparent migration away from dense cities, the *Financial Times* reported that the US National Association of Home Builders' housing market index reached the highest level in its history and that 'demand for single-family homes has also increased as people working from home depart crowded cities and seek to socially distance during the pandemic' (Anon 2020a). For New York City alone, by August 2020 rates of relocation were reported to have increased by 50% over the previous year (Satow 2020).

The idea that cities could be sites of increased risk during pandemics is supported by historical and contemporary evidence. Historically, dense settlements have been associated with increased disease risk and it is argued that virtually all human infectious diseases due to microorganisms arose with the emergence of urbanism (Scott 2017). The connection between urban density and disease transmission is also supported by some biomedical research. Studies have shown that population density can be positively associated with transmission rates for diseases transmitted via faecal–oral and respiratory routes, including influenza (Alirol et al. 2011; Xiao et al. 2014). The connection between density and infectious disease transmission—referred to as the 'urban penalty' in public health—is seen particularly clearly when looking at how urban residents responded to past pandemics, with flight from cities often being viewed as an effective response to infectious diseases.

In late medieval times, wealthy residents of European cities often retreated from urban areas during plague outbreaks (Carmichael 1986). Mirroring efforts of universities to 'de-densify' during the COVID-19 pandemic, students and faculty at Oxford University in the medieval period moved to rural areas during disease outbreaks, and by the fifteenth century, escape plans to countryside manors were well established (Courtenay 1980). In 1721, when a smallpox epidemic reached Boston, a variety of interventions were undertaken to contain an outbreak that ultimately infected more than 50% of the population, killed approximately 8%, and was responsible for three-quarters of all deaths that year (Blake 1952). As the outbreak grew, the legislature was relocated from Boston to more rural Cambridge and approximately 1,000 people, almost 10% of the population, and particularly the wealthy, fled the city for the countryside (Coss 2016). The widely accepted connection between urban density and perceptions of disease risk can likewise be seen in late nineteenth-century and early twentieth-century public health publications (Figure 7.1), which frequently represented cities as squalid and unhealthy

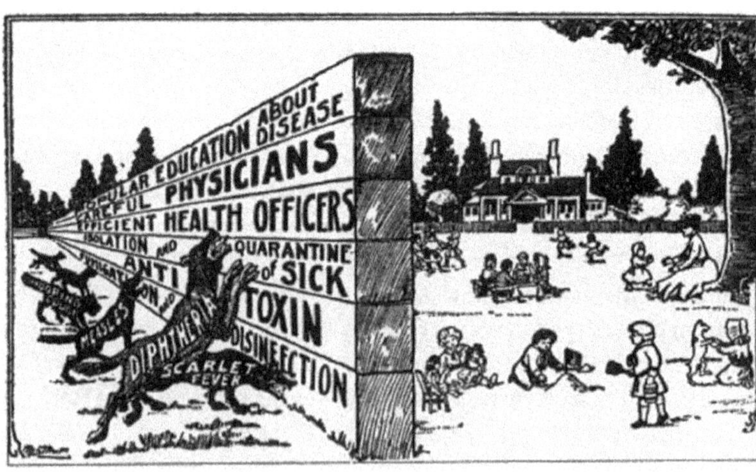

Fig. 7.1 A 1908 illustration from the *Virginia Health Bulletin* shows urban diseases threatening the hygienic conditions of suburban life
Source: Image by the Virginia Health Bulletin, licensed under CC BY-NC 2.0.

and contrasted them with the suburbs, which were viewed as bucolic and healthy (Virginia Department of Health 1908).

Despite the many stories published in the media during the COVID-19 pandemic about the perceived dangers of dense cities, the evidence is much more complex. Research shows, provocative news stories to the contrary, that while some relatively dense cities have been hard hit, others, and indeed some of the densest, have fared well. Furthermore, on a per capita basis, some of the places hardest-hit by COVID-19 have been rural or sparcely populated areas. Highlighting this complexity, the experiences of the United States' first and second most densely populated cities provide useful nuance. As of May 2020, New York City had more than 195,000 confirmed cases and 19,000 deaths, while San Francisco had approximately 2,000 confirmed cases and 36 deaths (Wiener and Iton 2020).

Many highly dense cities, ranging from Taipei, Taiwan, to Seoul, South Korea, have fared better in the current pandemic than many far less dense cities. Looking at China specifically, Fang and Wahba (2020) argue that the relationship between urban density and confirmed COVID-19 cases is weak. Comparing 284 cities, they found that many cities with high urban densities, including Shanghai and Beijing, had relatively few confirmed cases, while cities with the highest infection rates had relatively low densities (Fang and Wahba 2020). In the United States, on a per capita basis, many of the places hardest hit have been small and medium-sized metro areas in the country's Southwest, including those with large Native American or Hispanic populations (Anon 2020b).

A further layer of complexity emerges when we examine who in cities is at greatest risk of both contracting COVID-19 and of dying. As in other pandemics, considerable evidence has emerged that risks are not borne equally by urban residents. In this respect, the arguments in this chapter show considerable overlap with other contributions in this volume in emphasizing issues of inequality as pivotal to understanding the impacts of pandemics. Highlighting this, the United States' Centers for Disease Control (CDC) has argued that there 'is increasing evidence that some racial and ethnic minority groups are being disproportionately affected by COVID-19' (CDC 2020). Studies in the United States have shown that considerably higher percentages of African American and Latino populations have contracted COVID-19 with, as of June 2020, 21.8% of cases being African American and 33.8% Latino, despite making up only 13% and 18% of the population, respectively (Tai et al. 2020). In cities, minorities and racialized residents have likewise been found to have higher rates of COVID-19 infection and death. For example, in a study of New York City, positive associations were found between positive COVID-19 status and Black race, Hispanic ethnicity, and poverty (Cordes and Castro 2020). Similar results have been found in the UK, including in London, where Black, Asian and minority ethnic (BAME) people had higher risk of dying from COVID-19 (Aldridge et al. 2020; Faleiro 2020).

The results mentioned above regarding differential impacts suggest that, across cities, there is no consistent relationship between urban density and pandemic impacts and that, within relatively dense cities, not all residents bear the same risks. This contrasts with the tone adopted by many of the articles that have been written, particularly in the popular media, about cities and density. These commonly assume that a denser city, like New York, differs in a consistent way from a less dense city, like Houston. In fact, the nature of density varies considerably across any given city, as does the distribution of risks faced by the public. Given this complexity in the actual picture of pandemic risks and the way they intersect with density, the question then is not, why is density bad, but rather, under what conditions can density be good? Or, put another way, what can be done to mitigate the possible risks posed by urban density in pandemics? This is a vitally important question, particularly in light of the growing support for density and densification that had accumulated prior to the current pandemic. The COVID-19 crisis usefully helps us understand that not all dense cities are equally at risk, and neither are all residents of dense cities equally vulnerable. This chapter now turns to asking how we can reduce the risks associated with density and ensure that these are not borne unequally, and particularly by those who are already marginalized or vulnerable.

Planning for 'Good' Density: The Role of Infrastructure and Services

If density itself is not the culprit in pandemics, but rather certain kinds of dense settings, how can we be sure to create density that is good, or at least that is less bad? The policies that governments adopt have profound effects on the health of urban residents and this includes government policies related to density, which is too often treated as a single, homogenous idea, rather than as a highly variegated condition that is a function of complex private and public decisions. The fact that minority and racialized residents often face greater risk in dense settings is in part because they often have lower access to infrastructure and services and also experience some of the greatest crowding with respect to housing.

While areas with high built densities often have relatively high population densities, the relationship between the two can vary considerably, for example, due to differences in the average number of people per household (Churchman 1999). With respect to residential crowding, an analysis in Chicago showed that crowding within homes, rather than the density of housing units, was more likely to be the cause of increased COVID-19 infection rates, particularly among African American and Hispanic residents (Coryne 2020). Similarly, in the UK, the former head of the UK Civil Service, Lord Kerslake, has argued that overcrowding was one of the key drivers of COVID-19 infections (Gardiner 2020).

Like crowding, provision of, and access to, infrastructure and services can vary starkly across urban areas. This includes forms of hard infrastructure such as roads, highways, open space, water and sewer systems, and railways as well as soft infrastructure, such as education, health care, cultural activities, and financial services (Filion and Keil 2017). The poor and minorities typically have lower levels of access to these supports, all of which become even more vital in a crisis. Such differences in infrastructure and service provision across socio-economic groups and neighbourhoods have been identified in a wide range of urban settings ranging from the United States (Swanstrom et al. 2002) to China (Sun et al. 2017) and India (Saroj et al. 2020). For instance, as just one example from the large body of research showing that infrastructure and service provision often varies markedly, a study of water, sanitation, and hygiene services in India found that intra-city variation was actually higher than inter-city differences and that intra-city inequality was associated with differences in housing conditions, economic status, educational level, socio-religious affiliation and occupational status (Saroj et al. 2020).

One barrier to supporting urban residents in pandemics is the often overburdened nature of city governments. City governments have, in many countries, found themselves taking on increasing responsibilities in the face of declining budgets. This means that the vital services that could keep dense settlements safe, particularly during pandemics and other disasters, are often stretched thin. Differences in the financial resources available to cities have been posited as an important factor in the degree to which they are able to effectively respond to crises. In the United States, Swanstrom et al. (2002) argue that a major factor in differences in service provision across municipalities in a metro area or county are the very different tax bases and fiscal resources available to local governments. Comparing Chicago and Stockholm, Sampson (2014) argues that one reason for the lower levels of municipal inequality in the latter is the more equal provision of public goods. In the case of China, Fang and Wahba (2020) have argued that the reason larger cities fared better in the COVID-19 pandemic is that they were better able to mobilize financial resources to undertake interventions that reduce infection rates.

Notwithstanding that some places have more equal provision of public goods than others, there has been a widespread trend, in both the Global North and Global South, towards reduced urban resources for tackling inequality. There have been both widespread reductions in urban budgets and a rescaling of responsibility to local authorities for service delivery. In the UK, for example, policy shifts have seen major reductions in welfare spending, as well as a downloading of service provision responsibilities to local governments. The combination of these changes hit the poor and children particularly hard, especially following the financial crisis of 2007–2008, with as many as 1.4 million families made worse off as a result (Donald et al. 2014). Similar trends can be seen in many other countries, with South Africa providing a particularly striking example. As a result of that country's

GEAR initiative, focused on Growth, Employment and Redistribution, central-to-local transfers declined by 85% in real terms between 1991 and 1997 and an additional 55% between 1997 and 2000 (McDonald and Pape 2002). This left many, if not all, South African municipalities with radically reduced budgets with which to provide infrastructure and services.

There has been relatively little research on the role of governance in disaster risk reduction, including in pandemics. What is known, however, includes that effective governance is limited by the complex relationship between power and knowledge among diverse actors with very different control over key resources (Jones et al. 2014). Decisions over risk increasingly take place in a context where the state has been hollowed out and rolled back and its responsibilities devolved up to international organizations, down to local authorities, or out to non-state actors (Bulkeley and Jordan 2012). When the public sector fails to provide needed supports, such as in the form of safe public transportation, reliable health care, and quality education, those with private financial resources are likely to fill the void on their own. This leaves the poor and marginalized groups most vulnerable to the brunt of pandemics and disasters. Notably, it is very hard for resource-constrained and overburdened urban governments to retroactively create the social, economic, and infrastructural supports that would make cities safe after disaster strikes.

The often limited resources available to cities to fund infrastructure and service provision, combined with the well-established inequalities in their delivery, become particularly problematic in the context of considering how density might be implicated in pandemic-related risks. Infrastructure and services are particularly important, but too often under-considered, ingredients in determining whether the benefits and costs of densification are shared equitably. Supporting this, a study from Melbourne, Australia, argues that infrastructure and densification must go hand in hand to ensure that the poor do not end up bearing the burden of densification (Cook et al. 2018). The study authors argue that there has been relatively little examination of the densification–infrastructure nexus and that much resistance to densification efforts stems from disputes over how infrastructure and services are delivered to support development. In their analysis of Melbourne's inner suburbs, they highlight that, while there was particularly low investment in certain service categories (including, e.g. public transport, education, and public housing), these low levels of investment could be compensated for by the wealthy, through access to private alternatives, such as private schools (Cook et al. 2018). It is precisely this trade-off in cities that can put the poor at further disadvantage, particularly in a setting like a pandemic, where access to private alternatives are more limited. Ultimately, infrastructure and services are important elements in determining the carrying capacity of an urban area (Oh et al. 2005) and in many cases it is poorer areas in dense cities that exist above such carrying capacities and whose residents also lack the private resources to buy themselves out of risk.

Inequality in dense cities has also been enhanced by the way that densification has been undertaken. Density bonuses and other kinds of density-for-benefit agreements are a common strategy for increasing urban density. These are regulatory instruments that allow cities to secure benefits from developers in exchange for increases in project densities (Moore 2013). The delivery of such benefits have been found to be influenced by the interaction of interest groups, including developers and local political institutions (Ramirez de la Cruz 2009). In studies of locations as diverse as Taipei, Taiwan (Shih and Shieh 2020) and Sydney, Australia (Searle 2003), such agreements have been found to often be discretionary, relatively untransparent, and to involve limited public participation. In studies of density-for-benefit agreements in Canada, research has shown that they are idiosyncratically devised and that the unequal skills and levels of involvement of key actors, particularly city councillors, can result in very different terms with developers and can enhance inequality (Biggar 2017; Moore 2013). For example, Biggar (2017) concludes that urban residents would be better served if Toronto's approach to density-for-benefit agreements were better aligned with broader public-sector strategies and distributed benefits more widely.

Looking at both Toronto and Vancouver, Moore (2013: 2) likewise found that negotiations with developers and the decisions regarding which benefits can be secured remain ad hoc and 'obscure at best'. The idea that density strategies adopted by cities may not invariably lead to good or equal outcomes is further emphasized by a report from the Urban Land Institute (ULI) (Pain et al. 2018). That report begins from the premise that some forms of density are 'good', while others are less so and then seeks to identify the features of 'good density'. The study finds that good density is typically reinforced by investments in infrastructure and services that can support residents and businesses. For example, they contend that when increasing density, policies are the need to safeguard open spaces, support a green urban environment, and promote public transportation. The ULI report states that regulations and management approaches 'need to be developed that support good density through built infrastructure appropriate to different political, economic, and cultural contexts' (Pain et al. 2018: 18). Such strategic, context-informed strategies for supporting density are considerably different from the ad-hoc and discretionary processes that often characterize current density-for-benefit agreements. This is important since, relevant to the context of pandemics, a key advantage of well-supported, 'good' density is that it is more resilient, sustainable, and prosperity-enhancing in the face of risk and over the long-term (Pain et al. 2018).

One further challenge confronting those hoping to increase urban densities is that some of the same agencies that increasingly push for density are also those that have argued for austerity in public service provision. Since, as I have argued, density depends on adequate provision of infrastructure and services and there is often inequality in who receives these goods, there has been some prudent scepticism that densification will be accompanied by sufficient provision of public goods and services. A good example of this can be found in Ulaanbaatar, Mongolia. There, a new plan for the city, the Masterplan 2020, was developed with the support of UN-Habitat, the World Bank, and the Japanese International Cooperation Agency (JICA) (Anderson et al. 2017). The plan and related upgrading strategy argue, in part, that increased densities will help to achieve savings in the provision of needed physical infrastructure (Cities Alliance 2010). As the World Bank states (2010: 81): 'high density development [in Ulaanbaatar] will make it easier to provide better urban services with higher efficiency and lower cost'. Such calls for densification in the Global South are increasing common, with UN-Habitat having strongly promoted inclusion of efforts to reduce sprawl in the United Nations' Sustainable Development Goals (UN-Habitat 2013).

Research on the Ulaanbaatar masterplan shows sharply divergent opinions regarding the desirability of densification. While 100% of interviewed officials from multilateral organizations based in Mongolia looked favourably on plans for densification, only 39% of local interviewees did so (Anderson et al. 2017). Part of the reason for local residents' and officials' scepticism was that some of the same organizations that support densification, and associated displacement, in Ulaanbaatar have also been highly supportive of austerity and reductions in public spending in the country (UNICEF, 2018). Much as in the United States, Canada, and other countries, Mongolian local authorities have found their resources declining. In addition, the increasing privatization of the Mongolian economy, following the 'shock-therapy' model, was also broadly encouraged by similar international actors to those who supported plans for densification, including the World Bank (Nixson and Walters 2006). Such privatization was undertaken with relatively little analysis or consideration of its possible impacts on poverty and income distribution (Nixson and Walters 2006). It is perhaps unsurprising that in a climate of fiscal austerity, local officials and residents were sceptical that the kinds of increased urban densities envisioned in the masterplan would be adequately supported with investments in infrastructure and services.

The challenge of ensuring that dense cities can support their populations is heightened by the push towards increased private-sector involvement in the planning of cities. As one prominent example, the much vaunted involvement of Google and its parent company, Alphabet, through their subsidiary Sidewalk Labs, in the design and planning of Toronto's waterfront Quayside project reached a crisis point during the COVID-19 pandemic. After having invested three years in their relationship with the city, the company simply pulled out of the partnership due to threats posed to its finances by the pandemic. The episode highlights a pivotal difference between the private and public sectors in a crisis. Private actors can, as happened in Toronto, simply walk away.

Sidewalk Labs' involvement in planning in Toronto is emblematic of the increasing role of private-sector organizations in urban planning, the retreat of public accountability in urban decision-making, and the challenges that face the public in ensuring that dense development is equitable and sustainable. In the case of Sidewalk Labs, its involvement began in 2017, when it partnered with Waterfront Toronto, a tri-partite public company in Ontario. The involvement of Sidewalk Labs met with growing concern because of the way it led planning and because of the way that public officials retreated from processes designed to both inform the public of developments and solicit public input. Reports revealed that Sidewalk Labs led public consultations and that Waterfront Toronto officials did not involve themselves in these public processes (Flynn and Valverde 2019). The remarkably private-sector driven and seemingly unaccountable nature of the planning process raised concerns and generated considerable press (Carr and Hesse 2020). Describing Sidewalk Labs' foray into planning in Toronto, Flynn and Valverde (2019: 774) state: '[it] calls into question the degree to which smart city pioneers like [Sidewalk Labs], who have a tremendous amount of lobbying power and funding, make a play not only for more data or more money, but for the power to plan public space'.

Ultimately, the Sidewalks Labs project collapsed in May 2020. The company named the COVID-19 pandemic as the reason for the project's cancellation (O'Kane 2020). Daniel Doctoroff, Chairman and CEO of Sidewalk Labs, made the announcement public in a blog post in which he argued that the pandemic and resulting uncertainty over the city's real estate market made it impossible for the company to proceed (Vincent and Rider 2020). Of course, it is precisely under conditions of uncertainty, like a pandemic, that residents most need confidence that stable, high-functioning institutions can support the planning, operation, and resilience of dense urban systems.

As the example of Sidewalk Labs highlights, there are a variety of forces that can undermine the ability of dense urban environments to provide for the needs of residents during pandemics and other crises. These include the fact that infrastructure and services are already inequitably distributed in cities and that approaches that are commonly employed to increase urban densities, such as density-for-benefit agreements, can further enhance spatial inequality and lead to some areas being better resourced than others. These factors interact with patterns of crowding, which see racialized and other marginalized communities often experiencing higher levels of personal proximity in densely built urban environments. Inadequate support for density is exacerbated by the declining resources of many urban governments and increased private-sector leadership in planning. Together these factors mean that not all dense environments face similar risks in pandemics. Unfortunately, the unequal distribution of these risks is not the result of happenstance, but rather of past planning and policy decisions. On a more positive note, awareness of these patterns of inequality and their genesis can enable better decisions in the future. By planning in ways that ensure that urban residents fare well in pandemics, we can create cities where the benefits and costs of density are better shared across all residents and resident well-being and resilience are enhanced.

Conclusion

This chapter has argued that while pandemics are unlikely to lead to the decline of cities as sites of habitation and economic activity, as many popular articles have suggested, the current COVID-19 pandemic has clearly shown that the burdens of density are not borne equally. In this respect, the COVID-19 pandemic and its urban impacts mirror findings from past disease outbreaks and will, unless urban planning practices change, foreshadow those to be experienced in the future. The unequal distribution of pandemic risk is in part a function of long-standing inequalities in the way that infrastructure and services are provided in cities, which have been exacerbated by both declining resources available to cities and downloading of responsibilities to local authorities. Furthermore, the way that densification has been undertaken, often relying on untransparent and relatively unequal density-for-benefit agreements, has further meant that not all areas of dense cities face similar risks in times of crisis. Finally, the COVID-19 pandemic has shed light on the risks posed by the increasingly private-sector-led planning of cities. As seen in the case of Sidewalk Labs, in Toronto, at a time of crisis, this company left its planning responsibilities on short notice, precisely the opposite of the kind of resilient, stable engagement needed from planning agencies in times of peril. The chapter concludes by calling for greater attention to the unequal distribution of infrastructure and services in cities, to ensure that the benefits and costs of density are more fairly shared. Better and more equitably supported models of density would have many benefits, including limiting the risks borne by the most vulnerable, improving the receptiveness of residents to densification, and ensuring that costly retroactive interventions aren't needed to make cities and neighbourhoods liveable when disasters strike.

References

Aldridge, Robert W., Dan Lewer, Srinivasa Vittal Katikireddi, et al. 2020. 'Black, Asian and Minority Ethnic Groups in England Are at Increased Risk of Death from COVID-19: Indirect Standardisation of NHS Mortality Data'. *Wellcome Open Research 5* (88): p. 88.

Alirol, Emilie, Laurent Getaz, Beat Stoll, Francois Chappuis, and Louis Loutan. 2011. 'Urbanisation and Infectious Diseases in a Globalized World'. *The Lancet Infectious Diseases 11* (2): pp. 131–41.

Álvarez, Inmaculada C., Ángel M. Prieto, and José L. Zofío. 2014. 'Cost Efficiency, Urban Patterns and Population Density When Providing Public Infrastructure: A Stochastic Frontier Approach'. *European Planning Studies 22* (6): pp. 1235–58.

Anderson, Raven, and Michael Hooper. 2017. 'Competing Organisational Perspectives on Rapid Urbanisation and its Management: A Case Study of Ulaanbaatar, Mongolia'. *International Development Planning Review 39* (2): pp. 187–207.

Anderson, Raven, Michael Hooper, and Aldarsaikhan Tuvshinbat. 2017. 'Towers on the Steppe: Compact City Plans and Local Perceptions of Urban Densification in Ulaanbaatar, Mongolia'. *Journal of Urbanism 10* (2): pp. 217–30.

Anon. 2020a. 'US Homebuilder Confidence in August Climbs to Highest since 1998'. *Financial Times*, 17 August.

Anon. 2020b. 'COVID in the US: Latest Map and Case Count'. *New York Times*, 23 September.

Atkinson-Palombo, Carol. 2010. 'Comparing the Capitalisation Benefits of Light-Rail Transit and Overlay Zoning for Single-Family Houses and Condos by Neighbourhood Type in Metropolitan Phoenix, Arizona'. *Urban Studies 47* (11): pp. 2409–26.

Biggar, Jeff. 2017. 'Between Public Goals and Private Projects: Negotiating Community Benefits for Density from Toronto's Urban Redevelopment'. PhD dissertation, University of Toronto.

Blake, John. 1952. 'The Inoculation Controversy in Boston: 1721–1722'. *New England Quarterly 25* (4): pp. 489–506.

Boddy, Trevor. 2004. 'New Urbanism: The Vancouver Model'. *Places 16* (2): pp. 14–21.

Bulkeley, Harriet, and Andy Jordan. 2012. 'Transnational Environmental Governance: New Findings and Emerging Research Agendas'. *Environment and Planning C 30* (4): pp. 556–70.

Burton, Elizabeth. 2000. 'The Compact City: Just or Just Compact? A Preliminary Analysis'. *Urban Studies 37* (11): pp. 1969–2006.

Carmichael, Ann. 1986. *Plague and the Poor in Renaissance Florence*. Cambridge: Cambridge University Press.

Carr, Constance, and Markus Hesse. 2020. 'When Alphabet Inc. Plans Toronto's Waterfront: New Post-Political Modes of Urban Governance'. *Urban Planning 5* (1): pp. 69–83.

Centers for Disease Control and Prevention (CDC). 2020. 'Healthy Equity Considerations and Racial and Ethnic Minority Groups'. *Coronavirus Disease 2019 (COVID-19)*, 24 July. https://www.cdc.gov/coronavirus/2019-ncov/community/health-equity/race-ethnicity.html.

Charmes, Eric, and Roger Keil. 2015. 'The Politics of Post-Suburban Densification in Canada and France'. *International Journal of Urban and Regional Research 39* (3): pp. 581–602.

Churchman, Azra. 1999. 'Disentangling the Concept of Density'. *Journal of Planning Literature 13* (4): pp. 289–411.

Cities Alliance. 2010. 'Citywide Pro-poor Ger Area Upgrading Strategy of Ulaanbaatar City'. Cities Alliance Project Output Document Number P098471. Ulaanbaatar, Mongolia: UN-Habitat.

City of Vancouver. 2020. 'Laneway Housing How-To Guide'. Vancouver: City of Vancouver.

Cook, Nicole, Elizabeth Taylor, and Joe Hurley. 2013. 'At Home with Strategic Planning: Reconciling Resident Attachments to Home with Policies of Residential Densification'. *Australian Planner 50* (2): pp. 130–7.

Cook, Nicole T., Ilan Wiesel, and Fanqi Liu. 2018. 'Are Urban Development and Densification Patterns Aligned with Infrastructure Funding Allocation? Examining Data from Melbourne 1999–2015'. Faculty of Social Sciences Paper, University of Melbourne.

Cordes, Jack, and Marcia C. Castro. 2020. 'Spatial Analysis of COVID-19 Clusters and Contextual Factors in New York City'. *Spatial and Spatio-Temporal Epidemiology 34*: 100355.

Coryne, Haru. 2020. 'In Chicago, Urban Density May Not Be to Blame for the Spread of the Coronavirus'. *ProPublica Illinois*. 30 April.

Coss, Stephen. 2016. *The Fever of 1721: The Epidemic That Revolutionized Medicine and American Politics*. New York: Simon and Schuster.

Courtenay, William J. 1980. 'The Effect of the Black Death on English Higher Education'. *Speculum 55* (4): pp. 696–714.

Dave, Seema. 2010. 'High Urban Densities in Developing Countries: A Sustainable Solution?' *Built Environment 36* (1): pp. 9–27.

Delmelle, Elizabeth C., Yuhong Zhou, and Jean-Claude Thill. 2014. 'Densification without Growth Management? Evidence from Local Land Development and Housing Trends in Charlotte, North Carolina, USA'. *Sustainability 6* (6): pp. 3975–90.

Delves-Broughton, Philip. 2020. 'As New Yorkers Flee, the Suburbs Are under Siege'. *The Spectator*, 5 September.

Dempsey, Nicola, Glen Bramley, Sinéad Power, and Caroline Brown. 2011. 'The Social Dimension of Sustainable Development: Defining Urban Social Sustainability'. *Sustainable Development 19* (5): pp. 289–300.

Dillon, Liam. 2019. 'California Could Bring Radical Change to Single Family Home Neighborhoods'. *Los Angeles Times*, 13 May.

Donald, Betsy, Amy Glasmeier, Miam Gray, and Linda Lobao. 2014. 'Austerity in the City: Economic Crisis and Urban Service Decline?' *Cambridge Journal of Regions, Economy and Society 7* (1): pp. 3–15.

Dougherty, Conor. 2017. 'The Great American Single Family Home Problem'. *New York Times*, 1 December.

Faleiro, Sonia. 2020. 'British Ethnic Minorities Are Being Left for Dead'. *New York Times*, 22 May.

Fang, Wanli, and Sameh Wahba. 2020. 'Urban Density Is Not an Enemy in Coronavirus Fight: Evidence from China'. World Bank Blog, 20 April. https://blogs.worldbank.org/sustainablecities/urban-density-not-enemy-coronavirus-fight-evidence-china.

Filion, Pierre. 2003. 'Towards Smart Growth? The Difficult Implementation of Alternatives to Urban Dispersion'. *Canadian Journal of Urban Research 12* (1): pp. 48–70.

Filion, Pierre, and Roger Keil. 2017. 'Contested Infrastructures: Tension, Inequity and Innovation in the Global Suburb'. *Urban Policy and Research 35* (1): pp. 7–19.

Flynn, Alexandra, and Mariana Valverde. 2019. 'Planning on the Waterfront: Setting the Agenda for Toronto's "Smart City" Project'. *Planning Theory & Practice 20* (5): pp. 769–75.

Gardiner, Joey. 2020. 'Inadequate UK Housing Blamed for Spread of COVID-19'. *Housing Today*, 8 June.

Hassan, Carma, and Brian Ries. 2020. 'Harvard Wants Students to Move Out in Five Days in Bid to "De-Densify" Campus over Coronavirus'. *CNN*, 10 March. https://www.cnn.com/2020/03/10/us/harvard-students-coronavirus-trnd/index.html.

Holpuch, Amanda. 2020. 'Luxury Resorts Face Coronavirus Crisis as the 1% Flee Cities for Holiday Hideaways'. *The Guardian*, 4 April.

Jones, Samantha, Katie J. Oven, Bernard Manyena, and Komal Aryal. 2014. 'Governance Struggles and Policy Processes in Disaster Risk Reduction: A Case Study from Nepal'. *Geoforum 57*: pp. 78–90.

Lehmann, Steffen. 2019. 'Urban Density'. In *Wiley-Blackwell Encyclopaedia of Urban and Regional Studies*, edited by Anthony M. Orum, pp. 1–9. Hoboken, NJ: John Wiley and Sons.

Luckhoff, Paula. 2020. 'Urgent Plans Being Made to De-Densify Du-Noon and Kosovo amid Covid-19 Spread'. *DW.com*, 29 March. https://www.capetalk.co.za/articles/379188/urgent-plans-being-made-to-de-densify-du-noon-and-kosovo-amid-covid-19-spread.

Manville, Michael, Paavo Monkkonen, and Michael Lens. 2020. 'It's Time to End Single-Family Zoning'. *Journal of the American Planning Association 86* (1): pp. 106–12.

McDonald, David A., and John Pape. 2002. *Cost Recovery and the Crisis of Service Delivery in South Africa*. Cape Town: HSRC publishers.

Miller, Mark. 2019. 'State Lawmakers Hash Out Housing Legislation'. *The Astorian*, 22 April.

Moore, Aaron A. 2013. *Trading Density for Benefits: Toronto and Vancouver Compared*. Toronto: Institute on Municipal Finance and Governance.

Mukhija, Vinit. 2014. 'Outlaw In-Laws: Informal Second Units and the Stealth Reinvention of Single-Family Housing'. In *The Informal American City: Beyond Taco Trucks and Day Labor*, edited by Vinit Mukhija and Anastasia Loukaitou-Sideris, pp. 39–59. Cambridge, MA: MIT Press.

Nixson, Frederick, and Bernard Walters. 2006. 'Privatization, Income Distribution, and Poverty: the Mongolian Experience'. *World Development 34* (9): pp. 1557–79.

O'Kane, Josh. 2020. 'Sidewalk's End: How the Downfall of a Toronto "Smart City" Plan Began Long before COVID-19'. *Globe and Mail*, 24 May.

Oh, Kyushik, Yeunwoo Jeong, Dongkun Lee, Wangkey Lee, and Jaeyong Choi. 2005. 'Determining Development Density Using the Urban Carrying Capacity Assessment System'. *Landscape and Urban Planning, 73* (1): pp. 1–15.

Organisation for Economic Co-operation and Development (OECD). 2012. *Compact City Policies: A Comparative Assessment*. Paris: OECD.

Pain, Kathy, Daniel Black, John Blower, et al. 2018. *Supporting Smart Urban Development: Successful Investing in Density*. London: Urban Land Institute and the Coalition for Urban Transitions.

Peirce, Sean. 2002. 'Selling Urban Housing in London. Can High-Density Urban Living be Sold to a Sceptical British Public? Distinction, Mobility, and Control over Environment'. *European Planning Studies 10* (8): pp. 955–70.

Peters, Deike. 2016. 'Density Wars in Silicon Beach'. In *Protest and Resistance in the Tourist City*, edited by Claire Colomb and Johannes Novy, pp. 90–106. London: Routledge.

Quastel, Noah, Markus Moos, and Nicholas Lynch. 2012. 'Sustainability-as-Density and the Return of the Social: The Case of Vancouver, British Columbia'. *Urban Geography 33* (7): pp. 1055–84.

Ramirez de la Cruz, Edgar E. 2009. 'Local Political Institutions and Smart Growth: An Empirical Study of the Politics of Compact Development'. *Urban Affairs Review 45* (2): pp. 218–46.

Rousseau, Max. 2015. '"Many Rivers to Cross": Suburban Densification and the Social Status Quo in Greater Lyon'. *International Journal of Urban and Regional Research 39* (3): pp. 622–32.

Sampson, Robert. 2014. 'Notes on Neighborhood Inequality and Urban Design'. *The Cities Papers, SSRC*. http://citiespapers.ssrc.org/notes-on-neighborhood-inequality-and-urban-design.

Saroj, Shashi Kala, Srinivas Goli, Md Juel Rana, and Bikramaditya K. Choudhary. 2020. 'Availability, Accessibility, and Inequalities of Water, Sanitation, and Hygiene (WASH) Services in Indian Metro Cities'. *Sustainable Cities and Society 54*: p. 101878.

Satow, Julie. 2020. 'Movers in N.Y.C. Are So Busy They're Turning People Away'. *New York Times*, 20 August.
Scott, James C. 2017. *Against the Grain: A Deep History of the Earliest States*. New Haven, CT: Yale University Press.
Scott, Lucy. 2015. 'Overcoming the Resistance to More Density'. *Urban Land Magazine*, 6 July.
Searle, Glen. 2003. 'Planning Under-Empowerment and Urban Over-Development in Inner Sydney'. Presentation made to the State of Australian Cities Conference, Parramatta, Australia, 3–5 December.
Shih, Mi, and Leslie Shieh. 2020. 'Negotiating Density and Financing Public Goods in Vancouver and New Taipei City: A Development Rights Perspective'. *Planning Practice and Research 1*: pp. 1–16.
Stahl, Kenneth. 2018. '"Yes in My Backyard": Can a New Pro-Housing Movement Overcome the Power of NIMBYs?' *Zoning & Planning Law Report 41* (3): pp. 1–16.
Sun, Weizeng, Yuming Fu, and Siqi Zheng. 2017. 'Local Public Service Provision and Spatial Inequality in Chinese Cities: The Role of Residential Income Sorting and Land-Use Conditions'. *Journal of Regional Science 57* (4): pp. 547–67.
Swanstrom, Todd, Peter Dreier, and John Mollenkopf. 2002. 'Economic Inequality and Public Policy: The Power of Place'. *City & Community 1* (4): pp. 349–72.
Tai, Don Bambino Geno, Aditya Shah, Chyke A. Doubeni, et al. 2020. 'The Disproportionate Impact of COVID-19 on Racial and Ethnic Minorities in the United States'. *Clinical Infectious Diseases 72* (4): pp.703-706.
UN-Habitat. 2013. 'Revised Compilation for Sustainable Cities and Human Settlements in the Sustainable Development Goals (SDGs) within the Post-2015 Development Agenda'. 20 December. http://urbansdg.org/wp-content/uploads/2014/01/Revised_Cities_SDG_Compilation_20_Dec_2013.pdf.
UN Habitat. 2016. *World Cities Report 2016*. Nairobi: UN Habitat.
United Nations International Children's Emergency Fund (UNICEF). 2018. 'Mongolia's Air Pollution Crisis: A Call to Action to Protect Children's Health'. Discussion paper. Ulaanbaatar, Mongolia: UNICEF.
Urban Task Force. 1999. *Towards an Urban Renaissance*. London: E&FN Spon.
Vallance, Suzanne, Harvey C. Perkins, and Kevin Moore. 2005. 'The Results of Making a City More Compact: Neighbours' Interpretation of Urban Infill'. *Environment and Planning B 32* (5): pp. 715–33.
Vincent, Donovan, and David Rider. 2020. 'Sidewalk Labs Pulls Out of Toronto Quayside Project, Blaming COVID-19'. *Toronto Star*, 7 May.
Virginia Department of Health. 1908. 'Scarlet Fever, Diphtheria, and Disinfection'. *Virginia Health Bulletin 1* (6): p. 216.
Wegmann, Jake. 2020. 'Death to Single-Family Zoning … and New Life to the Missing Middle'. *Journal of the American Planning Association 86* (1): pp. 113–9.
Wells, Jane, 2020. 'After Coronavirus: The Office of the Future is the Office of the Past'. CNBC, 27 April. https://www.cnbc.com/2020/04/27/after-coronavirus-the-office-of-the-future-is-the-office-of-the-past.html.
Wiener, Scott, and Anthony Iton. 2020. 'A Backlash against Cities Would be Dangerous'. *The Atlantic*, 17 May.
World Bank. 2010. *Managing Urban Expansion in Mongolia*. Washington, DC: World Bank.
Xiao, Hong, Xiaoling Lin, Gerardo Chowell, et al. 2014. 'Urban Structure and the Risk of Influenza A (H1N1) Outbreaks in Municipal Districts'. *Chinese Science Bulletin* 59 (5–6): pp. 554–62.

8

Pandemics and the Use of Exceptions in International Economic Law

One Step Forward, Two Steps Back?

Charles-Emmanuel Côté, Richard Ouellet, and Jean-Michel Marcoux

Over the past few decades, states have adopted several international agreements that are geared toward protecting the movement of goods, services, and capital among them. In addition to the agreements that constitute the legal framework of the World Trade Organization (WTO), several states have negotiated regional trade agreements with the objective of pursuing deeper economic integration. At the time of writing this chapter, 306 regional free trade agreements were in force (WTO 2020b). Moreover, states have negotiated international agreements that specifically focus on the protection and the promotion of foreign investment. When adding the investment chapters found in regional free trade agreements to bilateral investment treaties, a total of 3,284 international investment agreements emerge (UNCTAD 2020b: xii). This growing web of international agreements, as well as their interpretation by a variety of panels and tribunals, constitute the main sources of international economic law.

The liberalization of economic relations between states unavoidably implies a tension with a variety of societal values and interests. The protection of public health, consumer safety, the environment, employment, economic development, public morality, and national security all constitute 'core tasks of governments' that must be guaranteed in addition to the protection of trade and foreign investment (e.g. Van den Bossche and Zdouc 2017: 544). There is thus a need to reconcile the right of states to regulate for legitimate objectives of public policy with their obligations under international economic law. It is for this specific purpose that various exceptions are included in some international agreements. These exceptions can be used to justify a measure that would otherwise be found inconsistent with the obligations that are included in international agreements.

Like other issues of international law addressed in this book (Chapter 15 by Parent and Chapter 16 by Bjorklund), the significance of exceptions in international

Charles-Emmanuel Côté, Richard Ouellet, and Jean-Michel Marcoux, *Pandemics and the Use of Exceptions in International Economic Law*. In: *A Multidisciplinary Approach to Pandemics*. Edited by Philippe Bourbeau, Jean-Michel Marcoux, and Brooke A. Ackerly, Oxford University Press. © Oxford University Press (2022). DOI: 10.1093/oso/9780192897855.003.0009

agreements is even more vivid in the context of pandemics. When considering the magnitude of the economic shock unleashed by the global health crisis combined with a high demand for medical products, the COVID-19 outbreak clearly differs from previous pandemics (UNCTAD 2020c: 12–23). The United Nations Conference on Trade and Development highlighted the uniqueness of the COVID-19 pandemic in the following terms:

> Never before has nearly half of the world population endured lockdown conditions, and never before have so many people been asked to change their daily activities and routines so quickly, with such consequences. Changes to ways of working, producing and consuming have been sudden and dramatic. All of this will make 2020 a year to be remembered for a long time to come.
>
> (UNCTAD 2020c: 111)

The COVID-19 outbreak thus offers a crucially important moment to reflect upon the use of exceptions in international economic law.

Pandemics force states to adopt measures that can have a negative impact on international economic relations in order to keep their populations safe and to protect particularly sensitive sectors of their domestic economy. From export restrictions of medical equipment to foreign investment screening procedures and lockdowns, the COVID-19 outbreak resulted in several measures that profoundly disrupted business activities across borders. For international economic lawyers, the justification of these measures by exceptions included in international agreements bears implications that must be taken into consideration. Focusing on the broader implications of these exceptions in the context of COVID-19, some authors have already identified an acceleration of the use of exceptions that could ultimately threaten the stability and legitimacy of international trade and investment law (Arato et al. 2020). In contrast to exceptions that allow the imposition of trade barriers, it has also been suggested that requiring free trade might be a more promising solution to addressing a pandemic (Pinchis Paulssen 2020). The use of exceptions thus seems to prevent the alignment of incentives with an efficient production and allocation of key resources that are crucially needed to fight the pandemic.

This chapter builds on these contributions to address the relevance of exceptions in international economic law in a context of pandemics. By focusing on the provisions that can be used by states to justify the adoption of measures intended to protect public health and the economy at the national level, it highlights an important tension. On the one hand, the use of exceptions in the context of a global health crisis may call for an extended interpretation of concepts that can lead to easier justifications of trade and investment restrictions in the future. On the other hand, an effective reliance on exceptions can ultimately hinder efforts to fight the pandemic globally. In order to shed light on this tension, this chapter focuses on exceptions that can be raised by states both in the context of international trade law and international investment law.

Pandemics and Exceptions under WTO Law

Trade measures that have been applied by WTO Members in response to the COVID-19 pandemic seem to operate in a context that differs from what the multilateral trading system is used to coping with. The General Agreement on Tariffs and Trade (GATT) and the agreements that constitute the current legal framework of the WTO establish legal rules that generally seek to limit the ability of governments to impose barriers to market access (e.g. Kerr 2009: 2). Protectionist measures applied by WTO Members are often designed to restrict imports. Legitimate measures aimed at protecting human, animal, or plant life or health also usually take the form of a ban of imports or a restriction of access to the domestic market of the country that intends to prevent the entry of a peril to its territory. In the case of previous pandemics, governments have generally forbidden the entry of products that could spread the virus, the pest, or the disease. Trade restrictions on pork and other meat products during the A/H1N1 crisis of 2009 are a case in point (Lin 2010: 527).

By contrast, one of the main preoccupations of governments during the COVID-19 pandemic was geared towards avoiding shortages of critical products—medical devices, personal protective equipment (PPE), drugs, or vaccines—that were essential to fight the spread of the virus and to treat patients within their own territory. The majority of the measures notified to the WTO Secretariat in the context of the COVID-19 crisis thus included export restrictions of goods such as face masks, disposable gloves or gowns, test kits, respirators, hand sanitizer, or foodstuffs (WTO 2020a). Other measures suspended the application of tariff duties on the imports of the same categories of products. At the same time, several governments made clear that they did not intend to act inconsistently with their obligations under international trade law. As the ministers responsible for the WTO from 48 Members explicitly declared at the General Council on 31 July 2020:

> We stress that trade restrictive emergency measures aimed at protecting health, if deemed necessary, shall be targeted, proportionate, transparent and temporary, not create unnecessary barriers to trade or disruption to global supply chains, and be consistent with WTO rules.... A predictable, transparent, non-discriminatory and open global trading system will be essential for broad-based, sustainable economic recovery. We, therefore, strongly reaffirm our support for the rules-based multilateral trading system and the central role of the WTO. We will continue to act in a manner consistent with our WTO rights and obligations.
>
> (WTO 2020c)

Even though no clear protectionist impulse underlies the application of the COVID-19 trade-restricting measures, and no WTO Member seems to be ready to fight decisions made by other governments to protect their people in these troubled times, trade disputes remain entirely possible. It is in this context that exceptions found in the WTO agreements become particularly relevant. After exploring how the current pandemic constitutes a challenge to the WTO rules and jurisprudence, this section underscores that Article XX and Article XXI of the GATT are not fit to cope with a global challenge such as the current health crisis. COVID-19 thus opens a window of opportunity to revisit the use and abuse of those exceptions.

Pandemics as a Challenge to WTO Disciplines and Jurisprudence

Leaving aside the risk of shortages caused by a hording panic that can result from trade restrictions of a specific good, it is worth exploring how international trade rules apply to measures that have been recently adopted by states in the context of the COVID-19 pandemic. One of the trade disciplines that must be considered relates to the prohibition of quantitative restrictions (i.e. quotas). In addition to rules that ensure a non-discriminatory treatment of products sold across borders and obligations pertaining to tariff barriers, international trade law sets out specific rules that limit the ability of states to impose quantitative restrictions on the importation and the exportation of goods. Entitled 'General Elimination of Quantitative Restrictions', GATT Article XI:1 proscribes 'prohibitions or restrictions other than duties, taxes or other charges, whether made effective through quotas ... export licences or other measures ... on the exportation or sale for export of any product'. It is important to note that Article XI:1 only applies to quantitative restrictions. The wording is clear: the prohibition does not apply to export duties or charges. Interestingly enough, to the best of our knowledge, no WTO Member has notified the Secretariat of a COVID-related measure that restricts trade of goods by applying export duties or taxes.

The general prohibition on quantitative restrictions is immediately followed by a carve-out provision. Article XI:2 provides that the prohibition does not extend to '[e]xport prohibitions or restrictions temporarily applied to prevent or relieve critical shortages of foodstuffs or other products essential to the exporting contracting party'. The Appellate Body of the WTO, in the *China—Raw Materials* case (WTO 2012), interpreted and defined some of the terms and expressions used in this provision. While the dispute did not relate to measures adopted in the context of a pandemic, the interpretation provided by the Appellate Body could have important implications if a panel were asked to determine the legality of export restrictions adopted since the COVID-19 outbreak. More specifically, the Appellate Body found 'that Article XI:2 describes measures applied for a limited duration, adopted in order to bridge a passing need, irrespective of whether or not the temporal scope of the measure is fixed in advance' (WTO 2012: para. 331). It also defined a 'critical shortage' as 'deficiencies in quantity that are crucial, that amount to a situation of decisive importance, or that reach a vitally important or decisive stage, or a turning point' (WTO 2012: para. 324). In line with the jurisprudence already established, the Appellate Body defined the term 'essential' as 'absolutely indispensable or necessary' (WTO 2012: para. 326).

Scholars seem to disagree about the possibility for WTO members to justify COVID-related export restrictions under the regime provided by Article XI. According to some authors, the measures adopted by states could fall under the scope of the carve-out provision and not be considered as violating the prohibition of quantitative restriction. For example, Joost Pauwelyn (2020) considers that international law generally offers enough leeway to enact restrictions during a pandemic. With respect to disciplines on export restriction, he is of the opinion that:

> As long as pandemic related export restrictions are 'temporarily applied,' limited to foodstuffs or 'essential products' and demonstrated to 'prevent or relieve critical shortages,' GATT Article XI:2(a) should, therefore, exempt such restrictions from the general prohibition in Article XI:1.
>
> (Pauwelyn 2020: 736)

Similarly, for Ignacio Carrenõ and colleagues, 'the WTO Appellate Body's interpretation of Article XI:2 of the GATT appears to provide Members with the authority to restrict exports of food and medical supplies as long as necessary in order to prevent critical shortages' (2020: 407).

By contrast, instead of focusing on the carve-out provision of Article XI:2, other authors consider that export restrictions would need to be justified by relying on general exceptions that are included in the GATT. For Julian Arato, Kathleen Claussen, and J. Benton Heath:

> WTO panels generally do not consider regulatory aims when applying these disciplines. A state's justificatory aim is typically relevant only after a *prima facie* violation is established and an exception is in play. Thus, any pandemic-related measure that discriminates among trading partners *de jure* or *de facto*, or that burdens free transit or imposes export restrictions, would likely have to be justified by reference to some exception.
>
> (Arato et al. 2020: 629)

Viktoria Lapa expresses more or less the same opinion when she posits that '[s]ince most of [COVID-19 export] restrictions would be contrary to WTO Members' commitments under General Agreement on Tariffs and Trade (GATT) Article XI, the question arises how to justify them' (2020: 340).

When the most esteemed scholars in the field of international economic law differ on the effect and the limits of a fundamental rule of the world trading system, one must admit that this system is under challenge. The absence of an 'aim and effect' test of a measure when applying the rules of the GATT, coupled with the extensive analysis of its contribution to the achievement of a non-trade objective when applying an exception, reveal a certain shrinkage of the role of the GATT rules in the conciliation between freedom of trade and other current objectives of today's governments. More specifically, when strictly considering the obligations imposed on WTO Members by trade rules and disciplines, measures adopted by states in the context of a pandemic can be problematic. The extent to which states can limit exports of products used to fight a pandemic can potentially conflict with the prohibition of quantitative export restrictions, despite the existence of additional provisions authorizing temporary restrictions of products that are essential to the exporting states. It is in this context that reliance on exceptions appears to be a reliable tool from a legal perspective to justify a potential violation of these obligations imposed on WTO Members.

An Opportunity to Revisit the Role and the Effects of the Exceptions in WTO Law

The compliance of national trade measures related to COVID-19 with the GATT ultimately depends on the possibility of invoking exceptions to justify a potential violation of obligations imposed on states under the GATT. The fragile equilibrium between free trade and non-market values or legitimate objectives pursued by countries is found by applying the general exceptions of Article XX or the national security exception of Article XXI. More specifically, Article XX of the GATT allows WTO Members to adopt measures that seek to achieve various legitimate objectives, such as the protection of human, animal, or plant life or health. The adoption of these measures is nevertheless subject to an additional requirement found in the introductory paragraph of the Article, which provides that the measures 'are not applied in a manner which would constitute a means of arbitrary or unjustifiable discrimination between countries where the same conditions prevail, or a disguised restriction on international trade'. In addition to this regime of general exceptions, Article XXI(b) provides that the GATT shall not be construed 'to prevent any contracting party from taking any action which it considers necessary for the protection of its essential security interests'.

The coexistence of a general exception that relates to public health and an exception to protect essential security interests raises an important question in the context of the GATT. While the terms included in Article XXI arguably allow the state to have more discretion when applying the measure than the general exception regime, one wonders if extending the concept of national security to include a health crisis is allowed under the GATT. In other words, it could be argued that the express reference to the protection of 'human, animal or plant life and health' under Article XX ultimately prevents the reliance upon Article XXI to justify a measure taken in the context of a health crisis.

Most importantly, even if states could potentially use exceptions to justify measures intended to protect the health of their populations or their security interests, the broader implications of using exceptions in the context of a pandemic must be carefully considered. For example, Arato and colleagues reject the idea of 'exceptionalism'—'a paradigm of justification according to which deviations from primary rules are absolved by way of "exceptions" (express or implied), and in which claims of exception can be expected to proliferate' (Arato et al. 2020: 628). This phenomenon is a source of risks and perils, for international economic law in particular and for public international law in general. These authors summarize those risks by two formulas: the 'ossification of underlying rules' and the 'colonizing expansion of international economic law' over other fields of international law. Arato and colleagues are of the opinion that the regulatory aim of a national measure should always be taken into consideration, and they suggest resuscitating the 'aim-and-effect' test rejected by the Appellate Body in the *Japan—Alcoholic Beverages II* case (WTO 1996). Those ideas fit considerations that have been articulated beyond the consideration of measures adopted in the context of pandemics. In previously published papers, Claussen (2020) advocates for the 'de-exceptionalisation' of the relation between trade and security. Similarly, Heath (2020) argues that 'the relationship between trade and security appears to be undergoing a historic transformation', thus calling for models that reconcile expanded security interests with trade obligations (2020: 223).

In addition to questioning the abuse of exceptions in the WTO legal regime, other scholars shed light on the adverse effects of exceptions. Tracing a link between the basic right to food, the concept of food security, and the national security exception, and after analysing the report of the panel in the *Russia—Traffic in Transit* case (WTO 2019), Lapa (2020) concludes that 'one could claim that GATT Article XXI(b)iii might be used by WTO Members which want to justify their export restrictions on foodstuff during pandemics like COVID-19'. However, she apparently deplores the effect of the wording of Article XXI. Taking into consideration the inclusion of the terms 'it considers necessary', the necessity of such export restrictions lies within the full discretion of the Member that adopts the measure. This contrasts with the general exceptions provided under Article XX. For Lapa, leaving so much leeway to each WTO Member in a context of emergency is regrettable: 'Globalization and national resilience if not survival do not exclude each other. On the contrary, there is evidence that food export restrictions will make everybody worse off in the long term given the interconnection of global supply chains' (Lapa 2020: 340; see also Petetin 2020: 328). Jingyuan Zhou (2020), and Tsai-Yu Lin (2010) apply the same kind of reasoning to the public health field. Zhou (2020) affirms that the International Health Regulations of the World Health Organization and the WTO rules work together to promote 'collective actions based on scientific evidence, close communication, and against discriminatory measures'. For him, public health is better served by free trade than by national measures of restriction. If borders remain open in times of a public health emergency of international concern, 'labs and researchers work collectively, though located separately, to study novel viruses' (Zhou 2020).

Obviously, the time has come to question the role and the effects of the exceptions in the world trading system. Some even believe that the pandemic creates a rare opportunity for radical change (Petetin 2020: 336). The most innovative idea certainly comes from Mona Pinchis Paulsen (2020), who proposes the concept of 'inverse exception'. For her, GATT exceptions are not adapted to the global nature of COVID-19. Trading nations are not currently facing multiple threats to their own national security. Rather, it is humanity that is facing one global threat. What is crucial is 'maintaining open trade to ensur[e] necessary supplies can go where needed'. Pinchis Paulsen concedes that the functioning of this proposal would not be easy and would depend on the creation of a new WTO specialized body resting on cooperation, transparency, and political will. It is ambitious, especially in the context of the institutional crisis the WTO is going through right now.

In summary, reliance on exceptions included in international trade agreements to justify measures adopted during a pandemic can be problematic on several fronts. International trade rules are challenged by the pandemic, and exceptions lead to the exact opposite of what the community of trading nations needs. The exceptions articulated in GATT Article XX and Article XXI allow each Member State to apply a national public policy to protect its own population. However, an extensive use of these exceptions can have deeper impacts on the primary rules that currently underlie the multilateral trade regime. Moreover, those exceptions could allow for discrimination and quantitative restrictions in times when fairness and free flow of essential products to fight the pandemic are needed more than ever.

Before turning to the use of exceptions in international investment law, it is worth emphasizing that reliance on exceptions significantly differs from the adoption of a waiver under WTO law. Such a distinction is particularly important in light of efforts deployed by some states to address barriers created by intellectual property rights to access vaccines and medicines. In a communication submitted in October 2020, India and South Africa requested that the Council for Trade-Related Aspects of Intellectual Property Rights (TRIPS) recommends to the General Council a waiver from the application of several provisions of the TRIPS Agreement (WTO 2020d). Such a waiver can be adopted pursuant to Article IX:3–4 of the Marrakesh Agreement Establishing the World Trade Organization to waive an obligation imposed on Member States for a specific period of time. Moreover, recent treaty practice excludes measures affecting intellectual property rights, such as compulsory licenses for vaccines, from the purview of international investment law as long as they are consistent with WTO law (e.g. Canada–United States–Mexico Agreement Articles 14.8.6, 14.10.3, and 14.12.4; Comprehensive Economic and Trade Agreement Articles 8.12.5, 8.12.6, and 8.15.4). By contrast, exceptions are used by states to justify a measure that would otherwise be inconsistent with their obligations under a specific agreement. While the role of intellectual property rights is a key and highly contentious aspect regarding the fight of pandemics, it has not been addressed through exceptions as far as COVID-19 is concerned.

Foreign Investment and Exceptions in Times of Global Pandemic

In addition to challenges related to international trade, the health crisis has shed light on problems associated with the free flow of capital. Under the framework of investment agreements, foreign investors can freely enter host states to purchase or establish businesses in sensitive sectors such as medical equipment or other health-related goods or services, export their production at their will to global markets, or shut down their plants and leave with valuable technological knowledge. They can also abandon less lucrative activities, despite their importance for the health authorities of the host state. It is no surprise that most states engaged in tightening their grip on foreign investors in the wake of the COVID-19 pandemic, whether by restricting admission into the national economy or interfering with the free operation of their businesses (UNCTAD 2020a). Investment made by foreign states also came under increased suspicion in this context, within a climate where state-owned enterprises and sovereign wealth funds had already been under much scrutiny in many parts of the world (Organisation for Economic Co-operation and Development (OECD) 2008). All these measures taken hastily are designed to preserve the capacity of host state health authorities to fight the pandemic and protect their population, without much coordination or care for the international community.

International investment agreements go well beyond the basic protection offered by customary international law to foreign residents and their property, and by diplomatic protection of their home state. Typically, they include guarantees in favour of foreign investors and their investment for non-discriminatory treatment (i.e. national treatment and most-favoured-nation treatment), fair and equitable treatment, and expropriation with compensation, as well as freedom to move capital in and out of the host state. In some cases, investment agreements even grant a right of admission to foreign investors, extending protection at the pre-investment stage. Various reservations, carve-outs, and exceptions, including a national security exception, may be provided to balance foreign investor protection with the right of the host state to regulate for legitimate purposes of public concern. In the context of the COVID-19 pandemic, states have instinctively assumed that measures taken to fight the pandemic must be allowed, despite this stringent legal framework, whether under treaty exceptions or customary international law defences. By doing so, and in this context of emergency, not much analysis has been given to the legal justification of these extraordinary measures.

A Quick Survey of Measures to Fight the COVID-19 Pandemic: The Affected Foreign Investors

In addition to causing a significant backlash on the global flow of foreign investment in the world (UNCTAD 2020b: 3–6), the COVID-19 pandemic slowed the pace of conclusion of new investment agreements (UNCTAD 2020a: 11). On the national level, two types of measures that may affect or directly concern foreign investment were taken. Specific measures forcing businesses to alter their production or exports were imposed in order to prioritize supplying the host state's market with medical equipment or other goods needed by health authorities. Screening of new foreign investment was also enhanced in many states, especially in the health sector or regarding businesses that became more vulnerable to foreign takeover due to the disruption of the economy. These measures may conflict with basic protection guaranteed by investment agreements.

Some countries adopted new restrictions on the free operation of businesses in the health sector, without specifically targeting foreign investors (UNCTAD 2020a: 9). One of the first restrictions was a mandatory order to produce goods needed to fight the pandemic. Switzerland adopted new legislation allowing the government to order mandatory production of public health-related goods. The US government ordered a car manufacturer to switch production to medical equipment on the basis of existing legislation. A second restriction related to the temporary confiscation by governments of production facilities or goods needed to protect public health. Both Spain and Switzerland enacted new legislation for that purpose. A third restriction consisted of an imposition by over 47 countries of export bans or export licensing for medical equipment and other public health-related goods, such as PPE, sanitizer products, medical ventilators, or drugs and pharmaceutical ingredients.

Many countries strengthened their screening procedure to prevent new foreign investment in the health sector or the takeover of vulnerable businesses in other sectors of the economy (UNCTAD 2020a: 7–8). To do so, they either announced more robust application of existing screening mechanisms or created new ones. It must be emphasized, however, that a steady trend in creating or intensifying screening of new foreign investment was already well under way in OECD countries before the COVID-19 pandemic (OECD 2020a: 3–4). Foreign investment screening mechanisms vary significantly from one country to the other, but they generally aim to prevent investment that is contrary to national security and subject the admission of new foreign investment to governmental approval. In rarer cases, they subject approval more broadly to a positive contribution to the economy of the host state, a policy that is not well regarded by the OECD, as it is too restrictive for the free movement of capital (OECD 2020b: Article 3).

The COVID-19 pandemic led to an expanded interpretation of the concept of national security by many countries to include a public health emergency (UNCTAD 2020a: 7). Prior to the health crisis, at least 29 countries already had a screening mechanism in place, including Canada, China, and the United States. Australia lowered the monetary threshold of its mechanism to cover all new foreign investment and extended the applicable delays. The European Union (EU), for its part, urged all member states to make full use of their existing screening mechanisms, or to set one up to preserve the capacity of the EU to protect the health of its citizens. Italy enlarged the scope of its mechanism to cover additional sectors like finance, credit, and insurances, and even to screen intra-EU investment. Spain adopted a new mechanism subjecting all new foreign acquisitions of at least 10% of stocks of any business to government approval.

The case of Canada is informative in this regard. Its screening mechanism remains one of the most restrictive among OECD members (Côté 2012: 252–67; Frigon 2011). Two different mechanisms coexist in Canada to screen new foreign investments by virtue of the Investment Canada Act. First, a general mechanism allows screening of all foreign acquisitions of Canadian businesses over a certain monetary threshold to analyse their economic contribution. This threshold varies according to the nationality of the foreign investor, the nature of its ownership, or the industry in which it seeks to invest. The legal test that must be met for the foreign takeover to be authorized is one assessing the 'net benefit' for the Canadian economy in light of a series of general factors that are examined. The minister responsible for the mechanism usually negotiates binding undertakings with the foreign investor to help tip the balance in favour of the authorization. Despite its shortcomings in terms of cumbersomeness, lack of transparency, and enforceability of undertakings, only two foreign takeovers have been blocked since the creation of the general screening mechanism in 1985.

A second mechanism was added in 2009 to screen all new foreign investments, both acquisitions and the creation of new Canadian businesses, for national security purposes. No monetary threshold exists, and any foreign investment may be subjected to a security screening at the will of the minister. It can even be applied retroactively to foreign investment up to 45 days after the establishment of a business, and no general factors are used to streamline the examination. The final decision is made at the highest political level, by decree, and at the total discretion of the federal government, and there is no transparency to the process. Since its entry into force, more foreign investment projects have been blocked under this new national security screening mechanism than under the general one (Canada 2019: 16–17).

In a policy statement issued shortly after the outbreak of the COVID-19 pandemic, the Canadian government announced that the screening of foreign investment would be more severe (Canada 2020). The policy statement affirms in the clearest possible manner that national security includes the individual health and safety of Canadians. It points to the two main problems caused by the pandemic: the abrupt loss in value of Canadian businesses and the importance of keeping control over businesses in the public health sector. Consequently, all acquisitions of businesses in that sector, as well as others supplying goods and services critical to Canadians or the government, will be screened, notwithstanding their value or the effective control gained by the foreign investor over a business. Moreover, all acquisitions by foreign state-owned enterprises will be systematically reviewed, notwithstanding their value, given the amplified risk they pose to the economy and national security in the current crisis. Timelines applicable to the national security mechanism were extended accordingly by ministerial order pursuant to the Time Limits and Other Periods Act (COVID-19). This strict scrutiny of new foreign investment will be applied temporarily until the Canadian economy has fully recovered from the COVID-19 pandemic.

The Use of Exceptions in International Investment Law

The risk of foreign investor claims in the current context of the COVID-19 pandemic is serious enough for observers to have called for the suspension of investor–state dispute settlement regarding all measures taken to fight the pandemic (Bernasconi-Osterwalder et al. 2020). All the measures affecting foreign investment adopted by states to fight the pandemic may potentially be inconsistent with the legal guarantees offered by investment agreements, unless they are justified under applicable exceptions. When looking at the first category of measures restricting the free operation of businesses, potential breaches could include prohibited performance requirements, although export bans or compulsory production of goods are usually not forbidden specifically by investment agreements. Another potential violation could be the discriminatory application of such measures, overwhelmingly targeting businesses owned by foreign investors (in breach of national treatment) or of a specific foreign nationality (in breach of most-favoured-nation treatment). Problems with compensation in cases of temporary confiscation of production facilities or goods could also breach clauses regarding compensation of losses in cases of crisis or state of emergency. The fair and equitable treatment clause could also be violated in cases where there is an arbitrary application of these measures. When considering the intensification of screening of foreign investment, consistency with investment agreements depends on the granting of a right of admission to foreign investors. If provisions of the applicable investment agreement cover the pre-establishment phase of the investment, subjecting foreigners to a screening mechanism could potentially constitute a breach of national treatment (unless the right of admission is made conditional on conformity to national legislation or is subject to reservations).

Again, the case of Canada is illuminating in this regard. International investment agreements signed by Canada usually grant a right of admission to foreign investors, including national treatment at the pre-investment stage. Canada's screening mechanisms are nevertheless protected by a grandfather clause that is included in these agreements. While ensuring the legality of the screening mechanisms as they existed at the time the investment agreement entered into force, this clause is of limited relevance when considering additional restrictions to the admission of foreign investment adopted in the context of the COVID-19 pandemic. In fact, new restrictions that did not exist at the time of the entry into force cannot be added to the mechanisms under this reservation and must be justified under an applicable exception in order not to be in breach of the agreement. Because the general screening mechanism cannot be altered to make it more restrictive, the robust measures announced by Canada will be enforced through the far more flexible and discretionary national security mechanism. The lawfulness of these measures thus ultimately depends on the consistency of this mechanism and its application with the national security exception. The claim made by Canada that national security includes human health and safety goes to the heart of this issue and shows how the COVID-19 pandemic has informed the understanding of this exception in international investment law.

A minority of investment agreements include a national security exception, designed to justify measures otherwise inconsistent with the legal protection of foreign investors and their investment (UNCTAD 2009: xviii). It is found mostly in agreements that apply at the pre-investment stage and that grant a right of admission to foreign investors. In the absence of an exception, states are left with customary international law justifications, most notably with the state of necessity, as a circumstance excluding wrongfulness of their measure (International Law Commission (ILC) 2001: Article 25). Justifications based on customary international law may prove difficult to apply, if applicable at all, given their strict criteria or controversial coexistence with investment agreements (Paddeu and Parlett 2020; Ranjan 2016: 295–8).

Rarely, investment agreements also include a general exception concerning measures necessary to protect human health, which are akin to general exceptions found in GATT Article XX. General exceptions are difficult to successfully invoke because they are, as already mentioned, subjected to an additional test of legitimacy that is non-existent with the national security exception. This additional test requires that the measures are not 'applied in a manner that constitutes arbitrary or unjustifiable discrimination between investments or between investors' or a 'disguised restriction on international trade or investment' (Canada 2014: Article 18). Canada used to be until recently a strong proponent of this approach, but most states refrain from extending exceptions beyond national security. An issue that is raised is whether measures taken to fight the pandemic must be exclusively channelled through the general exception for human health. As mentioned above in the context of the GATT, the provision of general exceptions could have the unexpected result of preventing the extension of the national security exception to cover health safety and sanitary security in those agreements. Having to resort to general exceptions instead of the national security exception would make it more difficult to justify a measure adopted to fight the COVID-19 pandemic.

The national security exception appears to be easier to apply, given the absence of a legitimacy test. However, the great diversity in the wording of the exception in investment agreements requires us to be cautious when making generalizations about their interpretation (Mantilla Blanco and Pehl 2020: 40; UNCTAD 2009: xviii). A critical issue raised by the pandemic is whether national security can be interpreted to include health and safety considerations. Traditionally, the exception has been primarily concerned with national defence and state security, but it was recently raised in investment disputes in the context of the Argentinean economic crisis (Mantilla Blanco and Pehl 2020: 39) or to justify screening of foreign investment in strategic industries or critical infrastructures (UNCTAD 2009: xiv). As already mentioned, the current trend is for states to expand this interpretation to cover measures adopted to fight the COVID-19 pandemic. In the absence of a general exception on public health, this appears to be a legitimate claim and the national security exception seems sufficiently flexible to accommodate such interpretation (Ranjan 2016: 298). This practice could, in turn, constitute subsequent practice of the state parties when interpreting investment agreements, which would have to be taken into consideration when interpreting the exception.

In a way that echoes the concerns raised by the use of the national security exception in international trade law, a controversial issue in international investment law is whether it is self-judging or not for the state wishing to invoke it. A self-judging exception would provide wide discretion to the state, and it has been argued that it could even prevent arbitral tribunals from reviewing their application. However, national security exceptions in investment agreements appear to provide less flexibility to states and are generally interpreted as being non-self-judging (Mantilla Blanco and Pehl 2020: 36; OECD 2007: 105). Arbitral awards have considered that the self-judging character of a clause must be explicit. Even self-judging clauses should not by themselves prevent arbitral tribunals from having jurisdiction. Application of national security exceptions can therefore be reviewed by arbitral tribunals. The issue then becomes one of determining under which standard they may do so. Another controversy emerges concerning the use of the strict criteria of the state of necessity defence of customary international law in determining the standard of review arbitral tribunals could use (Mantilla Blanco and Pehl 2020: 57–60). The conclusion is that autonomous criteria should be used, but their exact content will depend on the wording of the specific agreement at hand. The application of national security exceptions in investment agreements is thus normally reviewable by arbitral tribunals, but the test to be met by the state to justify a measure remains easier than with general exceptions or customary international law defences. Despite the wide regulatory space left to governments by the national security exception, an emerging trend in treaty practice consists of explicitly removing its application from the scope of investor–state dispute settlement (Mantilla Blanco and Pehl 2020: 63).

The great flexibility of the national security exception points to the question of whether it actually leaves too much room of manoeuvre for states. First, voluntary or involuntary abuses during the pandemic to infringe on the rights of foreign investors remain possible. Second, restrictions on much-needed foreign investment might prove counterproductive for a state's economic recovery (OECD 2020a: 5–7; Nimac 2020). Third, no consideration of the interests of the global community seems to be taken into account in the application of the national security exception. Absent a legitimacy test, the arbitrary or discriminatory application of unilateral measures seems to be beyond question, even if they frustrate global efforts to fight the pandemic or coordinate initiatives to fairly allocate medical equipment or other goods needed across the world. This situation could particularly harm developing and least developed countries. The absence of consideration for multilateral efforts to fight pandemics may prove to be a downside of the use of the national security exception in international investment law revealed by the COVID-19 crisis.

Conclusion

The extent to which states can rely on exceptions provided in international economic agreements geared towards the protection of free trade and foreign investment has important implications in the context of a pandemic. On the one hand, reliance on these exceptions suggests a step forward. States can potentially rely upon these exceptions if another state or a foreign investor seeks to challenge measures adopted to protect public health or the national economy at the domestic level. The exceptions should provide enough room to justify these measures adopted in the context of a pandemic. On the other hand, justifying these same measures by relying on exceptions can also be considered as two steps backward. First, some of these exceptions have not been crafted for the specific context of pandemics. While invoking the national security exception might be welcome in order to justify a measure adopted in the context of a global health crisis, a broader interpretation of this specific exception might lead to unforeseen results in other areas. Second, allowing states to individually adopt measures to protect their populations can harm global efforts to fight the pandemic. The use of export restrictions for PPE and the screening of foreign investment are examples of measures that, while potentially justifiable by exceptions provided in international agreements, could prevent efforts to counter the pandemic at a broader scale or negatively affect post-pandemic economic recovery.

By allowing states to adopt measures that are geared towards the protection of their population and economy rather than contributing to multilateral efforts to fight pandemics, exceptions found in international agreements can exclude other countries from enjoying a world without pandemics and even jeopardize efforts deployed by them to control the outbreak. In other words, reliance upon exceptions could ultimately lead to inefficient and unjust outcomes (see the Introduction to this volume by Ackerly et al.). The support for the unilateral fight against pandemics underlying exceptionalism might ultimately defeat multilateral, cooperative global solutions. Bearing in mind the need to consider pandemics as opportunities to reach equitable solutions, a careful approach to the use of exceptions in international economic law must be sought.

References

Arato, Julian, Kathleen Claussen, and J. Benton Heath. 2020. 'The Perils of Pandemic Exceptionalism'. *American Journal of International Law* 114: p. 627.

Bernasconi-Osterwalder, Nathalie, Sarah Brewin, and Nyaguthii Maina. 2020. 'Protecting against Investor–State Claims amidst COVID-19: A Call to Action for Governments'. *IISD Commentary*, 14 April. https://www.iisd.org/articles/protecting-against-investor-state-claims-amidst-covid-19-call-action-governments.

Canada. 2014. 'Model Foreign Investment Promotion and Protection Agreement'. 25 August. https://www.italaw.com/sites/default/files/files/italaw8236.pdf.

Canada. 2019. *Investment Canada Act: Annual Report 2018–2019*. Ottawa: Innovation, Science and Economic Development Canada. https://www.ic.gc.ca/eic/site/ica-lic.nsf/eng/h_lk81126.html.

Canada. 2020. 'Policy Statement on Foreign Investment Review and COVID-19'. 18 April. https://www.ic.gc.ca/eic/site/ica-lic.nsf/eng/lk81224.html.

Carreño, Ignacio, Tobias Dolle, Lourdes Medina, and Moritz Brandenburger. 2020. 'The Implications of COVID-19 Pandemic on Trade'. *European Journal of Risk Regulation 11* (Special Issue 2): p. 402.

Claussen, Kathleen. 2020. 'Trade's Security Exceptionalism'. *Stanford Law Review* 72: p. 1097.

Côté, Charles-Emmanuel. 2012. 'Le Canada et l'investissement étranger: entre ouverture et inquiétude'. In *L'investissement et la nouvelle économie mondiale: trajectoires nationales, réseaux mondiaux et normes internationales*, edited by Mathieu Arès and Éric Boulanger, pp. 241–313. Brussels: Bruylant.

Frigon, Mathieu. 2011. 'The Foreign Investment Review Process in Canada'. Library of Parliament. https://lop.parl.ca/sites/PublicWebsite/default/en_CA/ResearchPublications/201142E.

Heath, J. Benton. 2020. 'Trade and Security among the Ruins'. *Duke Journal of Comparative and International Law 30* (2): p. 223.

International Law Commission (ILC). 2001. 'Draft Articles on Responsibility of States for Internationally Wrongful Acts'. *Yearbook of the International Law Commission 2*: part 2.

Kerr, William A. 2009. 'Political Precaution, Pandemics and Protectionism'. *Estey Centre Journal of International Law and Trade Policy 10* (2): p. 1.

Lapa, Viktoria. 2020. 'GATT Article XXI as a Way to Justify Food Prohibitions Adopted as a Response to COVID-19?' Global Trade and Customs Journal 15 (7): p. 340.

Lin, Tsai-Yu. 2010. 'The Forgotten Role of WHO/IHR in Trade Responses to 2009 A/H1N1 Influenza Outbreak'. *Journal of World Trade 44* (3): p. 515.

Mantilla Blanco, Sebastián, and Alexander Pehl. 2020. *National Security Exceptions in International Trade and Investment Agreements: Justiciability and Standards of Review*. Cham, Switzerland: Springer.

Nimac, Ivan Anton. 2020. 'COVID-19 and FDI: How Should Governments Respond?' Columbia FDI Perspectives, No. 288, 5 October. http://ccsi.columbia.edu/files/2020/10/No-288-Nimac-FINAL.pdf.

Organisation for Economic Co-operation and Development (OECD). 2007. 'Essential Security Interests under International Investment Law'. In *International Investment Perspectives: Freedom of Investment in a Changing World*, edited by OECD, pp. 93–134. Paris: OECD. https://www.oecd.org/daf/inv/investment-policy/40243411.pdf.

OECD. 2008. 'Sovereign Wealth Funds and Recipient Countries Policies'. Report by the OECD Investment Committee. Paris: OECD. https://www.oecd.org/daf/inv/investment-policy/40408735.pdf.

OECD. 2020a. 'Investment Screening in Times of COVID—and Beyond'. Paris: OECD. www.oecd.org/coronavirus/policy-responses/investment-screening-in-times-of-covid-19-and-beyond-aa60af47.

OECD. 2020b. 'OECD Code of Liberalisation of Capital Movements'. Paris: OECD. www.oecd.org/daf/inv/investment-policy/Code-capital-movements-EN.pdf.

Paddeu, Federica, and Kate Parlett. 2020. 'COVID-19 and Investment Treaty Claims'. *Kluwer Arbitration Blog*, 30 March. http://arbitrationblog.kluwerarbitration.com/2020/03/30/covid-19-and-investment-treaty-claims.

Pauwelyn, Joost. 2020. 'Export Restrictions in Times of Pandemic: Options and Limits under International Trade Agreements'. *Journal of World Trade 54* (5): p. 727.

Petetin, Ludivine. 2020. 'The COVID-19 Crisis: An Opportunity to Integrate Food Democracy into Post-Pandemic Food Systems'. *European Journal of Risk Regulation 11*: p. 326.

Pinchis Paulsen, Mona. 2020. 'COVID-19 Symposium: Thinking Creatively and Learning from COVID-19—How the WTO Can Maintain Open Trade on Critical Supplies'. *Opinio Juris*, 2 April. http://opiniojuris.org/2020/04/02/covid-19-symposium-thinking-creatively-and-learning-from-covid-19-how-the-wto-can-maintain-open-trade-on-critical-supplies.

Ranjan, Prabhash. 2016. 'Protecting Security Interests in International Investment Law'. In *Security and International Law*, edited by Mary E. Footer, Julia Schmidt, and Nigel D. White, pp. 273–300. Oxford: Hart Publishing.

United Nations Conference on Trade and Development (UNCTAD). 2009. 'The Protection of National Security in IIAs'. UNCTAD Series on International Investment Policies for Development. New York and Geneva: United Nations. https://unctad.org/system/files/official-document/diaeia20085_en.pdf.

UNCTAD. 2020a. 'Investment Policy Responses to the COVID-19 Pandemic'. *Investment Policy Monitor*, Special Issue No 4, May. https://unctad.org/system/files/official-document/diaepcbinf2020d3_en.pdf.

UNCTAD. 2020b. 'World Investment Report 2020: International Production beyond the Pandemic'. New York: United Nations. https://unctad.org/system/files/official-document/wir2020_en.pdf.

UNCTAD. 2020c. *Impact of the COVID-19 Pandemic on International Trade and Development: Transitioning to a New Normal*. New York: United Nations.

Van den Bossche, Peter, and Werner Zdouc. 2017. *The Law and Policy of the World Trade Organization: Text, Cases and Materials*. 4th edn. Cambridge: Cambridge University Press.

World Trade Organization (WTO). 1996. 'Japan—Taxes on Alcoholic Beverages II'. Appellate Body Report WT/DS/8/AB/R, 4 October.

WTO. 2012. 'China—Measures Related to the Importation of Raw Materials'. Appellate Body Report WT/DS/394/AB/R; WT/DS/395/AB/R; WT/DS/398/AB/R, 30 January.

WTO. 2019. 'Russia—Measures Concerning Traffic in Transit'. Report of the Panel WT/DS512/R, 5 April.

WTO. 2020a. 'COVID-19: Measures Affecting Trade in Goods'. Updated 26 October 2021. https://www.wto.org/english/tratop_e/covid19_e/trade_related_goods_measure_e.htm.

WTO. 2020b. 'Regional Trade Agreements Database'. http://rtais.wto.org/UI/PublicMaintainRTAHome.aspx.

WTO. 2020c. 'Statement on COVID-19 and the Multilateral Trading System by Ministers Responsible for the WTO from Afghanistan; Australia; Barbados; Benin; Cambodia; Canada; Chile; Colombia; Costa Rica; Ecuador; El Salvador; Guatemala; Guyana; Hong Kong, China; Iceland; Israel; Jamaica; Japan; Kenya; Republic of Korea; the State of Kuwait; Liechtenstein; Madagascar; Mauritania; Mauritius; Mexico; Republic of Moldova; Montenegro; Nepal; New Zealand; Nigeria; North Macedonia; Norway; Papua New Guinea; Peru; Qatar; Saint Lucia; Kingdom of Saudi Arabia; Seychelles; Singapore; Solomon Islands; Switzerland; Ukraine; United Arab Emirates; United Kingdom; Uruguay and Viet Nam'. WTO doc. WT/GC/212/Rev.2, 31 July 2020.

WTO. 2020d. 'Waiver from Certain Provisions of the TRIPS Agreement for the Prevention, Containment and Treatment of COVID-19'. WTO doc. IP/C/W/669, 2 October 2020.

Zhou, Jingyuan. 2020. 'Guest Post: Facilitating WTO-Compliant Responses to International Public Health Emergencies'. *International Economic Law and Policy Blog*, 3 March. https://ielp.worldtradelaw.net/2020/03/guest-post-trade-policies-under-pandemic.html.

9

COVID-19

Exposing the Gender Gaps in Global Health

Julia Smith

A report to the United Nations (UN) Interagency Standing Committee, written in the midst of the 2014–2016 West African Ebola outbreak read, 'Vigilance against a repeat escalation—or future outbreak—of the disease (or any other similarly highly infectious virus) must incorporate the lessons learned on the significance of gender in the spread and control' (Inter-Agency Standing Committee (IASC) 2015). The report reflected upon a response within which gender experts were excluded from public health decision-making until after the fact and followed on reports from entities such as the World Bank, which failed to discuss gendered effects of the outbreak (Harman 2016). Even the World Health Organization (WHO) Ebola Response Roadmap (WHO 2014) included only one sentence about women. Academic outputs were not much better, with less than 1% of published research related to the Ebola outbreak discussing gender inequality (Davies and Bennett 2016).

Five years later, a very different kind of pandemic challenged the long-standing neglect of gender-based analysis in disease outbreak responses and scholarship. Like Ebola, and other previous outbreaks, COVID-19 exposed the increased vulnerability of women as frontline health workers and due to secondary impacts on sexual and reproductive health, differential economic impacts, reliance on the unpaid care economy, and rise in gender-based violence (Wenham et al. 2020a). Concurrently, a renewed momentum within global health called for greater gender balance in decision-making and pressurized national governments and global institutions to '#buildbackbetter', while generating rapid evidence on the gender effects of COVID-19. These combined forces exposed the fault lines in global health promises to act on gender inequality.

Gender equality can be defined as the equal access to and enjoyment of rights, responsibilities, and opportunities. While sex refers to the biological presence of male and female markers, gender refers to the socially constructed norms and roles that a given culture and society use to define men, women, and non-binary genders. The gender dimensions of disease outbreaks are both physical

Julia Smith, *COVID-19*. In: *A Multidisciplinary Approach to Pandemics*. Edited by Philippe Bourbeau, Jean-Michel Marcoux, and Brooke A. Ackerly, Oxford University Press.
 DOI: 10.1093/oso/9780192897855.003.0010

and socially constructed. Some diseases, by their nature, affect the sexes differently; for example, Zika may result in a relatively mild infection but is particularly risky during pregnancy, as it is linked to birth defects. Other dimensions are determined by social norms and gendered roles. For example, women may be more likely to experience infection due to their predominate role in health-care work and as caregivers in the home. The effects of pandemic responses, as opposed to the purely medical consequences of viral infection, are particularly gendered. For example, the closure of, or decline in, certain industries will affect men and women differently because of socialized gender roles which determine who is most likely to work where and under what conditions (see Chapter 14 in this volume by Herrmann and Isabelle for additional examples of the pandemic-induced gender gap in labour markets).

There are numerous models and approaches to gender-based analysis, but most share common characteristics of considering differential effects across genders, often including intersectional analysis related to race, ethnicity, sexuality, and other identity factors (Johnson et al. 2009). Gender-based policy analysis asks if, where, and how gender differences are taken into account within decision-making, and what are the intended and unintended differential gendered effects of policy responses. Assessments of decision-making ask what genders are present and if, and how, people of different genders are able to participate in and influence decision-making. Gender-based analysis is particularly suited to interdisciplinary inquiry as it seeks to expose the relationships between policy sectors, social phenomenon, and political processes, as well as to explore the relationships between the individual, household, state, and global context.

This chapter applies gender-based analysis to provide an overview of the gender dimensions of pandemics, as well as to analyse if, where, and how these have been responded to by governments and global health institutions. It draws on evidence from past outbreaks and emerging evidence from the COVID-19 pandemic. Reflecting the nature of pandemics, the focus is global, drawing on wide-ranging data and examples to illuminate how patterns and trends in inequality cut across geographies and population. Taken together, findings demonstrate that pandemics are more than global health crises; they are also gender equality crises.

This analysis draws on interdisciplinary feminist scholarship, which has particularly sought to expose masculine bias in governance and decision-making. As Elson explains, such bias is more than just personal perception, but is also a blindness to the policies and structures 'that operate in favour of men as a gender, and against women as a gender' (Elson 1993: 238). Davies and Bennett write that, 'male bias is very much present in thinking about disease outbreaks' (2016: 1043), pointing to the lack of consideration of how men, women, and non-binary genders experience health crises differently, persistent lack of gender and sex disaggregated data, and continuation of responses that disadvantage women and non-binary people compared to men. Applying a feminist lens illuminates opportunities to advance research of health crises by exposing the effects of bias within policy responses, inequities, and insecurities within the paid and unpaid labour that is central to responses, and how additional inequities interact to shape effects and responses.

Gendered Effects of Disease Outbreaks

Feminist frameworks outlined above challenge health, security, and economic assessments of outbreak effects to incorporate gender-based analysis by asking how non-binary people, women, and men are differentially affected by both outbreaks and the responses to them. Research on previous outbreaks, such as Ebola and Zika, provide evidence to inform gender questions to be asked about COVID-19. Effects differ not only by gender, but also by geographies (in terms of high-income and low- and middle-income countries and neighbourhoods, and in terms of urban and rural locations), as well as among specific population and identity groups. Across and among such differences, patterns of inequities can be traced, as well as the social, political, and economic structures that determine them.

Direct and Indirect Effects on Health

The direct health impacts of a pandemic are often gendered. The early HIV outbreak in North America and Western Europe primarily affected men who have sex with men. Subsequent outbreaks in sub-Saharan African (SSA) led to disproportionate infection rates among women of reproductive age, a trend that continues today. While sex and gender disaggregated evidence on the Ebola outbreak in Africa is inconclusive, there is some data to suggest more cases among women, possibly due to their role as caregivers (Harman 2016). Previous coronavirus outbreaks, such as Middle East respiratory syndrome (MERS), resulted in a higher number of cases and deaths among men compared to women (Chen et al. 2017). However, while such trends can be identified in many cases, evidence is also limited and often incomplete. Many countries still do not collect sex disaggregated data, and even fewer disaggregate by gender or other factors. Lack of data presents challenges in drawing conclusions regarding the reasons for sex and gender differences in cases and outcomes, particularly as these are often the result of mixed biological and social factors. For example, evidence suggests that female immune systems may offer increased protection against some viruses, while women's over-representation as frontline health-care workers increases their exposure to infection (Tadiri et al. 2020).

Early data on COVID-19 noted a higher rate of reported cases, morbidity, and mortality among men. However, six months into the epidemic, only 27% of confirmed COVID-19 cases reported to the WHO were disaggregated by sex and age (Heidari et al. 2020). Where disaggregated data was available, vast national differences were apparent. For example, while men made up approximately 75% of cases and deaths in Pakistan, they were only 45% of cases and deaths in Canada (UN Women 2020). Differences have been attributed to testing and contracting tracing approaches, as well as how gender roles and norms structure risk of exposure. Higher case numbers among men in Pakistan may be due to their larger social networks than women and to their role working outside the home. Higher cases and mortality among women in Canada may be the result of outbreaks in long-term care homes, where the majority of residents are women. One study found that those countries ranking lower on the gender equity index were more likely to have a greater proportion of male COVID-19-related deaths, suggesting that the gender inequities may be putting men particularly at risk (Tadiri et al. 2020). Women's dominant role in the health-care sector (women make up 70% of the health workforce worldwide) also increases their risk of infection. In Spain, Italy, and the United States, for example, COVID-19 infections among women health workers are between two and three times those of men health-care workers (Azcona et al. 2020). Infection rates also reflect racial and ethnic differences. Data from the city of New York show that COVID-19 deaths among black and Hispanic persons are significantly higher than those of white or Asian persons (Mays and Newman 2020). Data from England and Wales shows black women are 4.3 times more likely to die from a COVID-19-related death than white ethnicity women (Office of National Statistics 2020).

The health impacts of a pandemic are not isolated to infection. Surveys around the world report a rise in COVID-19-related mental health challenges in general, but with a disproportionate increase for women (notably, most surveys only include man or woman as gender categories). A US Centre for Disease Control (CDC) survey found that 32% of women reported suffering from anxiety as a result of COVID-19, in comparison to 24% for men (CDC 2020). In the UK, 22% of women reported insomnia related to COVID-19 worries, compared to 13% for men (Fawcett Society 2020). Similarly, surveys in Canada, China, and Hong Kong found that women were more likely than men to suffer from anxiety related to COVID-19 (Smith et al. 2020). One cause of this increased anxiety is women's position on the frontlines of the response as health-care workers and care providers within homes and families. Nurses, most of whom were women, who provided care during the severe acute respiratory syndrome (SARS) outbreak in Hong Kong reported high levels of anxiety related to their heightened likelihood of infecting family members and the challenges of managing work and family responsibilities during a crisis (Holroyd and McNaught 2008). Women providing care at home during the Ebola outbreak in West Africa reported suffering from long-term psychological trauma related to being solely responsible for the ill and from the fear of contracting and passing on the virus, particularly to their children (Abramowitz et al. 2015). Women's increased and disproportionate levels of anxiety are the logical reaction to their gender roles as health and care providers, as well as their increased responsibilities and risks during the COVID-19 crises.

Further secondary effects relate to changes in health services when the 'tyranny of the urgent' takes over and financial, human, and clinical resources are diverted to respond to a health emergency (Davies and Bennett 2016). Routine services are disrupted, causing a lack of health provision for other conditions beyond the outbreak. Such effects are particularly felt in lower-income countries and rural areas with already struggling and inadequate health systems. As limited resources are directed to pandemic testing, treatment, and care, choices about what to prioritize and what to neglect are explicitly gendered. For example, during the West African Ebola outbreak, sexual and reproductive health-care services were reduced as resources were diverted to the emergency response. Médecins Sans Frontières closed its obstetric and paediatric care facilities in affected areas, 'depriving the local population of essential services' (Stockhold Evaluation Unit 2016). Quarantine policies prevented pregnant women from accessing care and women suspected of being infected were denied care (Erland and Dahl 2017). Concurrently, the number of women giving birth in hospitals and health clinics dropped by 30%, and the maternal mortality rate increased by 75% (Davies and Bennett 2016: 1043).

While COVID-19 has, so far, primarily affected countries with low maternal and child mortality rates, and comparatively well-resourced health systems, the response had a negative impact on sexual and reproductive health (SRH) services and outcomes. Contraceptive supply chains were affected, as the majority of contraceptives are made in Asian countries, which were some of the first to be impacted by travel bans, disruption, and/or workforce shortages impacting factories and supplies. The United Nations Population Fund (UNFPA 2020) documented stockout risks in 46 countries. Marie Stopes International (MSI 2020), a non-governmental organization (NGO) providing contraceptive and family planning services, warned that, due to COVID-19-related disruptions, up to 9.5 million women and girls were at risk of losing access to contraception and safe abortion services, which could result in between 1.3 and 3 million unintended pregnancies, 1.2–2.7 million unsafe abortions, and an estimated 5,000–11,000 pregnancy-related deaths. Demand for contraception also reduced, as those in need either fear accessing a health provider, due to risk of infection, or are unable to access one due to interrupted services and required self-isolation (Friedrichs 2020). Access to abortion was restricted in countries where women require physician approval for an abortion and COVID-19-related quarantines restrict women's access to clinics. Some jurisdictions used COVID-19 to restrict abortion access by not designating it as an essential service (Wenham et al. 2020b). Various studies from around the world indicated a rise in stillbirths during the first half of 2020, which coincides with the first wave of the pandemic. The studies suggest that lack of access to routine screening and in-person health check-ups related to the lockdown inhibited preventative diagnosis and care, contributing to this increase (Watson 2020).

Transgender individuals—who already faced numerous barriers, related to discrimination and lack of specialized staff and services—also experienced reduced access to health services as resources were directed to the COVID-19 response. Many countries postponed medical gender transitions, deemed non-essential services, during the initial months of COVID-19. The impacts of these postponements were more than physical, as studies have showed that gender-affirming surgery greatly improves mental health outcomes (Wang et al. 2020). Lack of appropriate COVID-19-related services also reduced access by transgender individuals to COVID-19-related testing and care. For example, transgender women in the United States were hesitant to access COVID-19 testing due to past mistreatment from health-care providers (Poteat et al. 2020). Research from India found that transgender women were fearful of getting tested for COVID-19 in case they tested positive and were forced to stay in a COVID-19 ward for men (Pandya and Redcay 2020).

Labour and Economic Effects

Globally, women make up 70% of the health and social care workforce and are more likely to be front-line health workers, such as nurses, midwives, and community health workers (Global Health 50/50 2019). Women health-care workers also tend to earn less money than men and are more likely to work in precarious positions. An analysis across 25 countries found a wage gap where women on average made between 26% and 36% less than men (Shannon et al. 2019). This gap was greatest in lower-income countries. Across all 25 countries, a higher proportion of women in the health workforce was associated with an increased gender wage gap and more precarious work conditions. These women, working for low wages in precarious positions, became the front line of the COVID-19 response.

Despite their essential role, women are underrepresented in health systems leadership and decision-making bodies, which remain dominated by men. An analysis of 198 global health organizations found that only 30% have gender parity in management (Global Health 50/50 2019). This has led to a disregard for the needs of the majority of health-care workers, who are women. For example, when supplies were coordinated for health-care workers in Wuhan, China during the initial COVID-19 outbreak, personal cleaning products, food, and clothing was provided, but not menstrual supplies, leading to a social media campaign crowdsourcing these for women health-care workers (Xinhua 2020). In the UK, personal protective equipment (PPE) designed for men did not fit women health-care workers effectively, increasing their risk of infection (Sproul 2020).

The labour and economic effects of pandemics reach far beyond the health sector. Pandemic responses, such as border closures and the closing of all but essential businesses, can lead to economic downturns with distinctly gendered patterns. While other types of economic downturns often see increased layoffs and unemployment in male-dominated sectors such as manufacturing, pandemic-related economic crises are more likely to affect sectors that primarily employ women, such as the service industry. During the West Africa Ebola outbreak, women were particularly affected by the closure of informal markets, where mostly women entrepreneurs sold produce and other goods (United Nations Development Programme (UNDP) 2015). Not only did market women lose their source of income, but they also had few savings and lacked access to the credit and resources needed to absorb the outbreak's economic shock. Even after markets reopened, women struggled to achieve pre-outbreak income levels, while men's income recovered within a few months (UNDP 2015). Similar trends were noted during the 2015–2016 Zika outbreak in South America, where many women working in precarious positions within the hospitality and tourism sector lost their jobs and had limited access to financial supports (UNDP, International Federation of the Red Cross (IFRC) 2017). In such cases, the economic impacts of pandemics deepen pre-existing inequities related to pay and conditions of work.[1]

In the context of COVID-19, the majority of industries most affected by physical distancing policies, lockdowns, and reduced trade—such as tourism, the food and beverage sector, and the service sector—primarily employ women. Like health care, many of these feminized industries consist of low-paying, precarious work and often rely on migrant labour. For example, the majority of domestic workers, of whom there are over 67 million (mostly women) around the world, were at risk of losing their livelihood (International Labour Organization (ILO) 2020). While the demand for domestic services increased with school closures and new hygiene requirements, domestic workers were also unable to work remotely and those without formal contracts could be laid off without pay (UN Economic Commissoin for Latin America and the Caribbean (CEPAL) 2020). In Brazil, 39% of domestic workers were dismissed from employment, due to fears of COVID-19 transmission, without receiving any payment (Guimaraes 2020). In Hong Kong, foreign domestic workers were ineligible to receive government support, even as large numbers lost their jobs when their employers left the city (Milhaud 2020).

[1] Chapter 14 in this volume by Herrmann and Isabelle also highlights that this deepening gender gap may have longer-term health implications for women because of changes in both their absolute and relative income.

COVID-19 also increases the multidimensional risks faced by sex workers, the majority of whom are women or non-binary individuals. The closing of spaces where sex is often sold, such as bars and nightclubs, forces sex workers into less safe spaces, increasing the risk of violence and incarceration. Sex workers' ability to protect themselves from infection is limited by the nature of their work, particularly as a decrease in demand may prompt riskier behaviour in order to maintain clients (Azcona et al. 2020). Research on calculated risk in Zimbabwe related to HIV infection among young women who sell sex indicates that the immediate risk of loss of income often trumps the less immediate and unclear risk of infection (Crankshaw and Chareka 2019). It is likely that similar calculations go into decisions regarding sex work during COVID-19, particularly as sex workers are unlikely to be able to access government economic support programmes due to the informal, and often criminalized, nature of their work.

Due to gender norms and expectations around family roles, the majority of health and care work in the home is done by women. Globally, women do three times as much unpaid care and domestic work as men (Ferrant et al. 2014; ILO 2018). This feminized care economy includes the work of cooking, cleaning, and caring that is essential to others' participation in the formal economy and in social and political systems. During health crises, the burden of care work is exacerbated when health systems struggle to meet both outbreak-related and unrelated health needs, the overflow of which is then absorbed within the home. Similarly, when schools and childcare facilities are closed to prevent the spread of infection, education and childcare has to be provided at home, most often by women. In such cases, the care economy acts as a 'shock absorber' (Harman 2016: 525). Women sacrifice their own time (often at the cost of education and economic opportunities), well-being, and resources to care for those in their networks. While women may view care work as their duty and take pride in their essential role, this work also has costs in terms of opportunities and well-being, and usually goes unpaid and unrecognized. Assessments of the care work associated with the HIV epidemic in SSA demonstrate that women providing care often sacrifice their own health, safety, and resources (Ogden et al. 2006).

Social and Security Effects

The COVID-19 outbreak, and resulting closure of schools and childcare facilities, resulted in a global crisis within the care economy. In many highly affected countries, parents shifted to working from home while their children home schooled—a combination that often proved impossible to balance. While there is evidence that men took on a greater amount of care work in the context of COVID-19, the majority of work was still done by women. Research from the United States, the UK, Italy, Germany, and France found working women doing on average 15 hours more of unpaid care and domestic work a week compared to men (Azcona et al. 2020). Single parents, the majority of whom are women, were particularly expected to maintain the impossible balance of care and income-earning activities. The need to isolate from extended family and community members, particularly exacerbated care needs, as women could not rely on previous coping strategies, such as relying on grandparents to fill childcare gaps (Smith et al. 2020).

Women's engagement in paid employment dropped dramatically during the first six months of COVID-19. In Canada, fewer women returned to work following the COVID-19 lockdown compared to men (Deschamps 2020). In the United States, over three times the number of women (865,000) left the workforce than men (216,000), despite an additional 661,000 new jobs being added to the economy in September 2020 (Collins et al. 2020). Reasons for not returning to work related to financial rationales, including that the lowest-earning partner (most likely women) should stay home, being unable to participate in job searches because of the lack of childcare, and anxiety about the safety of sending children back to school/childcare (Smith et al. 2020).

School closures also had gendered impacts on children. Following school closures in Sierra Leone, Liberia, and Guinea during the 2014–2015 Ebola outbreak, more girls than boys did not return to school, exacerbating pre-pandemic inequities in educational attainment (Giannini 2020). Similarly, following the cholera outbreak in Yemen in 2017, fewer girls than boys returned to school (Office for the Coordination of Humanitarian Affairs (OCHA) 2018). Such disruptions not only affect children's educational development, but also their security. In Yemen, many boys who left school were recruited as child soldiers in the civil war, and girls were increasingly forced in to early marriages, leading to high rates of teenage pregnancies. Evidence from such cases suggests a relationship between school closures and increased sexual violence towards children and children engaging in transactional sex (Wenham et al., 2020b).

To contain the spread of COVID-19, 193 countries and areas around the world temporarily closed educational institutions, impacting over 1.54 billion children and youths. Over 111 million of these youths were girls living in the world's least developed countries, where access to education was already limited pre-COVID-19 (United Nations Educational, Scientific and Cultural Organization (UNESCO) 2020). The UN estimates that 24 million children will not return to school after the disruptions in their education (UN 2020). As a result of these disruptions, combined with economic insecurity, Save the Children (2020) predicts that up to 2.5 million more girls around the world are at risk of being forced into child marriage over the next five years.

COVID-19 lockdowns corresponded with a dramatic rise in gender-based violence (GBV) around the world. For example, in Malaysia and Lebanon calls to helplines doubled in March 2020, compared to March 2019, and in France they rose by 32% (UN News 2020). In China, police reports in Hubei province (the location of Wuhan city) documented a tripling of GBV incidents during the initial outbreak (UN News 2020). Notably, these figures reflect reporting, not incidence. Not only is domestic violence typically grossly underreported, but restrictions on movements and limited privacy due to COVID-19-related isolation measures indicate that many women were unable to phone or otherwise reach out for help or receive support from their social networks. In Canada, fear of the virus discouraged people from accessing shelters, even though 10% of women (and 6% of men) were concerned about violence in their home (Statistics Canada 2020).

COVID-19 policies further exacerbated the risk of violence for specific groups. Policies in Peru, Panama, and Columbia that dictated which days men and women could leave home (as a way of enforcing social distancing) led to increased violence towards transgender individuals (Perez-Brumer and Silva-Santisteban 2020). COVID-19-related lockdowns and recommended isolation orders particularly limited the ability of women living with disabilities (who are between two to three times more likely to experience GBV) to flee violence, as their connections to support people outside the home was reduced (Lund 2020). Institutionalized people with disabilities were further at risk of violence, as visitors and monitors had restricted access. The rise in GBV during the COVID-19 pandemic has been referred to as the 'shadow pandemic', caused not by the virus but by responses that exacerbated persistent insecurities.

Pandemic Responses

The multiple and unequal gendered impacts of pandemics, and the responses to them, documented above demonstrate the need for gender-based analysis and feminist policy development. However, responses to past pandemics, such as SARS, MERS, and swine flu (H1N1), have largely lacked gender-based dimensions. There is no mention of gender or women in any of the following global health policies related to pandemics: the World Health Assembly's International Health Regulations (2005); the Joint External Evaluations; the Global Health Security Agenda (and country action packages); the Biological Weapons Convention; and the WHO Research and Development Blueprint (Smith 2019). Most national policies, such as the United States Government's Global Health Security Strategy and the UK's Health is Global Strategy, also do not include gender analysis. Where gender or women's rights are mentioned, it is often limited to SRH. For example, Canada's Feminist International Assistance policy commits to strengthening health systems and fighting infectious diseases primarily by funding maternal, newborn, and child health initiatives (GAC 2018). Consequently, notable impacts of pandemics and outbreaks, such as increased unpaid care work conducted by women and gender-based violence, are often only considered after the fact. There has been even less consideration of the unequal impacts on women's mental health, the rights and needs of non-binary individuals, and the economic impacts related to precarious work (Wenham et al. 2020a).

Calls for more sustained and inclusive gender-based policy responses, though persistently put forward by advocates and activists for decades, began to be heard in earnest following the West African Ebola and South American Zika outbreaks. Ebola highlighted the impact on women care providers, particularly in a context of weak health systems (Harman 2016). Zika, as it primarily affected infected mothers and their children, drew attention to intersections with SRH, and led to renewed debate around access to contraception and abortion in highly affected contexts (Wenham et al. 2019). Concurrently, movements calling for greater action on gender equality gained momentum in global health governance spaces, where gender mainstreaming had been widely adopted within written policies, but resulted in fewer examples of change in practice and decision-making (Global Health 50/50 2019). Building on a growing recognition of this gap, Women in Global Health was founded in 2015 to promote gender transformative leadership in global health. Shortly after, Global Health 50/50 was formed at University College London to monitor gender composition and policies in global health organizations. These represent two emergent efforts to advance action towards gender equality within global health governance.

Within the context of limited gender analysis of health impacts in pandemics, early data on COVID-19 indicated sex differences in cases and mortality, as well as the multiple gendered effects (as described above). For the first time in decades, a disease outbreak was primarily affecting high-income and middle-income countries (in addition to low-income countries) where there were greater resources to support gender-based analysis and feminist responses. As a result, unprecedented attention was directed to the gendered effects of the pandemic, with a newly formed independent Gender and COVID-19 Working Group bringing together hundreds of academics, advocates, and health professionals around the world to mobilize research and inform responses (Wenham et al. 2020a). UN Women, and others, agitated for sex disaggregated reporting, created databases on gender relevant policies, and collated evidence on GBV incidents around the world (UN Women 2020). Following a civil society forum, coordinated by Women in Global Health (WiGH) in September 2020, the WHO committed to advancing its integration of gender-based analysis (WiGH 2020). Organizations ranging from the World Bank (2020) to the Global Vaccine Alliance (GAVI 2020) produced policy documents and guidance on mitigating the gendered effects of the outbreak. If and how these commitments are operationalized remains to be seen.

At the national level, by the end of 2020, UN Women found that of 206 countries, only 25 had implemented combined measures to address violence, support unpaid care workers, and strengthen women's economic security. Forty-two countries had no policies to support women, 135 had measures in place specifically to respond to GBV, and 61 had taken action to ease the care burden on women (Staab et al. 2020). An earlier study by CARE International of 30 countries reported that 76% had made at least one policy commitment that supported women, but, as the report pointed out, 'one policy cannot account for the tremendous implications of the pandemic on gender equality' (CARE 2020: 4). Despite global and national level mobilization, gender-based responses remained piecemeal.

Advocates also began tracking the gender composition of organizations within global health decision-making, as evidence suggests that organizations with greater representation of women are more supportive of gender-based analysis and responses. One analysis found that countries that have more women in leadership (as measured by the Council on Foreign Relations Women's Power Index) were more likely to deliver COVID-19 responses that considered the effects of the crisis on women and girls (Care 2020). On average, the higher the country's score on the index, the more likely it was to craft a gendered response. However, an analysis of 115 COVID-19-related decision-making bodies and task forces in 87 countries found that only 3.5% had gender parity in their membership (Van Daalen et al. 2020). Importantly, women are not the only gender excluded from decision-making. Non-binary people are rarely represented, particularly in countries that criminalize non-binary identities and homosexual behaviours. Decision-making bodies around pandemic responses are not only likely to primarily consist of men, but of men from dominant social, economic, and ethnic groups. However, at the time of writing, there is little nuanced analysis of how gender norms are shaping the COVID-19 response across countries beyond basic disaggregation along binary genders.

There are some notable examples of recovery plans that aim to not only include underrepresented groups in decision-making, but also to approach policy responses from a feminist perspective. As early as May 2020, the State of Hawaii produced a Feminist Economic Recovery Plan that stated, 'the road to economic recovery should not be across women's back' (Smith-Johnson et al. 2020) The plan cautioned against austerity measures and promoted a shift away from reliance on tourism, and associated precarious jobs, and towards investments in the health and care sectors. At the time of writing, the plan had yet to be approved by Senate, but was successfully passed in Kaua'i, Maui, and Hawai'i Island county councils.

In Canada, the Young Women's Christian Association (YWCA) produced a similar Feminist Economic Recovery Plan focused on recognizing care work as essential work, expanding investments in childcare, preventing GBV, and supporting those sectors where women were most impacted (Sultana and Ravanera 2020). Notably, following this report and further campaigns from civil society in Canada, the federal government described its COVID-19 response as 'an intersectional feminist recovery' and included a commitment to a national childcare programme (Government of Canada (GAC) 2020). The federal government also continued, throughout COVID-19, its commitment to gender-based analysis plus (GBA+), conducting gender assessments of almost all response emergency measures (Smith and Murage 2021). However, only two policies implemented during the first six months of the pandemic specifically aimed to address gender inequities: increasing funding for responses to gender-based violence and expansion of the Women's Entrepreneurship Strategy, and subsequent polls have found that women in Canada remained disillusioned with government responses as they struggled with the daily realities of care work and economic loss during the pandemic (Thompson 2020). At the time of writing, calls to '#buildbackbetter' are tempered by continued waves of outbreak and resulting economic and care crises, which are being disproportionately borne by women.

Conclusion

When applied to the study of pandemics, feminist gender analysis reveals gaps in global health responses and highlights the need to rethink the health, economic, and security implications of crises by asking who is most affected, in what (often less visible) ways, and why (see also the Introduction to this volume by Ackerly et al.). This requires in-depth interdisciplinary analysis. Such research from past and present pandemics has begun to reveal the differential gendered effects of health crises, demonstrating the particular direct and indirect health and security risks that people of different genders face. For example, pandemics have been shown to result in decreased economic security, elevated health risks, and increased care burdens for women. In addition to a health crisis, pandemics exacerbate gender inequities.

Evidence from the COVID-19 pandemic reveals gaps in pandemic responses. Despite progress since the West African Ebola outbreak five years ago, most governments and health-care organizations continue to fail to collect sex and gender disaggregated data and to exploit the paid and unpaid labour of women. National and global responses fail to protect individuals from increased gender-based violence and health risks structured by intersecting inequities. In particular, there is a need for further data and action on the experiences of non-binary individuals, as there is currently too little consideration of their needs within pandemic responses. Further identifying factors, such as age, ability, and race are also only sporadically considered alongside gender analysis, which too often still focuses primarily (as the examples in this chapter illustrate) on the experiences of women in general and on sexual and reproductive dimensions of health. Feminist recovery plans and the combined efforts of organizations, academics, and social movements around the world are beginning to fill these gaps, and it is past time for global health institutions and scholarship to catch up.

References

Abramowitz, Sharon, Kristen Mclean, Sarah McKune, Kevin Bardosh, Mosoka Fallah, Josephine Monger et al. 2015. 'Community-Centered Responses to Ebola in Urban Liberia: The View from Below'. *PLoS Neglected Tropical Diseases 9* (4): e0003706. doi:10.1371/journal.pntd.0003706.

Azcona, Ginette, Antra Bhatt, Sara Davies, Sophie Harman, Julia Smith and Clare Wenham. 2020. 'Will the Pandemic Derail Hard-Won Progress on Gender Equality? Spotlight on Gender, Covid-19 and the SDGS'. New York. https://www.unwomen.org/en/digital-library/publications/2020/07/spotlight-on-gender-covid-19-and-the-sdgs.

CARE. 2020. 'Where Are the Women? The Conspicuous Absence of Women in COVID-19 Response Teams and Plans, and Why We Need Them'. https://insights.careinternational.org.uk/publications/why-we-need-women-in-covid-19-response-teams-and-plans.

Centers for Disease Control and Prevention (CDC). 2020. 'Mental Health—Household Pulse Survey—COVID-19'. Washington. https://www.cdc.gov/nchs/covid19/pulse/mental-health.htm.

CEPAL. 2020. 'La Agenda 2030 para el Desarrollo Sostenible en el nuevo contexto mundial y regional: escenarios y proyecciones en la presente crisis'. April. https://www.cepal.org/es/publicaciones/45336-la-agenda-2030-desarrollo-sostenible-nuevo-contexto-mundial-regional-escenarios.

Chen, Xin, Abrar Ahmad Chughtai, Amalie Dyda and Chandini Raina MacIntyre. 2017. 'Comparative Epidemiology of Middle East Respiratory Syndrome Coronavirus (MERS-CoV) in Saudi Arabia and South Korea'. *Emerging Microbes and Infections 6* (6): e51. doi:10.1038/emi.2017.40.

Collins, Caitlyn, Liana Christin Landivar, Leah Ruppanner, and William Scarborough. 2020. 'COVID-19 and the Gender Gap in Work Hours'. *Gender, Work and Organization*. doi:10.1111/gwao.12506.

Crankshaw, Tamaryn, and Samantha Chareka. 2019. 'Selling Sex in a Precarious Economy: Increasing Vulnerabilities for Young Women Who Sell Sex in Zimbabwe'. HEARD. https://www.heard.org.za/publications-post/selling-sex-precarious-economy-increasing-vulnerabilities-young-woman-sell-sex-zimbabwe.

Davies, S. E., and Belinda Bennett. 2016. 'A Gendered Human Rights Analysis of Ebola and Zika: Locating Gender in Global Health Emergencies'. *International Affairs 92* (5): pp. 1041–60. doi:10.1111/1468-2346.12704.

Deschamps, Tara 2020. 'Women's Participation in Labour Force Reaches Lowest Level in 3 Decades due to COVID-19: RBC'. *CBC News*, 16 July. https://www.cbc.ca/news/canada/toronto/women-employment-canada-covid-19-1.5652788.

Elson, Dian 1993. 'Gender-Aware Analysis and Development Economics'. *Journal of International Development 5* (2): pp. 237–47. doi:10.1002/jid.3380050214.

Erland, Elin and Bente Dahl. 2017. 'Midwives' Experiences of Caring for Pregnant Women Admitted to Ebola Centres in Sierra Leone'. *Midwifery 55*: pp. 23–8. doi:10.1016/J.MIDW.2017.08.005.

Esplen, Emily. 2009. 'Gender and Care Overview Report'. https://gsdrc.org/document-library/gender-and-care-overview-report/.

Fawcett Society. 2020. 'Parenting and COVID-19—Research Evidence'. August. https://www.fawcettsociety.org.uk/Handlers/Download.ashx?IDMF=f1d5b1c3-d5e0-4497-8078-1bad6ca4eb5a.

Ferrant, Gaelle, Luca Maria Pesando, and Keiko Nowacka. 2014. 'Unpaid Care Work: The Missing Link in the Analysis of Gender Gaps in Labour Outcomes'. OECD, December. https://www.oecd.org/dev/development-gender/Unpaid_care_work.pdf.
Friedrichs, Ellen 2020. 'The COVID-19 Pandemic Exposes the Need for Over-the-Counter Birth Control'. *Rewire News Group*, 2 April. https://rewirenewsgroup.com/article/2020/04/02/the-covid-19-pandemic-exposes-the-need-for-otc-birth-control.
Giannini, Stephania 2020. 'COVID-19 School Closures around the World Will Hit Girls Hardest'. United Nations Educational, Scientific and Cultural Organization, 31 March. https://en.unesco.org/news/covid-19-school-closures-around-world-will-hit-girls-hardest.
Global Health 50/50. 2019. 'Equality Works'. University College London, 24 September. https://globalhealth5050.org/updates/document/gh5050-2019-report-equality-works.
Global Vaccine Alliance (GAVI). 2020. 'Why a Gender Lens Is Needed for the COVID-19 Response'. Gavi, the Vaccine Alliance, 16 April. https://www.gavi.org/vaccineswork/why-gender-lens-needed-covid19-response.
Government of Canada (GAC). 2018. 'Canada's Feminist International Assistance Policy'. Ottawa: Foreign Affairs. http://international.gc.ca/world-monde/issues_development-enjeux_developpement/priorities-priorites/policy-politique.aspx?lang=eng#5.2.
GAC. 2020. '2020 Speech from the Throne'. https://www.canada.ca/en/privy-council/campaigns/speech-throne/2020/speech-from-the-throne.html.
Guimaraes, Ligia 2020. 'Coronavírus no Brasil: 39% dos patrões dispensaram diaristas sem pagamento durante pandemia, aponta pesquisa'. *BBC News*, 22 April. https://www.bbc.com/portuguese/brasil-52375292?SThisFB&fbclid=IwAR23IUn1ml6ucxRIKc_HZIrJOj6bXYfIVChWTf4usiXsTE-LWlhsxLR_5rc.
Harman, Sophie 2016. 'Ebola, Gender and Conspicuously Invisible Women in Global Health Governance'. *Third World Quarterly 37*: pp. 524–41. doi:10.1080/01436597.2015.1108827.
Heidari, Shirin., Claudia Ahumada, and Ziyoda Kurbanova. 2020. 'Towards the Real-Time Inclusion of Sex- and Age-Disaggregated Data in Pandemic Responses'. *BMJ Global Health 5* (10): e003848. doi:10.1136/bmjgh-2020-003848.
Holroyd, Eleanor, and Carmel McNaught. 2008. 'The SARS Crisis: Reflections of Hong Kong Nurses'. *International Nursing Review 55* (1): pp. 27–33. doi:10.1111/j.1466-7657.2007.00586.x.
Inter-Agency Standing Committee (IASC). 2015. 'Humanitarian Crisis In West Africa (Ebola) Gender Alert: February 2015'. https://interagencystandingcommittee.org/system/files/iasc_gender_reference_group_-_gender_alert_west_africa_ebola_2_-_february_2015_0.pdf.
International Labour Organization (ILO). 2018. 'Women Do 4 Times More Unpaid Care Work than Men in Asia and the Pacific'. 27 June. www.ilo.org/asia/media-centre/news/WCMS_633284/lang--en/index.htm.
ILO. 2020. 'Impact of the COVID-19 Crisis on Loss of Jobs and Hours among Domestic Workers'. 15 June. www.ilo.org/global/topics/domestic-workers/publications/factsheets/WCMS_747961/lang--en/index.htm.
Johnson, Joy, Lorraine Greaves, and Robin Repta. 2009. 'Better Science with Sex and Gender: Facilitating the Use of a Sex and Gender-Based Analysis in Health Research'. *International Journal for Equity in Health 8* (1): p. 14. doi:10.1186/1475-9276-8-14.

Lund, Emily 2020. 'Interpersonal Violence against People with Disabilities: Additional Concerns and Considerations in the COVID-19 Pandemic'. *Rehabilitation Psychology 65* (3): pp. 199–205. doi:10.1037/rep0000347.

Marie Stopes International (MSI). 2020. '9.5 Million Women Could Lose Access to Our Services'. https://www.mariestopes.org/news/2020/4/95-million-women-could-lose-access-to-our-services.

Mays, Jeffery, and Andy Newman. 2020. 'Virus Is Twice as Deadly for Black and Latino People Than Whites in N.Y.C.'. *New York Times*, 26 June. https://www.nytimes.com/2020/04/08/nyregion/coronavirus-race-deaths.html.

Milhaud, Nina 2020. 'Stranded in Hong Kong: The Plight of Domestic Workers during COVID-19'. *Ariana*, 2 September. https://www.arianalife.com/topics/community/stranded-in-hong-kong-domestic-workers-covid-19.

Office for the Coordination of Humanitarian Affairs (OCHA). 2018. 'Gender Considerations in the Humanitarian Response in Yemen'. https://www.humanitarianresponse.info/en/operations/yemen/gender-considerations-humanitarian-response-yemen.

Office of National Statistics. 2020. 'Coronavirus (COVID-19) Related Deaths by Ethnic Group, England and Wales'. https://www.ons.gov.uk/peoplepopulationandcommunity/birthsdeathsandmarriages/deaths/articles/coronavirusrelateddeathsbyethnicgroupenglandandwales/2march2020to10april2020.

Ogden, Jessica, Simel Esim, and Caren Grown. 2006. 'Expanding the Care Continuum for HIV/AIDS: Bringing Carers into Focus'. *Health Policy and Planning 21* (5): pp. 333–42. doi:10.1093/heapol/czl025.

Pandya, Apurvakumar, and Alex Redcay. 2020. 'Impact of COVID-19 on Transgender Women & Hijra: Insights from Gujarat, India'. *Research Square*. doi:10.21203/rs.3.rs-44619/v1.

Perez-Brumer, Amaya, and Alfonso Silva-Santisteban. 2020. 'COVID-19 Policies Can Perpetuate Violence against Transgender Communities: Insights from Peru'. *AIDS and Behavior 24*: pp. 2477–9. doi:10.1007/s10461-020-02889-z.

Poteat, Tonia, Sari Reisner, Marissa Iller and Anrea Wirtz. 2020. 'COVID-19 Vulnerability of Transgender Women with and without HIV Infection in the Eastern and Southern U.S.'. *medRxiv*. doi:10.1101/2020.07.21.20159327.

Save the Children. 2020. 'COVID-19 Places Half a Million More Girls at Risk of Child Marriage in 2020'. 1 October. https://www.savethechildren.net/news/covid-19-places-half-million-more-girls-risk-child-marriage-2020.

Shannon, Geordan, Nicole Minckas, Des Tan, Hassan Haghparast-Bidgoli, Neha Batura,and Jenevieve Mannell 2019. 'Feminisation of the Health Workforce and Wage Conditions of Health Professions: An Exploratory Analysis'. *Human Resources for Health 17* (1): p. 72. doi:10.1186/s12960-019-0406-0.

Smith, Julia. 2019. 'Overcoming the "Tyranny of the Urgent": Integrating Gender into Disease Outbreak Preparedness and Response'. *Gender and Development 27* (2): pp. 355–69. doi:10.1080/13552074.2019.1615288.

Smith, Julia and Alice Murage. 2021. 'Integrating Gender-Based Analysis Plus (GBA+) into Policy Responses to COVID-19: Lived Experiences of Lockdown in British Columbia, Canada'. *Social Politics.* forthcoming

Smith, Julia, Sara E. Davies, Huiyn Fend, Connie Gan, Karen Grepin, Sophie Harman, et al. 2020. 'More than a Health Crisis: The Political Economy of the Gendered Effects of the Response to COVID-19'. *Global Public Health.* 16 (8): pp. 1364–1380.

Jabola-Carolus, Khara. 2020. 'Building Bridges, Not Walking on Backs: A Feminist Economic Recovery Plan for COVID-19'. Hawai'i State Commission on the Status of Women, 14 April. https://humanservices.hawaii.gov/wp-content/uploads/2020/04/4.13.20-Final-Cover-D2-Feminist-Economic-Recovery-D1.pdf.

Sproule, Lauren. 2020. 'From Pay Gap to Ill-Fitting PPE, Female Workers Highlight Challenges in U.K. Health Care'. *CBC News*, 4 October. https://www.cbc.ca/news/world/uk-health-care-gender-bias-1.5741670.

Staab, Silke, Constanza Tabbush, and Laura Turquet. 2020. 'Global Gender Response Tracker Assesses COVID-19 Measures for Women'. UN Women Data Hub, 28 September. https://data.unwomen.org/features/global-gender-response-tracker-assesses-covid-19-measures-women.

Statistics Canada. 2020. 'Impacts of COVID-19 on Canadians: First Results from Crowdsourcing'. *The Daily*, 23 April. https://www150.statcan.gc.ca/n1/daily-quotidien/200423/dq200423a-eng.htm.

Stockhold Evaluation Unit. 2016. 'OCB Ebola Review—Summary Report'. 30 April. https://reliefweb.int/report/guinea/ocb-ebola-review-summary-report-april-2016.

Sultana, Anjum, and Carmina Ravanera. 2020. 'A Feminist Economic Recovery Plan for Canada: Making the Economy Work for Everyone'. www.gendereconomy.org.

Tadiri, Christina, Teres Gisinger, Alexandra Kautzky-Willer, Karoline Kublickiene, Maria Trinidad Herrero, Valeria Raparelli, et al. 2020. 'The Influence of Sex and Gender Domains on COVID-19 Cases and Mortality'. *Canadian Medical Association Journal 192* (36): pp. E1041–5. doi:10.1503/cmaj.200971.

Thompson, Mitra. 2020. 'Canadian Women Are "Disillusioned and Disengaged" with COVID-19 Political Response'. *Global News*, 29 September. https://globalnews.ca/news/7363932/canadian-women-poll-covid-19.

United Nations (UN). 2020. *Education during COVID-19 and Beyond*. Geneva: UN.

UN News. 2020. 'UN Backs Global Action to End Violence against Women and Girls Amid COVID-19 Crisis'. 6 April. https://news.un.org/en/story/2020/04/1061132.

United Nations Development Programme (UNDP). 2015. 'Socio-Economic Impact of Ebola Virus Disease in West African Countries'. UNDP Regional Bureau for Africa. New York.

UNDP, International Federation of the Red Cross (IFRC). 2017. 'A Socio-Economic Impact Assessment of the Zika Virus in Latin America and the Caribbean: With a Focus on Brazil, Colombia and Suriname'. https://www.undp.org/content/undp/en/home/librarypage/hiv-aids/a-socio-economic-impact-assessment-of-the-zika-virus-in-latin-am.html.

United Nations Educational, Scientific and Cultural Organization (UNESCO). 2020. 'School Closures Caused by Coronavirus (COVID-19)'. https://en.unesco.org/covid19/educationresponse.

United Nations Population Fund (UNFPA). 2020. 'New UNFPA Projections Predict Calamitous Impact on Women's Health as COVID-19 Pandemic Continues'. 28 April. https://www.unfpa.org/press/new-unfpa-projections-predict-calamitous-impact-womens-health-covid-19-pandemic-continues.

UN Women. 2020. 'COVID-19 and Gender Monitor'. 26 June. https://data.unwomen.org/resources/covid-19-and-gender-monitor

Van Daalen, Kim, Csongor Bajnoczki, Maisoon Chowdhury, Sara Dada, Parnian Khorsand, Anna Socha, et al. 2020. 'Symptoms of a Broken System: The Gender Gaps in COVID-19 Decision-Making Handling'. *BMJ Global Health 5* (10): e003549. doi:10.1136/bmjgh-2020-003549.

Wang, Yuanyuan, Cailin Pan, Ye Liu, Amanda Wilson, Jianju Ou, Runsen Chen 2020. 'Health Care and Mental Health Challenges for Transgender Individuals during the COVID-19 Pandemic'. *The Lancet 8*: pp. 564–5. doi:10.1016/S2213-8587(20)30182-0.

Watson, Clare 2020. 'Stillbirth Rate Rises Dramatically during Pandemic'. *Nature*: pp. 490–1. doi:10.1038/d41586-020-02618-5.

Wenham, Clare, Amaral Arevalo, Ernestina Coast, Sonia Correa, Katherine Cuellar, Tiziana Leone and Sandra Valongueiro. 2019. 'Zika, Abortion and Health Emergencies: A Review of Contemporary Debates'. *Globalization and Health*: p. 49. doi:10.1186/s12992-019-0489-3.

Wenham, Clare, Julia Smith and Rosemary Morgan. 2020a. 'COVID-19: The Gendered Impacts of the Outbreak'. *The Lancet 395* (10227): pp. 846–8.

Wenham, C., Julia Smith, Sara E. Davies, Asha Herten-Crabb, Sophie Harman, Karen Grepin 2020b. 'Women Are Most Affected by Pandemics—Lessons from Past Outbreaks'. *Nature 583* (7815): pp. 194–8. doi:10.1038/d41586-020-02006-z.

Women in Global Health (WiGH). 2020. 'A High Level Digital Summit: Women in Global Health Security—Foreign Policy'. 17 September. https://foreignpolicy.com/events/women-in-global-health.

WHO. 2014. 'Ebola Response Roadmap'. www.who.int.

World Bank. 2020. 'Gender and COVID-19 (Coronavirus)'. 10 April. https://www.worldbank.org/en/topic/gender/brief/gender-and-covid-19-coronavirus.

Xinhua. 2020. 'Across China: Donations of Sanitary Products Aid Women in Fight against Virus'. 2 February. www.xinhuanet.com/english/2020-02/12/c_138777415.htm.

10

The COVID-19 Pandemic and the Shifting Opportunity Structure of Organized Crime

Robert Muggah[1]

The COVID-19 pandemic not only impacted population health, roiled politics and undermined economic stability, but it also profoundly disrupted globalization. In the process, the disease outbreak and government efforts to contain it generated a host of knock-on effects across the criminal underworld (Muggah 2020b). In the first few months of lockdown in spring 2020, when over two-thirds of the world's population faced some form of restricted mobility, most countries experienced a temporary lull in most forms of crime and victimization. A comparatively modest handful experienced sharp increases in violent organized crime and state repression (Semple and Ahmed 2020). These improvements faded when quarantines were eased. Meanwhile, analysts detected how several organized crime groups purposefully expanded their influence, taking advantage of over-extended governments and the stresses generated by the pandemic (Aziani et al. 2019). Policing agencies also reported a dramatic expansion in the digital footprint of crime groups as dependence on the internet and remote working ballooned (Europol 2020b).

Whether in the Americas, Africa, Asia, or Europe, large-scale disease outbreaks can alter the opportunity structure for organized criminal groups. On the one hand, fragmented supply chains disrupt the production, shipment, and sale of drugs. Increased border restrictions likewise slow the illegal movement of contraband and people. Fluctuations in supply and demand for certain high-value products—from drugs to personal protective equipment—ramps up (violent) competition over trafficking routes and territory. At the same time, deglobalization and the shortening of supply chains may force organized crime groups to diversify their business models, including into cyberspace. Meanwhile, the economic downturn and shortage of credit for many small and medium sized

[1] Thanks are due to Pedro Augusto Pereira for inputs into earlier versions of this chapter. Credit also to Jean-Michel Marcoux and Matthieu Guitton.

Robert Muggah, *The COVID-19 Pandemic and the Shifting Opportunity Structure of Organized Crime*. In: *A Multidisciplinary Approach to Pandemics*. Edited by Philippe Bourbeau, Jean-Michel Marcoux, and Brooke A. Ackerly, Oxford University Press. © Oxford University Press (2022). DOI: 10.1093/oso/9780192897855.003.0011

businesses can force some of them to turn to criminal syndicates to keep operations running. These interdependencies may generate longer-lasting effects on future trends in crime, not least money laundering and trafficking of goods (see also Chapter 4 in this volume by Guitton).

This chapter considers some of the far-reaching and multifaceted effects of the COVID-19 pandemic on organized crime. In this way, it offers preliminary reflections on three specific areas where pandemics can shift the opportunity structure for both perpetrators and prospective victims. First, it examines how certain forms of criminal violence have fluctuated during and after lockdowns came into effect throughout 2020. Second, it reflects on the ways in which the pandemic and associated digital onboarding of hundreds of millions of people has influenced the migration of many criminal actors to cyberspace. Third, it documents some of the ways in which organized crime has diversified operations. Crime groups are adept at gauging shifts in preferences and can rapidly respond to changes in supply and demand. Finally, the chapter highlights several emerging strategies to deter and dismantle organized crime in the wake of COVID-19. A particular focus is on global, national, and civil society-led responses. Owing to the novelty of COVID-19, these observations are necessarily preliminary and tentative. Indeed, there are significant data gaps with respect to reporting on recent crime trends.

Organized Crime and the Pandemic

Organized crime is often defined as a planned criminal activity undertaken by a group of individuals. The UN Convention against Transnational Organized Crime sets out four generic parameters of what constitutes a specific group: a structured entity of at least three people; a minimum duration of existence; the perpetration of serious crime; and the intended goal of acquiring a financial benefit (United Nations General Assembly (UNGA) 2000). According to the UN interpretation, organized crime is distinct from interpersonal crime involving a single individual motivated by profit or passion. Established organized crime groups range from Italian and Russian mafia to triads in Asia, wildlife smuggling rings in Africa, and drug-trafficking cartels and *mara* gangs in Latin America and the Caribbean. There are many grey areas when defining organized crime, including how it relates to militia, extremist, and terrorist organizations that may also engage in rent-seeking activities.

Major shocks such as pandemics, natural disasters, and armed conflict nearly always impact on the activities of organized crime groups. COVID-19 was no exception. While it is still too early to determine how deep the impacts of the pandemic have been, the slow-down in trade and the imposition of rigid border controls has distorted mainstay activities such as drug trafficking, people smuggling, the movement of sex workers, and the illicit trade in small arms and ammunition. Physical distancing has also limited the ability of crime groups to co-opt government officials and extort civilians. Yet COVID-19 has also generated an array of disruptions that have been readily exploited by organized crime. Many groups are identifying new sources of revenue, from fake medical supplies to the gaming of government relief packages. What is more, organized crime appears to be expanding its presence online, while also extending its governance closer to home.

Shifts in Criminal Violence

One of the more surprising outcomes of the COVID-19 pandemic was the decline in most types of crime shortly after the imposition of measures to slow and contain the virus (Dazio et al. 2020). In much of North America and Western Europe, for example, murder and violent assault plummeted as more people stayed at home. There are some straightforward hypotheses for why this was the case: the lack of physical and social contact likely reduced the opportunity for public misconduct or disputes that could escalate into violent confrontations. Meanwhile, reported domestic abuse and sexual violence exploded in most parts of the world (Ford 2020). Predictably, the confinement of people to their homes in situations of extreme stress and anxiety increased exposure to abusive family members and partners.

Some of the world's historically violent cities and countries recorded stunning declines in violent crime in the months following the onset of the pandemic. For example, Chicago's high crime rate dropped by 10% and drug-related arrests fell by over 40% shortly after lockdowns went into effect (Associated Press 2020). San Salvador, routinely considered among the most dangerous cities on the planet, reported a staggering decline in crime in March 2020 (Aleman 2020). From North America to most of Central and South America, the trend lines all pointed downward. Although welcome, these improvements in public security were temporary. Physical distancing and shelter-in-place orders did not deter drug cartels, gangs, and militia; to the contrary. The combination of police shortages and supply-and-demand shocks in the drug market triggered fresh waves of violence, especially in producer and transhipment countries such as Brazil, Colombia, and Mexico (Hope 2020).

For instance, Brazil's comparatively recent decline in murder came to a screeching halt even before restrictions were eased. In São Paulo, home to South America's most powerful drug trafficking faction, the Primary First Command, or PCC, murders rose by 10% over the three months of lockdown compared to the same period in 2019. Levels of reported domestic violence also surged in most states over the same period, including by more than 50% in Rio de Janeiro alone (Castro 2020). Police killings also soared, though some states stopped reporting them for fear of public rebuke (La Diaria Politica 2020). Mexico also registered a dramatic escalation in lethal violence during the first few months of the pandemic, especially in states dominated by drug cartels such as Chihuahua and Michoacan, and especially Guanajuato (Ernst 2020). Homicide rates reached an all-time high in the first 4 months of 2020, including 3,000 murders in March alone (Reuters 2020). With the armed forces and police distracted with pandemic control measures, Mexico's principal cartels and hundreds of criminal groups were fighting over control of drug routes and the siphoning of petrol (Agren 2020).

Even El Salvador's astonishing crime decline was ended by a sharp increase in gang violence as lockdowns were lifted. When dozens of people were slaughtered during a gang dispute over a single weekend, the country's president ramped up arrests and authorized lethal force to stem the bloodshed (BBC News 2020). Critics feared that these iron-fisted measures would make a bad situation worse: gangs already control the country's jails, and the mixing of rival factions is dangerous. In many of these countries, it is crime groups, and not the police, that are enforcing lock-down orders in informal settlements and slums. As explained below, organized crime groups—from cartels to gangs and militia—are reinforcing their soft power and extending their influence (Ernst 2020). Operating in full view of the local authorities, they are providing basic services and delivering basic goods and perishable food items to the poor, elderly, and infirm. Others are posting warnings online and off about abiding by curfews and social isolation (Fajardo 2020). Their appeal may be growing at a time when government leadership is being widely questioned.

The surge in drug-related violence partly comes down to changes underway in global markets (Hamilton and Stevens 2020). The slow-down in international trade means that cartels and gangs have fewer opportunities to push their product through global supply chains because there are simply fewer ways to move illegal merchandise by land, air, or sea. Meanwhile, drug producers in Bolivia (Morfini 2020), Colombia (Gomis 2020), Peru (Stargardter and Jorgic 2020), and Mexico (Weiss 2020) are struggling to source precursor chemicals to make methamphetamines, fentanyl, and even cocaine. The global economic crunch is triggering supply-and-demand shocks for the narcotics business as a whole (Hamilton and Stevens 2020). The COVID-19 crisis tamped down production, including in Peru, which produces 20% of the world's supply of cocaine. In Colombia, where 70% of global cocaine is manufactured, anti-narcotics police have taken advantage of the lockdowns to ramp up eradication efforts. Even before the imposition of lockdowns, cocaine and heroin prices surged on the assumption that there would be disruption in supply chains (Tagziria 2020).

Notwithstanding these challenges, the drugs business is an agile one. Anticipating a slow-down in global trade due to the pandemic, some Latin American traffickers ramped up shipments beforehand and warehoused cocaine before the outbreak hit (Guarascio 2020; Organized Crime and Corruption Reporting Project

(OCCRP) 2020). Cartels are adapting to the challenges presented by COVID-19 and government efforts to target them, and they are using new routes to sell their wares. Street prices in Europe reportedly increased by 30% in 2020, but cocaine and other drugs continue to flow from Mexico and South America to Europe and North America. Instead, users started to substitute in alternatives once their drug of choice was harder to source. Growing numbers of Europeans reportedly shifted from foreign-manufactured cocaine to home-grown marijuana or other synthetic alternatives. Meanwhile, some heroin users shifted to even more potent and dangerous opiates, such as fentanyl. Across the region, COVID-19 has accelerated the purchase of drugs online, including via the Dark Web (Cuthbertson 2020).

The Migration of Crime Online

Faced with economic uncertainty, closed borders, patchy communication, and difficulties accessing customers, organized crime groups are diversifying their income streams (Ahmed 2020). Some groups are shifting from drug trafficking to targeting banks, businesses, and high-net-worth individuals. In many parts of the world, crime groups are resorting to kidnapping, extortion, and protection rackets to keep the cash flowing. Most lucrative of all, however, is cybercrime, which shot up considerably as governments, businesses, and citizens started working remotely (IntSights 2020). Indeed, there has been a more than 40% surge in machines running remote desktop protocols, often without even minimal security precautions (Gately 2020). Rapid digital transformation accelerated by COVID-19 has created new opportunities for cybercrime: so-called brute force attacks against users increased over 400% and email scams grew by almost 700% in the first few months of the global pandemic (Climpani 2020; Shi 2020). Increased online dependencies coupled with poor cyber defences have dramatically increased cybercrime and the range of potential targets. Predictably, Interpol has reported a shift from individuals and small businesses being attacked to public agencies, large corporations, and critical infrastructure (Interpol 2020c).

There are several types of digital threats generated by organized criminal organizations in the wake of the pandemic. Among the most commonly reported are online scams and phishing schemes. These tend to consist of COVID-19-themed emails, typically impersonating public health authorities. The goal is to convince unsuspecting targets to relieve themselves of personal data and download malicious content. According to industry experts, phishing scams account for the vast majority of breaches (Verizon 2020). Disruptive malware—also known as ransomware—is another common technique used by cyber-criminals, often targeting hospitals, clinics, laboratories, financial institutions, technology companies and local governments.[2] In such cases, the private data and operating systems of selected targets are paralysed until a ransom is paid over (Muggah and Goodman 2019). Data-harvesting malware and malicious domains are also common, wherein trojans and spyware are used to compromise networks and access privileged information. There is also a surge in misinformation, channelled via SMS, email, and websites, some of it linked to illegal medical commodities.

Organized crime groups have successfully capitalized on the fear and anxiety associated with the global COVID-19 pandemic. Literally billions of people are searching the internet every day for news on the disease and ways to avoid it. A Google search reveals almost six billion pages with the expression 'COVID-19' at the time of this writing. Literally thousands of coronavirus-themed domains are being created every day, the vast majority of which are scams peddling misinformation and disinformation, fake cures, or containing malware. Illicit business is also thriving in the Dark Web, where zoom credentials are being sold, along with COVID-19-themed malware. Ransomware attacks, from a wide variety of attackers, have reportedly increased by at least 75% since the start of the pandemic (Skybox Security 2020). According to the European Union, for example, ransomware is considered one of the top threats facing the region (Europol 2020a).

A considerable proportion of the organized crime market has migrated online and is transacted using encrypted currencies in the Dark Web. The Dark Web was already fertile territory for money laundering and widely used by drug cartels, hackers, and state-sponsored attack groups to buy and sell goods and trade skills and expertise. While the average life cycle of Dark Web market sites appears to be shortening, there is still a preference among organized crime groups for so-called TOR infrastructure. Even so, there are signs of some criminal groups turning to other privacy-orientated distributed marketplaces to buy and sell illegal products—including digital tools to scam targets. Europol has singled out OpenBazaar, Samouraiwallet, Wasabiwallet, and a range of crypto-currency wallets as top threats. Decentralized marketplace protocols are classified as a 'high priority threat', since they facilitate the selling of illegal goods (Coindesk 2020).

Expanding into New Markets

Around the world, organized crime groups exploited the COVID-19 pandemic to expand their influence at home. In many areas, cartels and gangs already exert control over specific parts of government, the private sector, and civil society. Some may exert oversight over entire sections of cities and neighbourhoods. During

[2] Even before COVID-19, ransomware attacks were trending upwards. A 2018 report determined that 53% of executives experiencing such an attack admitted paying the ransom. On average, hackers are paid upwards of $24 billion a year.

periods of crisis, such as the outbreak of contagious disease, crime groups may seize the opportunity to deepen their control by providing relief assistance to areas in need (Laufs and Waseem 2020; UN Office on Drugs and Crime (UNODC) 2020c). In Mexico, for example, cartels provided aid marked with the logo of known cartel leaders. In Italy, mafia groups delivered food relief through fake charity organizations. In Japan, the Yakuza doled out masks and sanitary products to pharmacies and primary schools. Gangs in Cape Town called for a temporary 'truce', factions in Rio de Janerio imposed curfews on local residents, and militant extremist groups in parts of Syria distributed health information.

Organized crime groups rapidly moved to consolidate their governance in geographical territories during the early stages of the COVID-19 crisis. Italy's Cosa Nostra, for example, provided food to households in Palermo and Naples within days of the pandemic being declared (Di Donato and Lister 2020; Rosen 2020). In Mexico, the Jalisco New Generation, Gulf, and Sinaloa cartels distributed groceries and protective gear across their areas of control. Some food parcels distributed in Guadalajara were even emblazoned with the logo of 'El Chapo 701', the notorious jailed leader of the Sinaloa cartel. In Tamaulipas, aid was covered in stickers reading: 'Gulf Cartel, in support of Ciudad Victoria, Mr. 46, Vaquero'. For their part, the Japanese Yakuza even offered assistance to cruise liners docked in Yokohama (Cerantola 2020). From Italy and Japan to Central America and Mexico, organized crime groups extort local businesses and citizens to pay for said relief assistance and to subsidize future 'recovery' efforts (El Universal 2020; Ríos and Sapalú 2020).

A key goal of these influence operations is to strengthen the legitimacy of organized crime networks in areas where they operate. While often colluding with public and private entities, in some cases co-opting political elites, law enforcement agencies and the judiciary and customs officials, the ability of organized crime groups to influence residents provides an additional layer of protection (and a continued flow of recruits). This helps to explain the overt performative component of their aid delivery. Crime groups are quick to publicly enforce curfews, restrict the movement of people, and impose price controls on high-demand products. Such activities not only provide them with lucrative rents, but it also burnishes their credentials among the public. Much like aid agencies stamp their food relief with institutional logos, cartels and gangs are adamant that recipients know who is providing them with assistance. It also serves to underline the relative weakness of official state service providers. In some cases crime groups may publicize their good works—they understand that optics matter.

Many organized crime groups are remarkably adept at shifting their procurement networks and supply chains to meet changing demand (Gomis 2020). In the first few months of the pandemic, some of them reportedly struggled to move narcotics and people due to reduced demand, limited shipping options, and increased border restrictions (UNODC 2020a). Mindful of global demand for medical supplies (and associated challenges with trafficking in certain drugs), some groups pivoted to engage in production and trafficking of specialized (and often fraudulent) medical equipment and protective gear. Within weeks of the pandemic being announced, reports emerged of fake masks being seized in Western Europe, contraband equipment being impounded in Eastern Europe, and falsified pharmaceuticals being captured in the Americas. Interpol, for example, reported the seizure of more than 4 million fake pharmaceutical products involving close to 40 organized crime groups.

Evidence from past crises indicate that organized crime groups are likely to extract rents from legitimate public and private entities involved in crisis response. In the case of the COVID-19 pandemic, a likely target includes public cash injections to support businesses and citizens that are facing massive deficits. An area that is rising to the top of the agenda is fraud, corruption, and embezzlement of COVID-19-related funds. Governments have committed trillions of dollars to recovery and bail-out packages to support citizens and businesses. International development banks have likewise committed hundreds of billions of dollars to help lower- and middle-income countries. In past health crises, such as Ebola, audits revealed considerable financial crimes. Organized crime groups are likely to seize opportunities to access these funds, including through ostensibly legitimate third-party vendors.

Criminal actors will almost certainly seek to syphon off financial assistance intended for small and medium enterprises or public works projects intended to improve health facilities and public works projects, such as water and waste management. A typical entry point is the tendering and procurement process, whereby fake and shadow vendors are awarded contracts for services that are never completed or poorly executed. Another target are recipients themselves, who may be extorted after receiving state subsidies. Similar dynamics have played out in the context of natural disasters in Mexico, when the Gulf and Sinaloa cartels supported hurricane recovery. Likewise, in Japan, the Yakuza and Yamaguchi-Gumi provided assistance following earthquakes there (Goi 2017; Jones 2011).

In the longer term, organized crime groups may seek to deepen their influence and reach by providing liquidity to cash-strapped businesses and effectively infiltrating the legal economy. In some cases, organized crime groups could be in a position to offer high-interest loans to services in high demand—especially the food industry, transportation sector, retail outlets, cleaning companies, and even funeral homes. In others, they may provide zero-interest loans, requesting 'favours' on demand. When firms and individuals are unable to pay back loans or undertake said favour, crime groups may effectively take their businesses over. Their goal will be to secure interests in companies that allow them to expand their criminal capacities, including laundering profits and shipping contraband. As noted above, an area already being widely exploited by organized crime is the trade in medical products and protective gear (GI-TOC 2020a; UNODC 2020b; Kumar and Tidey 2020).

Global Efforts to Disrupt Organized Crime

Several international organizations were quick to acknowledge the threats of organized crime in the wake of COVID-19. Global policing institutions, in particular, reported large-scale operations to disrupt drug-trafficking networks, paedophilia rings, online fraud, and the smuggling and sale of faulty medical equipment and supplies. Interpol coordinated several major operations in partnership with police, customs, and health regulatory authorities, including one stretching across 90 countries to crack down on the vending of illegal medicines and medical products (Interpol 2020b). Europol also created a dedicated unit to fight COVID-19-related crime—the European Financial and Economic Crime Centre, specifically to tackle fraud, counterfeit goods, and money laundering (Ljubas 2020). While some of these efforts suggest accelerated global action, a closer inspection of international responses reveals that they were more limited than advertised.

At the international level, the UN did not urge any clear or decisive action on the organized crime threat posed by the COVID-19 pandemic. While the United Nations Security Council has the authority to advise on threats to international peace and security, it issued no firm statements or resolutions on the organized crime dimensions or conflict escalation potential of the pandemic in 2020. The lack of engagement of key UN bodies is surprising, given the fact that organized crime actors have clearly impeded global efforts to respond to the pandemic. As noted above, reports of illegal trafficking of medicine and supplies, digital extortion, and fraud in relation to economic recovery funding are widespread. Moreover, the potential for criminal activity arising from prolonged lockdowns, weakened service provision, and economic duress is also very real. To his credit, the UN Secretary General issued several calls for increased attention to the risks of COVID-19-related misinformation, including a 'communications for solidarity' initiative (UN 2020).

Meanwhile, UN intergovernmental bodies that are expected to galvanize action by member states against organized crime, especially illicit markets, also failed to take concerted action. In this case, there was not so much a lack of political will as very real logistical constraints associated with the pandemic—not least, restrictions on international travel. For example, planned gatherings of the UN Congress on Crime Prevention and Criminal Justice were postponed in 2020. Meetings of the UN Convention against Transnational Organized Crime and the UN Convention against Corruption were likewise pushed back. When these entities do reconvene, they will be forced to adjust their work plans to accommodate dramatic changes in the international landscape, including the growth of financial crimes related to COVID-19 relief, as well as surging cybercrime in a more digitalized world.

Despite the limited engagement of the UN Security Council and intergovernmental bodies, some UN agencies took steps to address the threat of organized crime in the wake of COVID-19 (Walker 2020). The World Health Organization (WHO), for example, was itself exposed to a phishing scam early in the crisis, with hackers sending false alerts requesting personal information. The organization initiated a project with social media companies to highlight the risks of digital malfeasance and specific cyber risks to health facilities. The UNODC issued materials on the impacts of organized crime, including the ways in which illegal wildlife smuggling contributes to disease outbreaks. The United Nations Interregional Crime and Justice Research Institute (UNICRI) also highlighted the ways in which terrorist and criminal groups exploited social media and digital tools during the pandemic. Other agencies such as the UN Children's Fund (UNICEF), the UN High Commissioner for Refugees (UNHCR), the UN Office of the Rule of Law and Security Institution (OROLSI), the United Nations Development Program (UNDP), and others weighed in with programs to monitor digital harms.

One issue where UN agencies were determined to make an impact related to prisons and detention centres. The UN Office of the High Commissioner for Human Rights (OHCHR) was one of the first agencies to address the issue, drawing attention to the risk of outbreaks of prison violence and urging the release of pre-trial detainees (OHCHR 2020; WHO 2020). Its director eventually called on member states to reduce the number of detainees, an appeal that was adopted by several, but not all, governments. The OHCHR likewise signed a joint statement with other organizations, such as the UN Programme on HIV/AIDS (UNAIDS), UNODC, and the WHO, emphasizing the importance of reducing overcrowding, ensuring access to health services, and implementing physical distancing measures. Likewise, the OROLSI set out guidance on ways that penal institutions could adapt to the health crisis. The issue of prison overcrowding and inhumane conditions issues have long been of concern to UN agencies, and COVID-19 generated opportunities to address them.

National Responses to Fighting Organized Crime

More or less every national government around the world prepared for a potential crime surge in the wake of the COVID-19 pandemic. An overriding concern was the risk of social unrest and disorder in the event of deep economic setbacks and the fragmentation of food supply chains. Yet with notable exceptions, nonviolent crime rates remained comparatively stable and even declined during the lockdown period (Eisner and Nivette 2020; Abt et al. 2020; Muggah and Pinker 2020). Where police adopted overly aggressive enforcement, however, the risk of protest and riots often increased. A priority for many countries, especially those in Latin America and the Caribbean, was keeping violence from spreading within and outside the prison system. Another worry for police agencies was the diversification of organized crime into new revenue streams and their taking advantage of the weaknesses of law enforcement agencies that were also at risk of reduced staffing due to COVID-19.

Sky-rocketing international demand for medical supplies and personal protective equipment triggered a parallel jump in criminal activity. As previously noted, several organized crime groups seized the opportunity to divert supplies, launch online fraud schemes, and sell counterfeit goods. Many governments launched operations to take down such criminal networks, from Iran (Eqbali and Rasmussen 2020) and Nigeria (Interpol 2020d) to the UK (Chowdhury 2020) and the United States (Neal and Gagne-Acoulon 2020). Interpol issued guidelines to support law enforcement agencies (Interpol 2020a), including recommendations on how to address the issue of fake and counterfeit medical products, such as disposable surgical masks, hand sanitizers, antiviral medication, and test kids. They advocated for high-powered communications strategies to educate the public about false and misleading adverts, as well as hotlines to detect scams at an early stage.

Several governments also used the COVID-19 pandemic as a strategic opportunity to shore up influence or advance new, potentially controversial, policies. For example, early on in the pandemic, the Chinese government modified its legislation related to wildlife trade (Cochrane 2020). Sensitive that illegal wet markets may be a source of viral outbreaks, China banned all wet markets across the country. Meanwhile, the United States also used COVID-19 as a pretext to redirect military assets into the Caribbean Sea. The move, according to the US president, was intended to prevent drug cartels from exploiting the pandemic and served to reinforce US efforts to combat narcotics trafficking in the region (Chalfant 2020). More benignly, Canada also pushed through money-laundering guidelines through the Financial Transactions and Reports Analysis Centre of Canada (FINTRAC) to assist accountants, banks, casinos, and real estate brokers to identify and prioritize reports of suspicious transactions (Humphreys 2020).

Many countries and companies also sped up processes to safeguard their digital assets. The UK government, for example, issued a wide range of advisories related to cyber threats, including notices warning the public of the nature of cyber-attacks that exploit the fear of COVID-19. As in many other countries, it highlighted the danger of phishing emails posing as official communications from health officials (Martin 2020). The UK's National Cyber Security Centre (NCSC) issued streamlined guidance for how public and private entities could mitigate malware and ransomware attacks (Antcheva 2020). Most governments encouraged citizens to avoid opening suspicious emails, to back up their online data, and to use strong passwords and two-stage authentication, and to improve their own digital literacy.

Non-Governmental Approaches to Tackling Organized Crime

A significant number of non-governmental organizations, media outlets, and private firms have also issued guidance to prevent and reduce the risk of organized crime. A prime example of this is the Global Initiative against Transnational Organized Crime (GI-TOC), which has produced a host of reports on the many ways COVID-19 has contributed to changes in criminal markets and behaviour (see GI-TOC 2020a, 2020b). Like the UNODC, it has created a resource page for COVID-related material and provides regular updates of news reporting on the issue. Other organizations ranging from Brookings and the International Crisis Group (ICG) to the International Committee of the Red Cross and the Royal United Services Institute have issued reports on the dangers posed by organized crime in the wake of COVID-19 (Felbab-Brown and Martinez 2020; Mačák et al. 2020; ICG 2020; Ditcham 2020).

Most of these institutions recommend deeper analysis of the dynamic nature of organized crime as it diversifies into new income streams and consolidates its governance in areas of low state control. Some also recommend the close monitoring of the supply chains of illicit products and patterns of consumption to determine whether COVID-19-related shifts are temporary or longer term. While independent media platforms such as InSight Crime are closely tracking what is happening in the Americas, there is less evidence of dynamics in parts of Africa, where information is scarce. According to the GI-TOC (2020a), it is critical to track 'second-order' security impacts of COVID-19, especially those in which criminal organizations are exploiting vulnerabilities.

A recurring concern among non-governmental organizations is that the risks posed by organized crime will not be redressed without international cooperation, enhanced investment in law enforcement and prevention, and more concerted involvement of non-state actors. A key focus, they contend, must be on concerted action to disrupt different points in the criminal network. Some human rights organizations advocate strongly against militarizing responses, urging governments to be particularly mindful of human rights considerations. Others urge more support for lower-income countries, with more limited resources, and where the impacts of organized crime are potentially more consequential for vulnerable populations. In these and other settings, civil society and the private sector has a role to play in helping governments to engage with communities at the neighbourhood scale, with a view of re-asserting governance and territorial control (Shaw and Reitano 2020).

COVID-19 has also exposed chronic frailties and, in some cases, corruption within police forces. It has also required police to take on roles that may entail more repression than is normal, alienating them from local communities. The prolonged lockdowns have also restricted more positive police–citizen engagement, which is so essential to ensuring real and perceived public security. These disconnects have been exploited by some organized crime groups, some of them offering 'protection' in the absence of law enforcement. By contrast, state-led measures that have involved deploying military and police assets have also often backfired, in some cases generating resentment and frustration. Non-governmental organizations have a role to play in highlighting the flaws of under- and over-policing, as well as encouraging transparency, accountability, and oversight (Vittori 2020).

Conclusion

The COVID-19 pandemic and the associated lockdowns are transforming organized crime. In addition to influencing the risk of various types of criminal violence, the pandemic has also indirectly strengthened the social, economic, and political clout of several criminal organizations in the same way that the Italian mafia and Japanese Yakuza emerged stronger after the great dislocations of the Second World War. Crime kingpins know full well that law enforcement and criminal justice systems are overstretched and that prisons are bursting at the seams. They also know that severe economic disruption could increase the risk of disequilibrium in illicit markets and violent competition as groups establish new pacts. The extent to which these shifts are temporary or permanent depend in large part on the timing and distribution of vaccines and other pharmaceutical measures and the ways in which governments respond.

In the short term, governments, international agencies, and civil society groups should focus on disrupting organized crime's exploitation of the health sector, as well as the runaway trade in illegal forestry and wildlife products. Partnerships with conventional and social media platforms to reduce the risk of digital malfeasance are critical, as are investments in protecting those most vulnerable to the fall-out of criminal activities. In the longer term, a priority is to curb opportunities for collusion and corruption between state entities and organized crime, strengthen state capacities to exert law and order in areas of low state presence, and build unified political and economic responses to deprived areas that undermine the credibility of organized crime.

Ultimately, the trajectories of organized crime will be shaped not just by regional and domestic factors, but also by the global political and economic environment. And just as pandemics shape the nature of organized crime networks, they also typically reconfigure how law enforcement and criminal justice agencies respond to counter them. The realignment of state resources—including police and criminal justice services—will profoundly influence the way both state agencies and organized crime evolve. Heavy-handed responses may generate counterproductive outcomes if they erode trust and confidence among citizens (Muggah 2018). By contrast, measures that adhere to the highest standards of professionalism and that nurture community support can deprive criminal groups of their legitimacy.

A distinctly twenty-first-century challenge is minimizing the threats of cybercriminals preying on communities during incidents such as pandemics. Strategies that build public awareness and improved cooperation between police forces at national and international levels are key. With hundreds of millions of people forced to work, purchase, and communicate online, cybercriminals are deft at exploiting digital loopholes and undermining data protection. Governments and citizens will need to invest heavily in promoting digital literacy and fostering digital resilience (Muggah 2020a). National computer emergency response teams (CSIRTs) will play an even more critical role in protecting cyberinfrastructure. CSIRTs can also improve information sharing with qualified private response teams. In the absence of internationally agreed rules and standards to manage cyber threats, multi-stakeholder cyber security governance will need to become the standard operating procedure for societies around the world.

References

Abt, Thomas, Richard Rosenfeld, and Ernesto Lopez. 2020. 'COVID-19 and Homicide: Final Report to Arnold Ventures'. https://craftmediabucket.s3.amazonaws.com/uploads/COVID-19-Homicide_061520_Final.pdf.

Agren, David. 2020. 'Mexico Murder Rate Reaches New High as Violence Rages amid COVID-19 Spread'. *The Guardian*, 3 April. https://www.theguardian.com/world/2020/apr/03/mexico-murder-rate-homicide-coronavirus-covid-19.

Ahmed, Jamal. 2020. 'Lockdowns Have Been Hard on Organized Crime Too'. *Foreign Policy*, 7 October. https://foreignpolicy.com/2020/10/07/ransom-hacking-cybercrime-pandemic-lockdowns-organized-crime.

Aleman, Marcos. 2020. 'El Salvador Homicides Drop; Experts Point to Virus Lock-Down'. *ABC News*, 1 April. https://abcnews.go.com/International/wireStory/el-salvador-homicides-drop-experts-point-virus-lock-69925070.

Antcheva, Ioanna. 2020. 'Keeping Ransomware at Bay: UK NCSC Updates Its Malware and Ransomware Guidance'. Slaughter and May, 24 March. https://thelens.slaughterandmay.com/post/102g2nw/keeping-ransomware-at-bay-uk-ncsc-updates-its-malware-and-ransomware-guidance.

Associated Press. 2020. 'Crime Falls Sharply in Even the Most Violence US Cities'. *The Guardian*, 11 April. https://www.theguardian.com/us-news/2020/apr/11/crime-falls-sharply-in-even-the-most-violent-us-cities.

Aziani, Alberto, Serena Favarin, and Gian Maria Campedelli. 2019. 'Security Governance: Mafia Control over Ordinary Crimes'. *Journal of Research in Crime and Delinquency 57* (4): pp. 444–92.

BBC News. 2020. 'El Salvador Gangs: "No Ray of Sunlight for Inmates"'. 28 April. https://www.bbc.com/news/world-latin-america-52454519.

Castro, Luiz Felipe. 2020. 'Subnotificação e gatilhos: o drama da violência doméstica na quarentena'. *Veja*, 29 March. https://veja.abril.com.br/brasil/subnotificacao-e-gatilhos-o-drama-da-violencia-domestica-na-quarentena.

Cerantola, Alessia. 2020 'Japanese Gangs Vie for Power amid Pandemic'. Organized Crime and Corruption Reporting Project (OCCRP), 22 April. https://www.occrp.org/en/coronavirus/japanese-gangs-vie-for-power-amid-pandemic.

Chalfant, Morgan. 2020. 'Trump Announces Enhanced Counternarcotics Operation at Coronavirus Briefing'. *The Hill*, 1 April. https://thehill.com/homenews/administration/490704-trump-announces-enhanced-counternarcotics-operation-at-coronavirus.

Chowdhury, Hasan. 2020. 'Almost 200 Fraudulent Coronavirus Sites Taken Down in UK'. *The Telegraph*, 30 March. https://www.telegraph.co.uk/technology/2020/03/30/almost-200-fraudulent-coronavirus-sites-taken-uk.

Climpani, Catalin. 2020. 'Kaspersky: RDP Brute-Force Attacks Have Gone Up since Start of COVID-19'. *ZDNet*, 29 April. https://www.zdnet.com/article/kaspersky-rdp-brute-force-attacks-have-gone-up-since-start-of-covid-19.

Cochrane, Jacqueline. 2020. 'China to Revise Wildlife Laws Following COVID-19 Outbreak'. *GI-TOC*, 24 February. https://globalinitiative.net/analysis/china-to-revise-wildlife-laws-following-covid-19-outbreak.

Coindesk. 2020. 'Europol Names Privacy Wallets, Coins, Open Marketplaces as "Top Threats" in Internet Crime Report'. 5 October. https://www.coindesk.com/europol-samurai-wasabi-wallet-openbazaar-monero-zcash-crime.

Cuthbertson, Anthony. 2020. 'Coronavirus: Dark Web Market Bans Drug Dealers Selling Fake COVID-19 Vaccines'. *The Independent*, 3 April. https://www.independent.co.uk/life-style/gadgets-and-tech/news/coronavirus-vaccine-cure-dark-web-drugs-market-covid-19-a9442671.html.

Dazio, Stefanie, Franklin Briceno, and Michael Tarm. 2020. 'Crime Drops around the World as COVID-19 Keeps People Inside'. *ABC News*, 11 April. https://abcnews.go.com/Health/wireStory/crime-drops-world-covid-19-people-inside-70098369.

Di Donato, Valentina, and Tim Lister. 2020. 'The Mafia Is Poised to Exploit Coronavirus, and Not Just in Italy'. *CNN*, 19 April. https://www.cnn.com/2020/04/19/europe/italy-mafia-exploiting-coronavirus-crisis-aid-intl/index.html.

Ditcham, Keith. 2020. 'How COVID-19 Is Changing the Organised Crime Threat'. Commentary, RUSI, 24 March. https://rusi.org/commentary/how-covid-19-changing-organised-crime-threat.

Eisner, Manuel, and Amy Nivette. 2020. 'Violence and the Pandemic: Urgent Questions for Research'. HFG Research and Policy Brief, April. https://www.hfg.org/hfg_reports/violence-and-the-pandemic-urgent-questions-for-research/.

El Universal. 2020. 'The Unión Tepito Cartel Is Providing Loans to Small Businesses in Mexico City'. 25 May. https://www.eluniversal.com.mx/english/union-tepito-cartel-providing-loans-small-business-owners-mexico-city.

Eqbali, Aresu, and Sune Engel Rasmussen. 2020. 'Iran Battles Coronavirus—and the Black Market for Medical Supplies'. *Wall Street Journal*, 1 March. https://www.wsj.com/articles/iran-battles-coronavirusand-the-black-market-for-medical-supplies-11583081174.

Ernst, Falko. 2020. 'Mexican Criminal Groups See COVID-19 Crisis as Opportunity to Gain More Power'. *The Guardian*, 20 April. https://www.theguardian.com/world/2020/apr/20/mexico-criminal-groups-covid-19-crisis-opportunity-gain-power.

Europol. 2020a. 'COVID-19 Sparks Upward Trend in Cybercrime'. Press release, 5 October. https://www.europol.europa.eu/newsroom/news/covid-19-sparks-upward-trend-in-cybercrime.

Europol. 2020b. 'How Criminals Profit from the COVID-19 Pandemic'. Press release, 27 March. https://www.europol.europa.eu/newsroom/news/how-criminals-profit-covid-19-pandemic.

Fajardo, Luis. 2020. 'Coronavirus: Latin American Crime Gangs Adapt to Pandemic'. *BBC News*, 21 April. https://www.bbc.com/news/world-latin-america-52367898.

Felbab-Brown, Vanda, and Ariel Fernando Ávila Martinez. 2020. 'COVID-19 and Organized Crime: Latin American Governments Are In a State-Making Competition with Crime'. Brookings Institute, 12 May. https://www.brookings.edu/on-the-record/covid-19-and-organized-crime-latin-american-governments-are-in-a-state-making-competition-with-crime.

Ford, Liz. 2020. '"Calamitous": Domestic Violence Set to Soar by 20% during Global Lockdown'. *The Guardian*, 28 April. https://www.theguardian.com/global-development/2020/apr/28/calamitous-domestic-violence-set-to-soar-by-20-during-global-lockdown-coronavirus.

Gately, Edward. 2020. '10 Destructive COVID-19 Data Breaches'. *Channel Futures*, 20 July. https://www.channelfutures.com/mssp-insider/10-seriously-destructive-covid-19-data-breaches.

GI-TOC. 2020a. 'Crime and Contagion: Impact of a Pandemic on Organized Crime'. March. https://globalinitiative.net/wp-content/uploads/2020/03/GI-TOC-Crime-and-Contagion-The-impact-of-a-pandemic-on-organized-crime-1.pdf.

GI-TOC. 2020b. 'The Impact: Coronavirus and Organized Crime Podcast'. 14 April. https://foreignpolicy.com/2020/04/14/we-can-make-the-post-coronavirus-world-much-less-violent.

Goi, Leonardo. 2017. 'Honduras Crime Group Used Natural Disaster to Launder Money'. *InSight Crime*, 29 March.

Gomis, Benoît. 2020. 'How the Illicit Drug Trade Is Adapting to the Coronavirus Pandemic'. *Work Politics Review*, 20 April. https://www.worldpoliticsreview.com/articles/28696/how-the-illicit-drug-trade-is-adapting-to-the-coronavirus-pandemic.

Guarascio, Francesco. 2020. 'COVID-19: Latin American Cocaine Floods Europe during Pandemic—Some of It Stashed in Squid'. *National Post*, 30 April. https://nationalpost.com/news/world/covid-19-latin-american-cocaine-floods-europe-during-pandemic-some-of-it-stashed-in-squid.

Hamilton, Ian, and Alex Stevens. 2020. 'How Coronavirus Is Changing the Market for Illegal Drugs'. *The Conversation*, 26 March. https://theconversation.com/how-coronavirus-is-changing-the-market-for-illegal-drugs-134753.

Hope, Alejandro. 2020. 'Narcos Are Suffering from the COVID-19 Lockdown Too'. *Financial Times*, 20 April. https://www.ft.com/content/42341ce6-82e5-11ea-b555-37a289098206.

Humphreys, Adrian. 2020. 'Canada's Money-Laundering Monitor Now Triaging Reporting Process by COVID-19-Hit Businesses'. *National Post*, 26 March. https://nationalpost.com/news/canadas-dirty-money-and-terrorist-financing-monitor-now-triaging-reporting-process-by-covid-19-hit-businesses.

International Crisis Group (ICG). 2020. 'COVID-19 and Conflict: Seven Trends to Watch'. Special briefing, March. https://www.crisisgroup.org/global/sb4-covid-19-and-conflict-seven-trends-watch.

Interpol. 2020a. 'COVID-19 Pandemic: Guidelines for Law Enforcement'. 26 March. https://www.interpol.int/content/download/15014/file/COVID19_LE_Guidelines_PUBLIC_26mar2020.pdf?inLanguage=eng-GB.

Interpol. 2020b. 'Global Operation Seems a Rise in Fake Medical Products Related to COVID-19'. 19 March. https://www.interpol.int/en/News-and-Events/News/2020/Global-operation-sees-a-rise-in-fake-medical-products-related-to-COVID-19.

Interpol. 2020c. 'Interpol Report Shows Alarming Rate of Cyberattacks during COVID-19'. Press release, 4 August. https://www.interpol.int/en/News-and-Events/News/2020/INTERPOL-report-shows-alarming-rate-of-cyberattacks-during-COVID-19.

Interpol. 2020d. 'Nigeria Arrests Two Suspects Linked to Massive Mask Fraud'. 9 September. https://www.interpol.int/en/News-and-Events/News/2020/Nigeria-arrests-two-suspects-linked-to-massive-mask-fraud.

IntSights. 2020. 'The Cyber Threat Impact of COVID-19 to Global Business'. https://intsights.com/resources/covid-19-cyber-threat-impact-report.

Jones, Terril Yue. 2011. 'Yakuza among First with Relief Supplies in Japan'. *Reuters*, 25 March. https://www.reuters.com/article/us-yakuza-idUSTRE72O6TF20110325.

Kumar Isabelle, and Alice Tidey. 2020. 'COVID-19: Organised Crime Group "Adapting" with "New Crime Trends," Interpol Warns'. *Euronews*, 30 March. https://www.euronews.com/2020/03/30/covid-19-organised-crime-group-adapting-with-new-crime-trends-interpol-warns.

La Diaria Politica. 2020. 'Brasil excluye del informe annual sobre violaciones a los derechos humanos los datos de violencia policial'. 13 June. https://ladiaria.com.uy/politica/articulo/2020/6/brasil-excluye-del-informe-anual-sobre-violaciones-a-los-derechos-humanos-los-datos-de-violencia-policial.

Laufs, Julian, and Zoha Waseem. 2020. 'Policing in Pandemics: A Systemic Review and Response to COVID-19'. *Journal of Disaster Risk Reduction 51*: 101812. https://www.ncbi.nlm.nih.gov/pmc/articles/PMC7439012.

Ljubas, Zdravko. 2020. 'Europol Launches New Unit to Address Crime Related to COVID-19'. OCCRP, 8 June. https://www.occrp.org/en/daily/12493-europol-launches-new-unit-to-address-crime-related-to-covid-19.

Mačák, Kubo, Tilman Rodenhäuser, and Laurent Gisel. 2020. 'Cyber Attacks against Hospitals and the COVID-19 Pandemic'. *Humanitarian Law and Policy Blog*, 2 April. https://blogs.icrc.org/law-and-policy/2020/04/02/cyber-attacks-hospitals-covid-19.

Martin, Alexander. 2020. 'Coronavirus: UK Intelligence Agency Issues Public Warning about Criminals Exploiting Outbreak'. *Sky News*, 16 March. https://news.sky.com/story/coronavirus-uk-intelligence-agency-issues-public-warning-about-criminals-exploiting-outbreak-11958113.

Morfini, Nicola. 2020. 'Coronavirus and Narcotics: Can Drug Cartels Survive COVID-19?'. *Al Jazeera*, 29 April. https://www.aljazeera.com/opinions/2020/4/29/coronavirus-and-narcotics-can-drug-cartels-survive-covid-19.

Muggah, Robert 2018. 'Reviewing the Costs and Benefits of Mano Dura versus Crime Prevention in the Americas'. In *Continuities and Change in IPE at the Start of the Twenty-First Century*, edited by Laura C. Mahrenbach and Timothy M. Shaw. London: Palgrave.

Muggah, Robert 2020a. 'Designing Digital Safety into the Smart City'. *European Cybersecurity Journal* 6 (1): pp. 36–43.

Muggah, Robert 2020b. 'The Pandemic Has Generated Dramatic Shifts in the Criminal Underworld'. *Foreign Policy*, 8 May. https://foreignpolicy.com/2020/05/08/coronavirus-drug-cartels-violence-smuggling.

Muggah, Robert, and Marc Goodman. 2019. 'Cities Are Easy Prey for Cybercriminals: Here's How They Can Fight Back'. *Agenda*, 30 September. https://www.weforum.org/agenda/2019/09/our-cities-are-increasingly-vulnerable-to-cyberattacks-heres-how-they-can-fight-back.

Muggah, Robert, and Steven Pinker. 2020. 'We Can Make the Post-Coronavirus World a Much less Violent Place'. *Foreign Policy*, 14 April. https://foreignpolicy.com/2020/04/14/we-can-make-the-post-coronavirus-world-much-less-violent.

Neal, Will, and Sandrine Gagne-Acoulon. 2020. 'US Files First Enforcement Act against COVID-19 Fraud'. OCCRP, 23 March. https://www.occrp.org/en/daily/11894-us-files-first-enforcement-act-against-covid-19-fraud.

Office of the High Commissioner for Human Rights (OHCHR). 2020. 'COVID-19 and Protection of Right to Life in Places of Detention'. Press release. https://www.ohchr.org/Documents/Issues/Executions/HumanRightsDispatch_2_PlacesofDetention.pdf.

Organized Crime and Corruption Reporting Project (OCCRP). 2020. 'What Lockdown? World's Cocaine Traffickers Sniff at Movement Restrictions'. *In-Sight Crime*, 26 May. https://www.insightcrime.org/news/analysis/world-cocaine-traffickers-lockdown.

Reuters. 2020. 'As Mexico Focuses on Coronavirus, Drug Gang Violence Escalates'. *International Business Times*, 18 June. https://www.ibtimes.sg/mexico-focuses-coronavirus-drug-gang-violence-escalates-47082.

Ríos, R., and L. Sapalú. 2020. 'Pandilleros conceden indulto en el cobro de extorsión'. *El Periodico*, 26 March. https://elperiodico.com.gt/nacionales/2020/03/26/pandilleros-conceden-indulto-en-el-cobro-de-extorsion/.

Rosen, Kenneth R. 2020. 'Stoking Unrest and Distributing Groceries: Italy's Mafias Gain Ground in Fight for Loyalty during Pandemic Lockdown'. *Newsweek*, 18 April.

Semple, Kirk, and Azam Ahmed. 2020. 'Murder Rates Were Staggering. The Virus Has Brought Some Quiet, for Now'. *New York Times*, 11 April. https://www.nytimes.com/2020/04/11/world/americas/coronavirus-murder-latin-america-crime.html.

Shaw, Mark, and Tuesday Reitano. 2020. 'COVID-19: Strengthen Civil Society in a Time of Unprecedented Change and Undermine Criminal Governance'. *GI-TOC*, 31 March. https://globalinitiative.net/analysis/covid-19-strengthen-civil-society-in-a-time-of-unprecedented-change-and-undermine-criminal-governance.

Shi, Fleming 2020. 'Threat Spotlight: Coronavirus-Related Phishing'. Blog post, 26 March. https://blog.barracuda.com/2020/03/26/threat-spotlight-coronavirus-related-phishing.

Skybox Security. 2020. 'Tear Up the Cybersecurity Rule Book'. https://www.skyboxsecurity.com/trends-report.

Stargardter, Gabriel, and Drazen Jorgic. 2020. 'Special Report: Peruvian Coca Farmers to Paris Pushers, Coronavirus Upends Global Narcotics Trade'. *Reuters*, 22 April. https://www.reuters.com/article/us-health-coronavirus-latam-narcotics-sp/special-report-peruvian-coca-farmers-to-paris-pushers-coronavirus-upends-global-narcotics-trade-idUSKCN2242ZI.

Tagziria, Lyes. 2020. '#CovidCrimeWatch—no. 6'. *GI-TOC*, 29 April. https://globalinitiative.net/analysis/covidcrimewatch-n6.

United Nations (UN). 2020. 'UN Tackles Infodemic of Misinformation and Cybercrime in COVID-19 Crisis'. Press release. https://www.un.org/en/un-coronavirus-communications-team/un-tackling-%E2%80%98infodemic%E2%80%99-misinformation-and-cybercrime-covid-19.

UN General Assembly (UNGA). 2000. 'UN Convention against Transnational Organized Crime'. Resolution 55/25, 15 November. https://www.unodc.org/unodc/en/organized-crime/intro/UNTOC.html.
UN Office on Drugs and Crime (UNODC). 2020a. 'COVID-19 and the Drug Supply Chain: From Production and Trafficking to Use'. Research brief, May. https://www.unodc.org/documents/data-and-analysis/covid/Covid-19-and-drug-supply-chain-Mai2020.pdf.
UNODC. 2020b. 'COVID-19-Related Trafficking of Medical Products as a Threat to Public Health'. Research brief. www.unodc.org/documents/data-and-analysis/covid/COVID-19_research_brief_trafficking_medical_products.pdf.
UNODC. 2020c. 'The Impact of COVID-19 on Organized Crime'. Research brief, July. https://www.unodc.org/documents/data-and-analysis/covid/RB_COVID_organized_crime_july13_web.pdf.
Verizon. 2020. '2020 Data Breach Investigations Report'. https://enterprise.verizon.com/resources/reports/dbir/?CMP=OOH_SMB_OTH_22222_MC_20200501_NA_NM20200079_00001.
Vittori, Jodi. 2020. 'Corruption Vulnerabilities in the U.S. Reponse to the Coronavirus'. Carnegie Endowment for International Peace, 20 March. https://carnegieendowment.org/2020/03/20/corruption-vulnerabilities-in-u.s.-response-to-coronavirus-pub-81336.
Walker, Summer. 2020. 'COVID-19 and Crime: A Response Develops at the UN'. *GI-TOC*, June. https://globalinitiative.net/wp-content/uploads/2020/06/Covid-19-and-crime-A-response-develops-at-the-UN.pdf.
Weiss, Sandra. 2020. 'How the Coronavirus Lockdown Is Hitting Mexico's Drug Cartels'. *DW*, 4 April. https://www.dw.com/en/how-the-coronavirus-lockdown-is-hitting-mexicos-drug-cartels/a-53001784.
World Health Organization (WHO). 2020. 'UNODC, WHO, UNAIDS and OHCHR Joint Statement on COVID-19 in Prisons and Other Closed Settings'. Press release, 13 May. https://www.who.int/news/item/13-05-2020-unodc-who-unaids-and-ohchr-joint-statement-on-covid-19-in-prisons-and-other-closed-settings.

11

The Pandemic Crisis

A Tragic Perspective

Christophe Roux Dufort and Mary-Lieta Clément

Many crisis management models and tools provide decision-makers and governments with effective means to prevent, manage, and learn from major catastrophes (Pauchant and Mitroff 1992; Williams et al. 2017; Waller et al. 2014). However, few studies have supported the effectiveness of these tools on the capacity of organizations to cope with these crises, especially since unthinkable events such as the 9/11 terrorist attacks of 2001 or major climatic episodes mostly made these tools and models inoperative (Dror 2001). Pandemics such as severe acute respiratory syndrome (SARS), swine flu (H1N1), Ebola, or COVID-19, for example, are examples of these unavoidable and inescapable episodes that put crisis management plans to the test and eventually exceed their limits. To cope with the number of victims and death, as in the COVID-19 pandemic, which resulted in more than 3 million deaths in spring 2021, governments hurriedly implemented curative measures that led to a major global economic weakening and revealed that health, economic, and social systems, previously thought to be robust, could collapse in a short period of time. While several governments believed that great epidemics were a thing of the past as a result of scientific progress in hygiene, medicine, and disease prevention, the experience of the COVID-19 pandemic has deeply challenged these assumptions and questioned the capacity of governments to cope with pandemics. From this point of view, we hypothesize that pandemics, COVID-19 among others, show similarities with the Greek tragedy model, where despite any plans heroes devise to escape a forthcoming catastrophic scenario, they are doomed to fail and eventually realize the extent of their debacle.

In keeping with the multidisciplinary perspective of this volume (see the Introduction by Ackerly et al.), in this chapter we attempt to analyse the management of pandemics, and, by extension, the management of major crises, through the lens of Greek tragedy literature. This angle opens up new avenues for defining crises and analysing the behaviours and strategies of government decision-makers in times of pandemics in particular (see Chapter 5 in this volume by Bickerton). Greek tragedy

Christophe Roux Dufort and Mary-Lieta Clément, *The Pandemic Crisis*. In: *A Multidisciplinary Approach to Pandemics*. Edited by Philippe Bourbeau, Jean-Michel Marcoux, and Brooke A. Ackerly, Oxford University Press.
 DOI: 10.1093/oso/9780192897855.003.0012

provides an opportunity to view crises under a new light, as it features characters grappling with forces beyond their control and conflicting dilemmas that can only be resolved by heart-breaking decisions that ultimately lead to despair and terror (De Romilly 2014; Judet de la Combe 2012). It also portrays the behaviours and the strategies implemented by heroes to cope with inescapable scenarios, and the inner emotional turmoil theses attempts may fuel for heroes torn between the search for freedom of action and the inescapable necessity of events (Denham 2014).

The investigation of pandemics and, more specifically, the COVID-19 pandemic, through the lens of Greek tragedy should thus be carried out at the crossroads of a point of no return triggered by the official declaration of the pandemic by the World Health Organization (WHO) and the government decision-makers' strategies. As we will show, viewed from the perspective of tragedy, the behaviours and strategies of decision-makers are not based on a rational management of events guided by plans and tools. They are rather built upon alternative and more desirable interpretations of reality, intuitions, and bets intended to maintain hope among the members of crisis teams and the general population. Greek tragedy also helps us to uncover how these decisions may precipitate a further worsening of the crisis and cause decision-makers to measure the full extent of their failures too late in most cases.

Tragedy and the Tragic Tone

Greek tragedy originated in Athens, Greece, in the first tragic competitions organized during the religious festivals in honour of Dionysus in the fifth century BC (De Romilly 2014). It is a theatrical genre that depicts heroes tormented by a struggle between freedom and necessity (Szondi 2003; Denham 2014). By revealing the ending at the very beginning of the play (De Romilly 2014), tragedy conveys the principle of imminent or already concluded annihilation that cannot be avoided. It manifests itself by way of a blindness that pushes the tragic hero to commit a fatal error while believing he is doing the right thing (Szondi 2003). Tragedy provides us with a rich perspective from which to understand the nature of crises and their development by highlighting the existence of a division between the hope of having a way to flee a situation and its inescapable nature (Comte-Sponville 2018). To sum up, we consider tragedy as a theatrical form that puts noble characters at the heart of an overdetermined scenario in which they have to make heart-breaking decisions that lead to a catastrophe. In particular, tragedy provides opportunities to reflect on the behaviour of decision-makers in a crisis and to understand their decision-making process.

Tragedy involves several intertwined events that suddenly emerge, causing a reversal of the normal course of the hero's life without giving him the possibility of changing anything in its trajectory (De Romilly 2009; Denham 2014). In the myth of Oedipus, the oracle announces the inevitable scenario to which the hero will be subjected. He will kill his father and marry his mother. These two announcements appear in a peaceful environment in which Oedipus lives in happiness. It is a complete upheaval of his previously balanced reality and a radical change of trajectory toward a destiny announced in advance. No matter what happens, Oedipus will not be able to avoid the prophecy proclaimed by the oracle. The first key dimension of tragedy thus lies in the nature of the scenario itself that is experienced by heroes as inevitable, insurmountable, and irreparable (Rosset 2014) and renders them incapable of reversing the course of events.

As mentioned above, the scenario is inescapable, but it is also fatal (Judet de la Combe 2013). In *Oedipus Rex*, for example, the ambiguity of the information provided by the oracle about the scenario makes it impossible for Oedipus to anticipate how he will fall (De Romilly 1998; Steiner 1993), which is the second dimension of tragedy. The hero is thus placed in a position of trying by all means available to divert the trajectory of events to make the oracle's prophecy a lie. To do so, he creates a second reality, one that is more acceptable to him and that gives him hope that the oracle's prediction can be circumvented (Rosset 1993). Rosset (1993) refers to this as the duplicate reality that illustrates the second key dimension of tragedy: the hero's capacity to change the scenario by creating a duplicate version of it in which he recovers his power to act and change fate. From that point forward, the hero takes a series of initiatives based on bets that give him the illusion of being free from his destiny and maintaining control over future events.

The hero's choices are not without high risks and severe consequences, however. In the myth of Oedipus, for example, the young hero, horrified by the oracle's prediction, tries to thwart the prophecy and save his parents by sacrificing his royal life in Corinth and travelling to Thebes. To a certain extent, the tragic hero is pushed towards a threshold beyond which he is forced to make heart-breaking choices involving sacrifice in the hopes of escaping his destiny (De Romilly 1998; Sewell-Rutter 2007). The third dimension of tragedy thus lies in the nature and consequences of the choices made by the hero to escape the inevitable outcome. These choices force the hero to sacrifice a crucial part of his life.

This third aspect of tragedy comes hand in hand with a fourth: the self-fulfilling nature of the hero's decisions. As explained above, the tragic hero makes decisions that allegedly free him from his fate (Rosset 2014). In doing so, however, studies on tragedy teach us that he unknowingly sets the stage for the prophecy to be fulfilled. His attempt to escape the scenario takes one more step towards the final, unavoidable outcome. In a nutshell, the fourth key dimension of tragedy is the self-fulfilling nature of the hero's choices, inasmuch as it is his attempts to alter the trajectory of the foretold scenario that actually create the conditions for the prophecy to be fulfilled (De Romilly 2014; Judet de la Combe 2012).

As time goes by and the hero pursues his strategy, he can still convince himself that he has made the right choice and he is in the process of changing fate until he realizes he has hit a dead end. At this point, it is too late. Therefore, temporality is central in tragedy but does not follow a chronological logic. For that reason, Rosset (2014) distinguishes chronological time from tragic time. Tragic time is the time when the hero retrospectively realizes his failure once the scenario has already come to an end. It is particularly well described in *Oedipus Rex*. As Rosset (2014) explains: 'The hero approaches tragic time in reverse …, the final event is the one Oedipus fears. As soon as he is made aware of this plague that needs an investigation, the tragic tension has already come to an end' (2014: 15–16 [our translation]). The fifth dimension of tragedy thus lies in the idea that tragedy only crops up at the end, when it is all over and the hero's ignorance and the irreparable nature of the scenario are retrospectively revealed to him.

To sum up, the five key dimensions of tragedy are the inevitable, insurmountable, and irreparable nature of the scenario; the incapacity to anticipate; the sacrificial decisions; the self-fulfilling nature of decisions; and the double temporality. In the next section of this chapter, we will use these five dimensions of tragedy to discuss the crisis management response to the COVID-19 pandemic and outline five proposals to explain how COVID-19 is a tragedy

The Tragic Dimension: Tragedy in the COVID-19 Crisis

In order to build a tragic reading of pandemics, we relate the five key dimensions of tragedy identified above with key aspects of crises and crisis management regularly found in the literature to draw research proposals from this cross-literature review. This set of research proposals offers a broader perspective on pandemics. It provides an alternative view to account for several aspects that must be taken into consideration to provide a comprehensive understanding of pandemics from a crisis management perspective.

Confiscation of Alternatives

In the same way that tragedy sets up a scenario that is beyond the hero's control, there is a fair degree of consensus among crisis management researchers that crises are sudden and unexpected episodes that disrupt the existing system of reference and the normal course of business (Pearson and Clair 1998). Definitions are also fairly close to the idea articulated by studies on tragedy that crises such as pandemics should be theorized as inevitable scenarios that pave the way for a tragic episode.

However, in management, crises are rarely viewed as insurmountable and irreparable, as they are portrayed in Greek tragedy. It is assumed that they are potentially controllable. Many studies have shown how organizations develop management routines to mitigate consequences as quickly as possible when crises emerge (Comfort 2007). The effectiveness of resilience capacities (Williams et al. 2017), the need for team coordination, crisis communication plans, and other activities are more often than not put forward to contain and resolve crises and disasters (Pearson and Clair 1998). These practices are usually formalized in emergency plans and procedures (Marcum et al. 2012) that serve as a basis for decision and action in times of crisis.

In terms of managing pandemics, on the heels of the H1N1 experience in 2009 many countries set up pandemic plans in order to be prepared to respond to potential future episodes. Leung and Nicoll (2010) have studied the major components of such plans, which were built upon key crisis management principles that include clear communication of public health messages that should not confuse what *could* happen with *what is most likely* to happen; evidence and fact-based decisions regarding the pandemic response; a review of national pandemic plans in coordination with the WHO to ensure that they are consistent; the collection of essential data, including epidemiological and immunological data, and the sharing of this information among countries; and greater and more timely access to antivirals and influenza vaccines worldwide.

Even though this planning approach to crisis management is widely shared among managers and government officials, some researchers argue that crises, and especially pandemics, are so unexpected that all plans and resources may instantly become obsolete and discarded (Perrow 1984; Byrne and Callaghan 2013; Dekker et al. 2011; Longstaff and Yang 2008). The absence of any plans to cope with unprecedented episodes such as COVID-19 further adds to the surprise and dismay of decision-makers, who are now faced with a double challenge: coping with an irremediable scenario in the absence of any alternatives or plans to escape it. In such circumstances, Greek tragedy teaches us that heroes feel powerless and are left with no adequate or adapted resources to change and reverse the course of events (Rosset 2014; De Romilly 2009; Bryce et al. 2020; Winston 2020).

In the same vein, unthinkable crises discard any possibility of a better scenario and remove all alternatives for action in the minds of decision-makers. As an example, what make the COVID-19 pandemic tragic, for instance, is not only the threatening onset of a deadly virus that leads to the realization that nothing will ever be the same again, but also the overwhelming sense that an inevitable, insurmountable, and irremediable scenario is occurring with no available plans to cope with it. The increasing numbers of infections and the absence of any vaccines or medications mean that the situation has reached a point of no return that suppresses any hope for a quick end to the pandemic (Agence France Presse 2020).

Proposal 1
Pandemics are tragic because they impose a crisis scenario that quickly appears inevitable, insurmountable, and irreparable and, as a result, confiscates the possibility of a more desirable scenario for decision-makers, thereby fuelling a sense of powerlessness.

Duplicating Reality

To cope with crises, decision-makers, like tragic heroes, are forced to resort to behaviours and strategies likely to help them overcome powerlessness and regain control. In crisis management, studies explore strategies such as denial of reality (Roux-Dufort 2009). Laughlin (1979) explains that managers deny reality by convincing themselves that the situation is not so serious and is still recoverable. Denial can also be seen in tragedy, when the hero creates a duplicate reality (Rosset 1993), which acts as a virtual scenario in which the hero imagines he may recover his freedom to make decisions and act according to his own will. We therefore suggest that decision-makers themselves resort to the construction of a more desirable reality in the hope that it creates a space in which response strategies leading to a positive outcome can be envisioned.

In the specific case of the COVID-19 pandemic, the differences in the sanitary responses implemented by various countries to cope with it illustrate how government officials have based their responses on differing scenarios. In Sweden, for example, the government accepted the inevitable scenario of a massive and deadly pandemic by attempting to create herd immunity. Other countries, such as many in the European Union, rejected this idea and saw a more desirable scenario in the option of mitigating the number of sick and dead from COVID-19 (Cazenave 2020). These two approaches to the management of the pandemic illustrate the extent to which each government was challenged to manage an inescapable scenario by building alternative virtual realities in which they envisioned an array of strategies that differed from one country to another.

Making decisions regardless of cost is another strategy to cope with powerlessness, at least in the early stages of a crisis. As in tragedy, crises require quick decisions that are also irreversible (Kouzmin 2008; De Romilly 2014). Researchers recommend that decisions be guided by a planned approach, with tools supported by analytical and conscious processes (Sayegh et al. 2004; Parnell and Crandall 2020). While many authors subscribe to this view, other scholars point out the shortcomings associated with rational decision-making models in times of crisis. They claim that crisis plans, procedures, and routines confine managers to a limited set of alternatives (Bourrier and Bieder 2013) and suggest that managers resort to intuition to enrich the rational decision strategies (Curnin et al. 2020; Okoli and Watt 2018; Parnell and Crandall 2020; Kahneman et al. 1982). As in tragedy, where the hero cannot but follow his intuition to envision a possible way out of his predicament (De Romilly 1998; Vernant and Vidal-Naquet 1982), we suggest that, in the absence of any plans, decision-makers use their intuition to guide them as they create their duplicate reality, thereby fuelling their own hope and trust about the positive outcomes of the strategies they implement.

Coming back to the COVID-19 pandemic, faced with a lack of any existing plans or updates since 2009, governments have had to improvise a response to cope with the early stages that was mainly based on an intuition that their preferred strategy would work. For instance, in many Western countries, government officials persuaded themselves that confinement would be the most efficient strategy to control the spread of the virus (Lacroix 2020), whereas in March 2020 very few scientific studies were available to support the effectiveness of such a strategy to mitigate a pandemic (St Onge and Campan 2020). Sweden, on the other hand, made the decision to provide education and commit its population to abiding by the sanitary measures in an effort to develop herd immunity. This strategy, however, was also not based on any empirical evidence that this approach would work (Sirois 2020). In both cases, governments followed their intuitions based on a construct that served as an argument to convince themselves of their ability to gain the upper hand over the pandemic. Beyond the search for effectiveness, we argue that these response strategies aimed to maintain trust and hope among the population and the decision-makers themselves. They should be viewed as bets on the positive outcomes of their response, which is the very nature of tragic decision-making.

Proposal 2

Pandemics are tragic when decision-makers design strategies based on a duplicate reality on the basis of which they convince themselves of their ability to reverse the worst-case scenario and fuel hope and trust about the success of their strategies.

Sacrifice

In tragedy, the hero consents to making heart-breaking choices in the hope of saving his life. In the same vein, crisis management literature reports that managers use sacrificial strategies in times of crisis as an ultimate solution to restore balance (Amiridis 2018; Kent and Boatwright 2018). In particular, Halverson and colleagues (2004) have shown how self-sacrifice by leaders in certain circumstances provides psychological comfort to subordinates who, as a result, assign a higher degree of charisma and organizational commitment to those leaders in situations of crisis. However, the reasons for the sacrifice must be clear to be approved of and understood by the subordinates. If there is ambiguity, the sacrifice will be perceived as irrational and dangerous and may cause decision-makers to lose credibility (Halverson et al. 2004).

We suggest that in a tragic crisis such as a pandemic, decisions entail a certain amount of sacrifice as a price to pay to overcome what appears to be inescapable. The purpose of this sacrifice should be clearly communicated to the population, which runs the risk of being misunderstood and raising suspicion towards the sanitary strategies implemented by governments. In the COVID-19 pandemic, for example, many governments made the decision to sacrifice economic growth to limit the spread of the virus, but had to face increasing defiance by their populations about the reasons for maintaining and extending the imposed sacrifice over a longer term (Lecavalier 2020).

Proposal 3

Pandemics are tragic when governments make decisions that sacrifice the core resources and assets of their countries to protect populations against viruses. If not properly communicated and shared with the population, sacrifices may backfire on the decision-makers, who may lose credibility and legitimacy.

Self-Fulfilling Decisions

As mentioned above, tragedy highlights the self-fulfilling nature of the hero's decisions (De Romilly 2013; Szondi 2003). Likewise, in crisis management the self-fulfilling nature of decisions has been observed in the relationship between downplaying reality and the escalation of consequences. When managers face serious events, they mobilize psychological defence mechanisms such as underestimating their magnitude or potential consequences that lead them to believe they can keep the situation under control (Lewis 2019; Roux-Dufort 2009). This is particularly the case when managers have to cope with high levels of uncertainty. They demonstrate a cognitive bias of illusion of control or optimism biases (Weinstien 1989) to nurture an illusionary sense of self-confidence. This perception affects their understanding of the situation and drives them to make decisions that are not based on a realistic measure of the situation (Weick 1988; Okoli and Watt 2018; Anderson and Sun 2017), thereby increasing the risk that their decisions will precipitate or escalate the crisis (Weick 1993; Lewis 2019). Management literature thus illustrates how a manager's myopia and attempts to downplay crises lead to an underestimation of the risks, a limited number of response options being considered, and a potential escalation of the consequences. In other words, while their intention is to mitigate the crisis, decision-makers may actually be in a position where they can precipitate or escalate it.

In the case of the COVID-19 pandemic, the controversy surrounding the lockdown as an amplifying factor (additional stress, increased violence, layoffs, etc.) partly exemplifies the self-fulfilling nature of decisions made in highly uncertain and ambiguous times (Orjollet 2020). The multiple side effects of the decision to impose confinement measures are now viewed as escalating the consequences of the COVID-19 pandemic. The underestimation of the risks of a pandemic in the months preceding its onset and the lack of scientific knowledge about the virus, in combination with the difficulty governments faced in exploring and evaluating alternative options to the lockdown, contributed to the implementation of an immediate short-term solution. However, the longer-term negative and devastating impacts of the decisions were not considered because of the nature of the emergency.

Proposal 4

Pandemics are tragic when decisions made by governments to prevent the escalation of virus actually end up precipitating and amplifying it.

The Retrospective Failure

As in tragedy, once again, crisis management research emphasizes the importance of time and, more specifically, the importance of acting within a limited time frame (Claeys and Cauberghe 2012). A quick response allows organizations to take control of the crisis and mitigate its severity (Williams et al. 2017). Reaction, prevention, or learning takes place within a specific window that, if not respected, could make the action ineffective.

Overall, crisis management research perceives time in a linear fashion—that is, minute by minute. In the event-based approach to crises, for example, a crisis is seen as a sudden and unique event that erupts abruptly within a specific time and space (Pearson and Clair 1998). In the process-based approach, however, a crisis is theorized as a process that develops over a long period of time (Roux-Dufort 2009). In both perspectives, time is chronological. In tragedy, however, we have argued that time was essentially retrospective and contains revealing information about how and why decision-makers were unable to prevent and stop the crisis. In the crisis management literature, this retrospective view is present particularly in the sense-making processes that decision-makers go through when they eventually see the consequences of their actions (Furey and Rixon 2018; Weick 1995) and realize the extent to which the catastrophe was inevitable, insurmountable, and irreparable. Both the manager and the tragic hero realize the ineffectiveness of these decisions once the scenario comes to its conclusion.

As long as time is running out, decision-makers overestimate their control over the crisis and assume they can reverse it by increasing their effort (Weick 1988; Okoli and Watt 2018; Anderson and Sun 2017). However, what eventually turns a crisis into a tragedy is the inability of decision-makers to realize the limitations and inadequacy of their decisions before the crisis comes to an end. They only understand the full magnitude of the chaos they have helped create after it is too late. This is where tragedy reveals its true essence. In the case of the COVID-19 pandemic, when governments opted for a lockdown strategy, they could not anticipate the magnitude of the side effects until they became apparent (Pilon-Larose 2020). Two months after the lockdown was ordered, governments started taking the real measure of the consequences of such a drastic decision. The economy had declined drastically. In the Canadian province of Quebec, senior citizens were dying in abnormal proportions in retirement homes. Many organizations had gone bankrupt, mental health was quickly becoming a major issue, and schoolchildren were falling behind in their studies, in addition to a number of other emerging social issues (Di Domenico et al. 2020). Although the lockdown was a response to control the pandemic, it plunged many countries into a major economic and social crisis, the consequences of which could not yet be seen.

Proposal 5
Pandemics are tragic when governments only take the measure of the consequences and side effects of their response after it is too late to reverse the scenario and adjust their decisions.

This comparative analysis of the literature on tragedy and crisis management and the development of research proposals about pandemics leads us to define a pandemic crisis as follows: a pandemic crisis results from the collision of an overdetermined scenario (the announced pandemic) that is perceived as inevitable, insurmountable, and irremediable and an attempt by decision-makers to free themselves from these constraints to control and reverse the trajectory of the pandemic. They design a more acceptable version of the pandemic scenario from which they hope to overcome it, and they make sacrificial decisions, while hoping to reap positive outcomes. The pandemic crisis is tragic when decision-makers discover that, despite decisions to mitigate the crisis, the dreaded catastrophic scenario has already come to pass and forced them to acknowledge at least a partial failure.

A Development Model of a Tragic Crisis

In this final section, we present a four-stage model of the evolution and development of crises based on the tragic perspective and illustrate this model with the example of Quebec government's responses to the COVID-19 crisis from March to September 2020. The following examples drawn from the Quebec experience do not constitute empirical testing. They exemplify and nurture certain points on which to reflect on the management of a pandemic crisis.

Phase 1: Emergence of the Catastrophic Scenario

As mentioned above, a pandemic crisis breaks out with the eruption of a catastrophic scenario perceived as inevitable, insurmountable, and irremediable. In the case of the COVID-19 pandemic in Quebec, Canada, as in many other countries, the disruption began in December 2019, when China alerted the WHO about an outbreak of atypical cases of pneumonia in Wuhan. The virus responsible for this hitherto unknown disease was a new virus of the coronavirus family. The symptoms of this contagious disease were fever, cough, severe fatigue, and respiratory discomfort, which in the most severe forms could lead to death. By March 2020, the number of people in the world with COVID-19 was increasing and spreading at a rapid rate. On 13 March 2020, there were 7,498 cases worldwide, including 4 cases in Quebec, according to the WHO (WHO 2020; INSPQ 2020).

At this point, for Quebec Premier François Legault and his government, it was difficult to fully grasp the situation and its scope. In March 2020, tests were still unreliable and insufficient to determine the total number of infections (Labbé 2020) and draw a reliable picture of the extent of the pandemic in the province. Above all, no one in Quebec knew how this trend would evolve. A major outbreak was in sight, but the worst was still to come (Bourgault Côté 2020). The government feared that the health-care system might not be robust enough to absorb the number of cases requiring medical treatment. Successive cuts in budgets and human resources in the past and the reorganization of the entire health-care system have resulted in an undercapacity issue among hospital infrastructures. The system should have been fully changed if they wanted to control and stem the epidemic as quickly as possible (Bourgault Côté 2020), but it was obviously too late for such considerations. The pandemic in Quebec started as a real tragedy, as government decision-makers who faced the announcement of an imminent catastrophe retrospectively discovered the consequences of past financial decisions made by previous governments on the capacity of the province to cope with the pandemic.

Phase 2: Negotiating with the Scenario

Trapped in the paradox of having to cope with a major pandemic with no plans and inadequate resources, Premier Legault and his government entered the second stage of the tragic process in which they had to negotiate with the terrifying reality to come up with responses and solutions to protect the population and stem the pandemic as quickly as possible. In this phase, they had to find their way towards freedom of action in the midst of chaos and uncertainty to cope with the fate of a pandemic crisis that appeared to be sealed.

As discussed above, the situation offered a limited set of options, all of which were considered a unique way to mitigate the consequences of the pandemic. However, with each option, the government had to make a sacrificial decision and put the province's core resources at risk. At this point, Premier Legault and his government were in the midst of the tragic dilemma. The first alternative lay in the creation of herd immunity by allowing the virus to circulate freely. However, this option required that 70% of the population become infected, which would mean that lives would have to be sacrificed (Institut Pasteur 2020). The second option called for a full or partial confinement of the population, in addition to closing the Canada–United States border to non-essential travel, in order to limit the spread of the virus. This strategy required that the province's economic growth be sacrificed at its peak period (Le Journal de Montreal 2020), with dramatic consequences on employment, education, social relations, and so on. Moreover, in the absence of solid scientific proof concerning the outcomes of confinement in times of pandemic, the effectiveness of this option was also uncertain. The final decision to order a full lockdown was certainly not made on the basis of entirely rational reasoning or through established procedures, but rather by hoping that the general lockdown would be the most desirable scenario (Bélair-Cirino 2020).

Although these response strategies seemed like bets on the future, they nurtured the illusion of having options, and therefore freedom. They nevertheless set the stage for a social, economic, and psychological crisis to erupt. From that point forward, each step to protect the population from the virus appeared to be one more step towards tragedy.

Phase 3: Measuring the Consequences of Early Decisions

As the crisis continued throughout the spring and summer (in September 2020, Quebec had reached 64,244 cases and 5,773 deaths (Santé et service sociaux Québec (SSSQ) 2020)), the Quebec government started to see the consequences of its early decisions by looking back on its actions (Furey and Rixon 2018). This retrospective sense-making was made possible through the feedback and reactions from a wide range of stakeholders, such as political opposition parties, the media, the judiciary, teachers, entrepreneurs, health-care personnel, and the general population, all of whom had to deal with the impacts of the lockdown.

Premier Legault and his government were initially viewed as heroes and praised by both the media and the public in the early stages of the pandemic (Custeau 2020), but were subsequently highly criticized by opponents for having ruined the province's economy; not having invested enough in the health-care system; not having implemented further prevention measures (Richer 2020); having created major social problems, such as stress and mental health issues (QMI 2020); having created a situation that saw an increase in cases of spousal abuse (Gagné 2020);

having not prevented the deaths of many seniors; and having allowed students to fall behind in their studies. In addition, Premier Legault's government was accused of having been too slow in its response and issuing contradictory messages, in particular regarding the wearing of masks, which damaged its credibility (Fortier 2020; St Onge and Campan 2020). The tragic irony is that the government was also criticized for not having chosen the other options it had considered earlier in March: mass screening and a targeted lockdown (Mercure 2020).

Despite all of its efforts and attempts to prevent the pandemic from escalating, the government's decisions had not been successful in sparing the province from a major crisis. As of October 2020, Quebec is still the Canadian province with the highest number of cases and deaths from COVID-19. To a certain extent, the stakeholders took a retrospective look at the pandemic scenario while the government remained stuck in a chronological time frame. This conflict of temporality made the crisis tragic because it was much too late to catch up with the turn of events. The government's leaders were then pushed into the last phase of the model.

Phase 4: Colliding with the Tragic

In the last phase of the COVID-19 tragedy, Quebec's leaders realized that the decisions to mitigate the pandemic had not prevented the province from experiencing a major crisis. In tragic terms, this highlights the insurmountable nature of events (Rosset 2014). No matter what the hero did, the situation could never be overcome. In this stage, there is no longer any hope that the situation will improve, as the tragedy has delivered its verdict. The dreaded disaster has occurred. The prophecy has been fulfilled. When the situation is this dire (Yin and Jing 2014), studies on tragic literature refer to this as an *irremediable situation* (Rosset 2014).

In the months after the event, the actions of Premier Legault and his government are being questioned. Once considered heroes, they are now viewed as responsible for inconsistent and disorganized decisions that have led to an unprecedented crisis (Richer 2020; Fortier 2020). Regardless of their choices and their legitimate search for the most efficient solutions, the pandemic and its consequences have taken an insurmountable and irremediable turn against which the government can no longer fight.

Conclusion

In this chapter, we analysed the tragic nature of crises through the angle of pandemics. In particular, we showed that strategies may become ineffective because the decisions taken to thwart the scenario actually precipitate, and even escalate, the crisis. The inevitable and irremediable nature of a tragic crisis causes any attempts to anticipate, prepare, or prevent it to be limited in scope and effectiveness.

However, our model of tragic crises provides avenues to reflect on how leaders could face a no-return situation such as a pandemic. In these circumstances, we proposed that decision-makers are likely to act from a duplicate version of reality that stimulates intuition and inspires a series of bets on the future. Bets aim to maintain a collective hope of escaping the worst-case scenario and may serve as a strong motivational process for both decision-makers and the general population, even though they involve making sacrifices to save what is most essential (i.e. in the case of COVID-19, sacrificing economic growth in the interests of public health).

A tragic approach to pandemics suggests that crisis management teams should train and prepare to evolve in circumstances where the time for preventative and planned interventions is behind them. On the one hand, they should learn to create and maintain hope over the long term to keep the population mobilized and motivated to continue abiding by the sanitary recommendations, for example. On the other hand, leaders need to learn how to insist on compliance when alternatives involve sacrificing important assets to safeguard the essentials. Such dilemmas are rarely discussed in crisis management literature, and even less so in practice.

Finally, we propose that any public response to pandemics should be composed of organizational measures that encourage team members, employees, and leaders to maintain internal coherence and prepare stakeholders to understand and accept the sacrifices that pandemics may inevitably require. The tragic essence of crises, and pandemics in particular, is unavoidable. We believe that acknowledging this fact sets the conditions for a more robust crisis management response to face such ruthless events.

References

Agence France Presse. 2020. 'Bilan de l' épidémie de Covid-19 dans le monde le 28 Mars: Plus de 30 000 morts'. 29 March. https://www.latribune.ca/covid-19/bilan-de-lepidemie-de-covid-19-dans-le-monde-le-28-mars-plus-de-30-000-morts-4c6e8869e5f28b89d721f337c25561b8.

Amiridis, Kostas. 2018. 'The Shadow of Sophocles: Tragedy and the Ethics of Leadership'. *Business Ethics Quarterly 28* (1): p. 15.

Anderson, Marc H., and Peter Y. T. Sun. 2017. 'Reviewing Leadership Styles: Overlaps and the Need for a New "Full-Range" Theory'. *International Journal of Management Reviews 19* (1): p. 76.

Bélair-Cirino, Marco. 2020. 'Le pari que fait François Legault'. *Le Devoir*, 25 March. https://www.ledevoir.com/politique/quebec/575647/coronavirus-point-de-presse-legault-arruda-24-mars.

Bourrier, Mathilde, and Corinne Bieder. 2013. *Trapping Safety into Rules: How Desirable or Avoidable Is Proceduralization?* Boca Raton: CRC Press.

Bourgault-Côté, Guillaume. 2020. 'Pour le gouvernement Legault, le plus difficile reste à venir'. *Le Devoir*, 21 March. https://www.ledevoir.com/politique/quebec/575482/une-crise-a-fragmentations.

Bryce, Cormac, Patrick Ring, Simon Ashby, and Jamie K. Wardman. 2020. "Resilience in the Face of Uncertainty: Early Lessons from the COVID-19 Pandemic'. *Journal of Risk Research 1* (8): p. 1.

Byrne, David and Gillian Callaghan. 2013. *Complexity theory and the social sciences: The state of the art*. London: Routledge

Cazenave, Fabien. 2020. 'Coronavirus: Quelles sont les mesures prises en Europe pour éviter la propagation du virus?'. *Ouest France*, 13 March. https://www.ouest-france.fr/sante/virus/coronavirus/coronavirus-quelles-sont-les-mesures-prises-en-europe-pour-eviter-la-propagation-du-virus-6778616.

Claeys, An-Sophie, and Verolien Cauberghe. 2012. 'Crisis Response and Crisis Timing Strategies: Two Sides of the Same Coin'. *Public Relations Review 38* (1): p. 83.

Comfort, Louise K. 2007. 'Crisis Management in Hindsight: Cognition, Communication, Coordination, and Control'. *Public Administration Review 67* (1): p. 189.

Comte-Sponville, André. 2018. *Du tragique au matérialisme (et retour): Vingt-six études sur. Montaigne, Pascal, Spinoza, Nietzsche et quelques autres*. Paris: PUF.

Curnin, Steven, Benjamin Brooks, and Christine Owen. 2020. 'A Case Study of Disaster Decision-Making in the Presence of Anomalies and Absence of Recognition'. *Journal of Contingencies and Crisis Management 28* (2): p. 110.

Custeau, Jonathan. 2020. 'Image des chefs en temps de crise: Legault fait mieux que Trudeau'. *La Tribune*, 20 March. https://www.latribune.ca/actualites/image-des-chefs-en-temps-de-crise--legault-fait-mieux-que-trudeau-34b48de48f0b4dda2573dcc35888f247.

Dekker, Sidney P., Paul Cilliers, and Jan-Hendrik Hofmeyr. 2011. 'The Complexity of Failure: Implications of Complexity Theory for Safety Investigations'. *Safety Science 49* (6): p. 939.

Denham, Alison. 2014. 'Tragedy without the Gods: Autonomy, Necessity and the Real Self'. *British Journal of Aesthetics 54* (2): p. 141.

De Romilly, Jacqueline. 1998. 'La prévision et la surprise dans la tragédie grecque'. In *Actes du 8ème colloque de la Villa Kérylos (Beaulieu-sur-Mer les 3 & 4 octobre 1997)*, pp. 1–9. Beaulieu-sur-mer: Publications de l'académie des inscription et Belles -Lettre.

De Romilly, Jacqueline. 2009. *Le temps dans la tragédie grecque: Eschyle, Sophocle, Euripide* (2nd edn). Paris: Vrin.

De Romilly, Jacqueline. 2013. *Magic and rhetoric in ancient Greece*. MA and London: Harvard University Press.

De Romilly, Jacqueline. 2014. *La tragédie grecque* (9th edn). Paris: Presses universitaires de France.

Di Domenico, Laura, Guilia Pullano, Chiara E. Sabbatini, Pierre-Yves Boëlle, and Vittoria Colizza. 2020. 'Impact of Lockdown on COVID-19 Epidemic in Île-de-France and Possible Exit Strategies'. *BMC Medicine 18* (1): p. 240.

Dror, Yehezkel. 2001. *The Capacity to Govern: A Report to the Club of Rome*. London: F.Class.

Fortier, Dominique. 2020. 'La critique libérale en santé Marie Montpetit reproche au gouvernement Legault sa gestion de la crise'. *Chaleurs Nouvelles*, 6 August.

https://www.chaleursnouvelles.com/article/2020/08/06/la-critique-liberale-en-sante-marie-montpetit-reproche-au-gouvernement-legault-sa-gestion-de-la-crise.

Furey, Mary, and Daphne Rixon. 2018. 'When Abnormal Becomes Normal: How Altered Perceptions Contributed to the Ocean Ranger Oil Rig Disaster'. *Journal of Management Policy and Practice 19* (3): p. 106.

Gagné, Louis. 2020. 'Les femmes violentées en mode "survie" durant le confinement'. *Radio-Canada*, 18 April. https://ici.radio-canada.ca/nouvelle/1695235/violence-conjugale-maisons-hebergement-femmes-confinement-ressources-aide-covid-19.

Halverson, Stefanie K., Courtney L. Holladay, Stephanie M. Kazama, and Miguel Quiñones. 2004. 'Self-Sacrificial Behaviour in Crisis Situations: The Competing Roles of Behavioural and Situational Factors'. *Leadership Quarterly 15* (2): p. 263.

Institut national de santé public du Quebec (INSPQ). 2020. 'Données COVID-19 au Québec'. *Institut national de santé public du Quebec*, 13 March. https://www.inspq.qc.ca/covid-19/donnees.

Institut Paster. 2020. 'Qu'est-ce que l'immunité collective?' 15 April. https://www.pasteur.fr/fr/espace-presse/documents-presse/qu-est-ce-que-immunite-collective.

Judet de La Combe, Pierre. 2012. 'Catastrophe et crise: De l'épopée à la tragédie grecques'. *Critique 783–784* (8): p. 642.

Judet de la Combe, Pierre. 2013. 'L'histoire dans l'essai tragique'. *Revue germanique internationale 17* (1): p. 67.

Kahneman, Daniel, Paul Slovic, and Amos Tversky. 1982. *Judgment under Uncertainty: Heuristics and Biases*. Cambridge: Cambridge University Press.

Kent, Michael L., and Brandon C. Boatwright. 2018. 'Ritualistic Sacrifice in Crisis Communication: A Case for Eliminating Scapegoating from the Crisis/Apologia Lexicon'. *Public Relations Review 44* (4): p. 514.

Kouzmin, Alexander. 2008. 'Crisis Management in Crisis?' *Administrative Theory & Praxis 30* (2): p. 155.

Labbé, Jérôme. 2020. 'Dépistage de la Covid-19: Quebec respectera dorénavant un ordre de priorité'. *Radio-Canada*, 26 March. https://ici.radio-canada.ca/nouvelle/1688208/coronavirus-covid-19-tests-priorites-quebec.

Lacroix, Guy. 2020. 'Les mesures du confinement sont-elles efficaces?' Cirano Allier savoir et décision, 30 April. https://cirano.qc.ca/files/publications/2020PE-11.pdf.

Laughlin, Henry P. 1979. *The Ego and Its Defenses*. New York: J. Aronson.

Lecavalier, Charles. 2020. 'Le écoles, les Cégepe et les universités seront fermés au Québec pour deux semaines'. *Le Journal de Québec*, 13 March. https://www.journaldequebec.com/2020/03/13/la-fermeture-de-toutes-les-ecoles-envisagee.

Le Journal de Montréal. 2020. 'Confinement, immunité collective, méthode coréenne: à la recherche de la bonne stratégie'. 23 April. https://www.journaldemontreal.com/2020/04/23/confinement-immunite-collective-methode-coreenne--a-la-recherche-de-la-bonne-strategie.

Lewis, James. 2019. 'The Fluidity of Risk'. *Disaster Prevention and Management 28* (5): p. 636.

Leung, Gabriel M., and Angus Nicoll. 2010. 'Reflections on Pandemic (H1N1) 2009 and the International Response'. *PLoS Med 7* (10): p. 1.

Longstaff, P. H., and Sung-Un Yang. 2008. 'Communication Management and Trust: Their Role in Building Resilience to "Surprises" such as Natural Disasters, Pandemic Flu, and Terrorism'. *Ecology and Society 13* (1): p. 3.

Marcum, Christopher S., Christine Bevc, and Carter T. Butts. 2012. 'Mechanisms of Control in Emergent Interorganizational Networks'. *Policy Studies Journal 40* (3): p. 516.

Mercure, Phillippe. 2020. 'Des chercheur remettent en question le "bien fondé du confinement"'. *La Presse*, 5 October. https://www.lapresse.ca/covid-19/2020-06-05/des-chercheurs-remettent-en-question-le-bien-fonde-du-confinement.

Okoli, Justin, and John Watt. 2018. 'Crisis Decision-Making: The Overlap between Intuitive and Analytical Strategies'. *Management Decision 56* (5): p. 1122.

Orjollet, Stephane. 2020. 'Confinement prolongé, santé mentale à surveiller'. *La Presse*, 4 October. https://www.lapresse.ca/actualites/sciences/2020-04-19/confinement-prolonge-sante-mentale-a-surveiller.

Parnell, John A., and Willian R. Crandall. 2020. 'The Contribution of Behavioural Economics to Crisis Management Decision-Making'. *Journal of Management & Organization 26* (4): p. 585.

Pauchant, Thierry C., and Ian I. Mitroff. 1992. 'Management by Nosing Around: Exposing the Dangerous Invisibility of Technologies'. *Journal of Management Inquiry 1* (1): p. 70.

Pearson, Christine M., and Clair Judith A. 1998. 'Reframing Crisis Management'. *Academy of Management Review 23* (1): p. 59.

Perrow, Charles. 1984. *Normal Accidents: Living with High Risk Technologies* (updated edn). Princeton, NJ: Princeton University Press.

Pilon-Larose, Hugo. 2020. 'Après la pandémie, la crise des finances publiques'. *La Presse*, 13 April. https://www.lapresse.ca/covid-19/2020-04-13/apres-la-pandemie-la-crise-des-finances-publiques.

QMI. 2020. 'Les effects du confinement sur soi'. *Le Journal de Montréal*, 19 April. https://www.journaldemontreal.com/2020/04/19/les-effets-du-confinement-sur-soi-1.

Richer, Jocelyne. 2020. '(Quebec) Au début exemplaire, la gestion de la crise sanitaire par le gouvernement Legault montre Désormais des ratés, selon la nouvelle cheffe du Parti Libéral du Quebec (PLQ), Dominique Anglade'. *La Presse*, 12 May. https://www.lapresse.ca/covid-19/2020-05-12/anglade-critique-legault-sur-sa-gestion-de-la-crise.

Rosset, Clément. 1993. *Le réel et son double: Essai sur l'illusion*. Paris: Galimard.

Rosset, Clément. 2014. *La philosophie tragique* (3rd edn). 'Quadrige'. Paris: Presses universitaires de France.

Roux-Dufort, Christophe. 2009. 'The Devil Lies in Details! How Crises Build Up within Organizations'. *Journal of Contingencies and Crisis Management 17* (1): p. 4.

Santé et service sociaux Québec (SSSQ). 2020. 'Pandémie de la COVID-19-Le gouvernement du Québec présente le bilan de la dernière journée'. 8 September. https://www.msss.gouv.qc.ca/ministere/salle-de-presse/communique-2303.

Sayegh, Lisa, William P. Anthony, and Pamela L. Perrewé. 2004. 'Managerial Decision-Making under Crisis: The Role of Emotion in an Intuitive Decision Process'. *Human Resource Management Review 14* (2): p. 179.

Sewell-Rutter, Neil James. 2007. *Guilt by Descent: Moral Inheritance and Decision Making in Greek Tragedy*. Oxford: Oxford University Press.

Sirois, Alexandre. 2020. 'Lâchez-nous avec la Suède!' *La Presse*, 4 October. https://www.lapresse.ca/debats/editoriaux/2020-10-04/lachez-nous-avec-la-suede.php.

Steiner, Georges. 1993. *La mort de la tragédie*. Paris: Galimard.

St Onge, Peter, and Gaël Campan. 2020. 'COVID-19: Le modèle défectueux qui confiné le Canada'. IEDM, 4 June. https://www.iedm.org/fr/covid-19-le-modele-defectueux-qui-a-confine-le-canada.

Szondi, Peter. 2003. *Essai sur le tragique*. Belval: Circé.

Vernant, Jean-Pierre, and Pierre Vidal-Naquet. 1982. *Mythe et tragédie en grèce ancienne*. Paris: Maspero (FM/Fondations).

Waller, Mary J., Zhike Lei, and Robert Partten. 2014. 'Focusing on Teams in Crisis Management Education: An Integration and Simulation-Based Approach'. *Academy of Management Learning and Education 13* (2): p. 208.

Weick, Karl E. 1988. 'Enacted Sensemaking in Crisis Situation'. *Journal of Management Studies 25* (4): p. 305.

Weick, Karl E. 1993. 'The Collapse of Sensemaking in Organizations: The Mann Gulch Disaster'. *Administrative Science Quarterly 38* (4): p. 628.

Weick, Karl E. 1995. *Sensemaking in Organizations*. Thousand Oaks, CA: Sage.

Weinstein, Neil D. 1989. 'Optimistic Biases about Personal Risks'. *Science 246* (935): p. 1232.

Williams, Trenton A., Daniel A. Gruber, Kathleen M. Sutcliffe, Dean A. Shepherd, and Yenfei Eric Zhao. 2017. 'Organizational Response to Adversity: Fusing Crisis Management and Resilience Research Steams'. *Academy of Management Annals 11* (2): p. 733.

Winston, A. 2020. 'Is the COVID-19 Outbreak a Black Swan or the New Normal?' *MIT Sloan Management Review*, 16 March. https://sloanreview.mit.edu/article/is-the-covid-19-outbreak-a-black-swan-or-the-new-normal.

World Health Organization (WHO). 2020. 'Number at a Glance'. 13 March. https://www.who.int/emergencies/diseases/novel-coronavirus-2019.

Yin, Shoujun, and Runtian Jing. 2014. 'A Schematic View of Crisis Threat Assessment'. *Journal of Contingencies and Crisis Management 22* (2): p. 97.

12

International and Global Cooperation in Response to COVID-19

The Past, the Present, and the Future

Sara E. Davies

The World Health Organization (WHO) received its first report of a suspect novel coronavirus (SARS-CoV-2) in Wuhan city, China, on 31 December 2019. The epidemiology reported 44 cases of pneumonia with a suspected link to a large seafood and live animal market. On 9 January 2020, the WHO announced that a novel coronavirus had been detected in patient samples from Wuhan city. The disease had spread by human-to-human transmission and self-isolation was recommended for 14 days for all persons who may have come into contact with persons infected with the virus or travelled in the affected area. The WHO Director-General declared the outbreak a Public Health Emergency of International Concern (PHEIC) on 30 January 2020 under the International Health Regulations (IHR). By the end of January, there had been 213 deaths, 9,682 confirmed cases (1,527 'severe' cases) and over 15,000 suspected cases of COVID-19 caused by SARS-CoV-2, across 31 provinces in China. On the same day as the declaration of the PHEIC, the IHR Emergency Committee provided advice to states on how to respond to the outbreak. It advised that countries prepare for early detection of the virus, to isolate infected individuals in accordance with international human rights standards, to put in place a contact tracing regime to prevent the spread of the virus, to regularly share national data on COVID-19 detection with the WHO, and to inform the WHO of travel restrictions—which the WHO did not recommend at the time.

Fourteen years earlier, states had agreed to establish an international legal framework to govern situations like the outbreak of COVID-19 (see Chapter 1 in this volume by Jacobsen for an understanding of the history of pandemics). The IHR had three aims to achieve better international cooperation in response to a PHEIC: build national capacities to detect, assess, and report public health events; invest in the WHO, the coordinating role to build this capacity; and, in the

Sara E. Davies, *International and Global Cooperation in Response to COVID-19.* In: *A Multidisciplinary Approach to Pandemics.* Edited by Philippe Bourbeau, Jean-Michel Marcoux, and Brooke A. Ackerly, Oxford University Press.
 DOI: 10.1093/oso/9780192897855.003.0013

event of a PHEIC, agree to specific measures at ports, airports, and ground crossings to limit the spread of health risks. These specific measures were intended to guide trade and travel restrictions so that the open reporting of outbreak events does not lead to unnecessary and punitive trade and travel restrictions. According to their proponents, the revised IHR provide 'rules and processes designed to increase compliance' with trade and travel measures that the WHO Director General could recommend on the basis on scientific evidence concerning the outbreak.

What does the international response to the COVID-19 pandemic tell us about the state of international health cooperation and its future? Drezner (2020) has argued that COVID-19 will be no more than a footnote in international relations scholarship and the status quo of international (dis)order will remain unchanged. In light of this argument, the predominant narrative that international cooperation 'failed' in response to COVID-19 (Clark 2020) may be understood from two competing points of view: first, that there was indeed a 'failure' in international cooperation stemming from the relationship between global health and global politics. A rival view, however, might suggest that COVID-19 reveals incremental progress in the area of global health cooperation and the emergence of thick networks of global health governance that includes both state and non-state actors. From this perspective, although COVID-19 presented an unexpected exogenous shock, global health cooperation continued—even multiplied—across various sectors and groups of actors. This suggests that for all the challenges it confronts, global health governance has been developing a complex agency that operates on multiple levels (state institutions, regional organizations, private for-profit actors, civil society, private–public partnerships) such that even when one political track is blocked, other tracks may continue to function (Lee et al. 2002: 274). This chapter examines this phenomenon.

The first section explores the historical evolution of concepts and practices of international health governance and health security. The most recent equivalent precedent to COVID-19 was the swine flu (H1N1) pandemic in 2009. This experience revealed that the concept of health security has always had a tenuous grip on states' commitment and attention, but global health cooperation continued to thrive across a network of actors.[1] The second section considers the shortfalls of international cooperation in response to COVID-19, considers to what extent the international cooperation 'failure' observed at the start of COVID-19 is a continuation of the status quo, and illustrates the need to pay more attention to acts

[1] Global is deliberately chosen here instead of international precisely because the networks involve state and non-state actors and transnational flows. Lee, Fustukian, and Buse (2002: 4–5) argued that international refers to the 'primacy of the state and state-defined actors that distinguishes international health'; international health becomes global when the 'causes and consequences of a health issue circumvent, undermine or are oblivious to the territorial boundaries of the states and, thus, beyond the capacity of states to address effectively through state institutions alone'.

of cooperation in functional areas such as health. The third section examines the alternative modes of global health cooperation that gained traction during the COVID-19 outbreak. Cooperation in the global health sector has occurred during COVID-19, but cooperation has not been sourced from the usual places or with the usual actors. States participated in, but did not lead, the vaccine discovery initiative; methods in detection benefitted from scientific networks; civil society networks united to protect human rights during the pandemic; and international disease surveillance networks kept track of states' information on testing, contract tracing, and fatalities. In global health, there is the international order to which Drezner refers and there is a global order comprising non-state actors working in complex collaborations with states and international organizations, performing functions in anticipation that more formal multilateral avenues will be blocked. These actors came to the fore during COVID-19 in complex and ad hoc fashions. Far from becoming a footnote in international relations, they will likely drive and influence global health governance into the future.

The Past: Global Health Security

Two decades ago, the concept of a cooperative global strategy towards infectious disease containment was novel (Fidler 2004; Price-Smith 2009). The (re)evolution of international infectious disease cooperation (Fidler 1999) was marked by the World Health Assembly (WHA) member states' unanimous agreement on revisions to the IHR in 2005. The IHR (predating to the mid-nineteenth century) is the formal framework that commits states to particular quarantine and outbreak response behaviours in the event of an infectious disease outbreak. It was the first—and for a long time only—treaty to be adopted by the World Health Assembly (1951). In 2005, this agreement was radically changed: from the scope of diseases to which the revised IHR applied to the incorporation of non-state actors into the framework; assessment of states' capacity to meet pandemic readiness criteria; guidelines for appropriate state behaviour after an outbreak concerning response, notification, travel, and trade restrictions; and new WHO administrative authority. There was the creation of the term 'public health emergency of international concern', a PHEIC, which if declared by the WHO was to trigger a number of alert notification requirements that states were to follow in response to WHO Director General advice. It was argued at the time that the IHR revisions were not just about formalizing new policy choices, but were also underpinned by a bigger shift of beliefs concerning what is appropriate *collective* state, international organization and non-state behaviour in the event of a PHEIC (Fidler 2004).

What were these beliefs that underpinned the shift from an individualist pursuit of infectious disease containment strategy to a collective pursuit of infectious disease containment? There were the material and reciprocal benefits from such a shift: early 'warning' and notification of disease outbreak events and the chance to share novel genomic and epidemiological data in readiness for testing and treatment (Davies 2008). This step towards collective behavioural expectations also entailed a number of political, capacity (scientific, financial, and bureaucratic), and trust demands on states. Mary Whelan, who chaired the negotiations of the revised IHR, doubted that states would ultimately follow through on these commitments:

> I am not at all sure that outside this very defined area, even, for example, in the case of a specific PHEIC, that it would be possible to recreate the unity of purpose. We can unite against the fear of the unknown, but it may be more difficult to unite against a real and present threat.
>
> (Whelan 2008: 16)

The collective fear generated from the outbreak of Severe Acute Respiratory Syndrome (SARS) in China in 2002, and the relief by the close of 2003 that this was not *the* pandemic to rival 1918 Spanish flu, was pivotal for achieving the international cooperation necessary to sign the revised treaty in 2005. The question, as Whelan posed, was whether fear would sustain international cooperation and collective enterprise over the years to follow; namely, would states commit to collective action or individualist pursuit of alert and containment procedures when the inevitable pandemic arrived?

Until the confirmation of SARS-Cov-2 in January 2020, there had been, since 2005 only one outbreak that achieved the title of being both a pandemic and a PHEIC: H1N1 (H1N1pdm09 Flu Virus) in 2009. The collective international response to H1N1 was found (as Whelan had suspected) to be wanting in the areas of cooperation. For example, only 78 million doses of vaccine were sent to 77 countries and, had the virus proved more deadly, this rate of supply and distribution was too little and too late. States promptly reported the virus, as encouraged to do so under the revised IHR, but experienced waves of trade and travel restrictions from other states when they did so; and the WHO came under attack. A World Health Assembly-appointed independent panel determined, in 2010, that: 'The world is ill prepared to respond to a severe influenza pandemic or to any similarly global, sustained and threatening public-health emergency' (Fineburg 2014). What proved particularly damaging for the WHO at the time was its decision to alert the international community to H1N1 as a pandemic. The WHO-led deliberations to declare H1N1 a PHEIC was relatively uncontroversial—this was a novel influenza. The declaration of the virus as a phase 6 health emergency—a pandemic—was controversial. The deliberations were confidential. The identities of the experts on the IHR Emergency Committee and the Global Strategic Advisory Group of Experts (SAGE) on Vaccines were not publicly disclosed. This sparked conspiracy theories that the WHO appointed experts who 'cashed in' from an 'unnecessary' phase 6 alert. For many national governments, a phase 6 pandemic alert triggers vaccine production orders. Journalists and politicians started to question potential conflict of interest between the SAGE experts and research grant incomes from vaccine manufacturing pharmaceutical companies. This kind of suspicion proved hard for the WHO to dispel, despite the fact that the declaration of phase 6 was delayed until there was sustained community spread in multiple countries in multiple WHO regions (Fineburg 2014). In years to come, it would be revealed that, while the mortality rate of H1N1 was lower than first feared, it was a particularly deadly virus strain for people younger than 65, which was unusual in typical seasonal influenza epidemics (Centers for Disease Control and Prevention 2019).

A series of recommendations were made to change the internal disclosure and transparency practices of the WHO, the functioning of the IHR and its Emergency Committee processes, the phasing of pandemic alerts, and the international cooperation frameworks for virus sharing, vaccine production, and distribution (which are not attached to the IHR mandate) (McInnes and Roemer-Mahler 2017). Fast forward to 2020, and the WHO's reputation and transparency has again come under question. This time, the WHO is not under suspicion for a false alert, but for not alerting states soon enough. The consistent factor is the international government organization blame game. As Tana Johnson (2020) has argued: 'Thus, although the pandemic may be extraordinary, its political patterns are quite ordinary.' The challenge, argues Johnson (2020) is to make sense of the ordinary political patterns that led to international cooperation around an area of expertise, such as infectious disease preparedness, to then trace why it is so easily undermined in crisis. It is also instructive to observe what cooperation is sustained, and who sustains it, during a crisis.

As the next section discusses, COVID-19 has demonstrated the power of states to ignore WHO-issued advisories on international cooperation and brought into question the legitimacy of the WHO issuing such orders. The H1N1 pandemic reveals that this is an ordinary political pattern; and if this was all there was to global health, the prospects would be bleak. However, if we look beyond international cooperation between states and the WHO, we can see a more complex dynamic global picture emerging, one where transnational cooperation and transnational networks played crucial roles in advancing efforts to detect, contain, and respond to the COVID-19 pandemic.

The Present: Global Health Security Stalled

On 22 January 2020, the IHR Emergency Committee for COVID-19 was convened to consider the outbreak of a novel coronavirus. By this stage, the virus had been detected in China and nine additional countries were testing suspect cases. The vote was split on whether the outbreak was yet a public health emergency of international concern (PHEIC) (Eccleston-Turner 2020). It is important to note that some Western public health experts at this meeting sided with the Chinese government representative and agreed that the novel coronavirus did not yet meet the conditions for a PHEIC (Borger 2020). A PHEIC declaration is the decision of the WHO Director General upon the advice of the convened expert Emergency Committee members. Committee members do not, technically, represent a government, but the affected country (in this case, China) is permitted to send a government representative to present the situation and answer questions posed by the Committee. The Emergency Committee agreed to convene a week later, and at this meeting, a PHEIC was declared. In his statement, Dr Tedros stated that the PHEIC decision was not linked to the risks posed by China to the international community, but the risk posed to low- and middle-income country settings with weak health systems unprepared to manage the demands of a major epidemic (WHO 2020a).

By March, the WHO was coming under increasing criticism from key donor states including the United States, Australia, and even the UK for its handling of the outbreak and suggestions of duplicity with China. This led to the WHA, in May 2020, proposing that an independent panel be established to evaluate the lessons to be learned from the international health response to COVID-19. In June 2020, the Associated Press published internal email communications revealing that there had been internal debates within the WHO during late December and most of January concerning the transparency of the Chinese government to the WHO's requests for more information (Associated Press 2020). These emails revealed that WHO staff believed they would face tremendous backlash however they handled this situation: they were trapped between 'The difficulty in endlessly trying to get updates from China about what was going on' and 'The danger now is that despite our good intent … especially if something does happen, there will be a lot of finger-pointing at WHO' (Mike Ryan emails in Associated Press (2020)).

During February and March, the WHO's praise for China's response to the outbreak jarred with the evidence emerging that the Chinese government may have made decisions that delayed detection and full disclosure. The WHO's praise also appeared at odds with its mandate to protect health as a human right, as it was revealed that the Chinese police had threatened medical staff with arrest for any online communication about the outbreak, there had been forced quarantine and lockdowns on cities, coupled with tragic failures to recognize and address the human and civil rights implications within such intervention (Kupferschmidt 2020). At the same time, however, Western countries had begun to adopt their own measures that contravened the IHR—in particular, the implementation of restrictive travel measures against China without justification (over 70 countries, including the United States, Australia, and New Zealand) (Pillinger 2020).

Four weeks after the PHEIC declaration, over 70 countries adopted travel restrictions that were against the WHO recommendations on 30 January 2020 (Pillinger 2020), and some of these states (New Zealand, Australia, Norway) have had relatively 'mild' pandemics. China has secured impressive public health security against surges of COVID-19 through mandatory ID and contact-tracing requirements through a geo-surveillance grid system. Vietnam imposed mandatory quarantine for those infected with COVID-19.

While the WHO was criticized for its failure to call out China for breaches of the IHR, the WHO Director General did not call out these individual states for their failure to heed the IHR and WHO advice on travel.

Cooperation was not the first instinct of most (if not all) states in the first months of COVID-19, including amongst the Permanent Five of the UN Security Council—China, France (exception noted below), Russia, the UK, and the United States. Between 30 January and 1 April, there was no resolution, or statement, from the UN General Assembly or UN Security Council. On 2 April, the UN General Assembly adopted Resolution A/RES/74/270, *Global solidarity to fight the coronavirus disease*; and on 20 April, A/RES/74/274, *International cooperation to ensure global access to medicines, vaccines and medical equipment to face COVID-19*. Neither of these resolutions however, established the financial mechanism that would secure international cooperation for distribution of vaccines, diagnostics, and treatments. It was the G20, in March 2020, that called for a mechanism which led to the creation of the Access to COVID-19 Tools (ACT) Accelerator on 26 April 2020 (see below). The UN Security Council Resolution (UNSCR) 2532 on COVID-19 was adopted on 1 July 2020 and it (finally) made all the right noises: ceasefires to secure humanitarian access, international cooperation, and a focus on fragile situations and marginalized populations, but it was scant on operative paragraphs.

It has been said that the threshold for the health securitization test is if a disease or health event has a Security Council resolution attached to it (Youde 2016). In the case of COVID-19, securitization proceeded without the need for a UN resolution. Many leaders adopted military metaphors and language in response to COVID-19 (Freedman 2020), and sought to secure their vaccine supply and their personal protective equipment (PPE) before looking out to see if the world needed help. The UN Security Council did not agree to a resolution in response to the pandemic (declared 11 March 2020) until 1 July 2020 (UNSCR 2532). To some, the slowness of the Security Council response was disappointing (Brown 2020; Clark 2020; Duong et al. 2020). However, what could an earlier UNSCR have been expected to achieve? No one thought an emergency response mission similar to that set up to address the Ebola outbreak in West Africa in 2014 was a viable option (Harman and Wenham 2018). Many—including those within the WHO—considered the Ebola mission an overreach of the UN Security Council and UN General Assembly that should not be repeated (Harman and Wenham 2018). Second, it was going to be logistically and financially impossible to mount such a response to a pandemic (which the Ebola outbreak was not). Eventually, the UN Secretary General's call for a ceasefire due to COVID-19 was the primary 'win' in the UNSCR 2532.

Beyond the call for a ceasefire and continued delivery of humanitarian aid, tragically, it is not clear what an earlier UNSCR could have delivered in this instance. From the onset of COVID-19, this was perhaps the most troubling aspect of the crisis of international order: the international was rendered meaningless and most states sought to protect themselves first and foremost (see Chapter 5 in this volume by Bickerton for an understanding of [absent] regional coordination in response to the pandemic). Multilateral organizations were not the first place to which states turned in January, February, and March 2020.

As the next section explains, although many of the most prominent avenues for state–state health cooperation became blocked, diverse global health governance networks continued to function and produce positive results. Actors across the sciences, civil society, philanthropic, and technology sectors continued to collaborate in ad hoc fashion alongside each other, and the global health governance architecture to which these networks belong continued to engage states and international organizations, and even to push them towards collaboration in some instances. Thus, global health governance during COVID-19 decidedly shifted from the traditional two-level system of international cooperation towards a more dynamic three-level system of global cooperation in response to the pandemic.

Multilateralism beyond the State

If we accept the premise that states always seek to maintain their sovereign independence over cooperation, greater insight is achieved into the few instances when states chose to delegate authority to separate organizations to build institutional capacity, encourage moral persuasion, or development enforce mechanisms (Johnson 2020). In other words, rather than explaining why cooperation is absent, it is more instructive to examine the few instances when states responded to problems with collective action, rather than 'going it alone' (Abbott et al. 2015). As such, with states diverging from the WHO's advice and traditional UN principal organs during COVID-19, we should ask how cooperation was possible at all and where it tended to happen.

The WHO's pre-COVID record of outbreak coordination or orchestrating state cooperation in response to health emergencies requires brief consideration (see Chapter 11 in this volume by Roux Dufort and Clément for an understanding of decision-makers' behaviour in times of crisis). Since the adoption of the revised IHR in 2005, the primary international instrument and governance mechanism that guides collective behaviour in the event of an outbreak, many publications have flagged implementation gaps. There was the H1N1 pandemic in 2009, and the findings from the independent panel that the WHO would struggle to gain authority under its existing funding, administrative, and regulatory arrangements. The review also found that the WHO Headquarters would struggle to bring cohesive commitment to the IHR core capacity building requirements. Attached to the IHR are 13 (originally 8) core capacity criteria that states are expected to meet through legislation, finance, training, laboratory preparedness, etc. Since 2010, the WHO has received State-Parties Self-Assessment Annual Reports (SPAR) considering progress with building IHR core capacities and measuring performance against 13 criteria and 24 indicators (WHO 2018: 7). In addition, since 2016, the WHO has coordinated over 60 Joint Evaluation Exercises (JEE), which, upon state invitation, send an external committee to evaluate how states are meeting their IHR obligations (Tsai and Katz 2018). A funding mechanism was set up in 2015 to support low- and middle-income states in meeting core capacity obligations, but the mechanism was chronically underfunded. As the Independent Panel for Pandemic Preparedness and Response (IPPPR) noted in their May 2021 final report: 'despite the consistent messages that significant change was needed to ensure global protection against pandemic threats, the majority of recommendations were never implemented. At best, there has been piecemeal implementation' (IPPPR 2021: 16).

The WHO has struggled to maximize on states 'prior consent to be advised according to the IHR during actual health emergencies. The organization in January 2020, as an Associated Press report describes, clearly struggled to know how to proactively act in the absence of state permission to do so (Associated Press 2020). The IPPPR investigation into the early response to the COVID-19 outbreak states that it does not set out to blame China or the WHO; but the report does, diplomatically, find that a key failing of all actors involved was too much adherence to the IHR alert matrix and not enough adherence to the precautionary principle. Specifically, the absence of proof of human-to-human transmission in December 2019 and January 2020 prevented issuing immediate protective action and recommendations which assumed that human-to-human transmission of the virus was occurring (IPPR 2021: 26).

However, we can identify three functional areas—surveillance, human rights, and scientific cooperation—where cooperation not only continued, but, in some cases, expanded in response to the COVID-19 pandemic. These areas have sometimes included state cooperation but, significantly, have not *depended* on state cooperation. Civil society, scientists, philanthropic, and technology sectors—with the WHO—have been building hybrid arrangements where state leaders are not the only actors upon whom cooperation needs to be sought. These networks have been important contributors to accelerating cooperation in the areas of surveillance, rights, and science during the COVID-19 pandemic. What these three cases reveal is that state-centred security language is not the only diplomatic and public health tool available to secure global cooperation. In fact, persistent reference to health security, and demanding UN General Assembly or Security Council resolutions in response to the COVID-19 pandemic could produce more diplomatic stagnation than diplomatic progress. COVID-19 reveals the shortfalls of existing international order, the pre-eminence of security, and the presumption that traditional UN organs such as the Security Council are the only forces for diplomatic gains in global health. Thus, within global health governance, we can identify cooperation proceeding outside the two-level game of domestic and international players (including international government organizations) in which international relations can study practices of diplomacy that thrive despite the narrative that states are 'going it alone'.

Surveillance

The COVID-19 outbreak has revealed that the majority of states are willing to detect, assess, and report public health emergencies. The high degree of surveillance and reporting for COVID-19 is similar to the high degree of states' observation of the need to detect and report cases during the H1N1 'swine flu' outbreak in 2009. The problem then, as with COVID-19 today, has been the minority of states that delay reporting or refuse to report cases at all (in the case of H1N1, some countries later confirmed H1N1 cases after the pandemic phase was lifted). On the whole, few states were 'beaten' to their public announcement of outbreak detection by a non-state public health information surveillance network such as PRO-Med Mail or the Johns Hopkins University COVID-19 Dashboard. The IHR was set up in the anticipation that states may fail to detect and report public health risk events. In that instance, the WHO would need access to information from non-state actors. In the IHR, under Article 11, it was a hard fought win to secure the right for the WHO Headquarters, Regional Offices, and Country Offices to receive and share 'unofficial' information about public health risks from reliable sources (non-state actors) without seeking agreement from the States Parties concerned. This Article is one of the unsung heroes of the IHR (Davies 2017), and it proved vital, yet again, at the onset of COVID-19 (World Health Authority 2021: 13).

The IPPPR investigation found that the Chinese government communicated through the Wuhan Municipal Health Commission about the suspicious outbreak of pneumonia of unknown origin on 31 December 2019. This public notice was picked up by a local publication, which was then picked up by several public health surveillance systems, including the Centre for Disease Control Taiwan and PRO-Med Mail. It was through these alerts, it seems, that the WHO Country Office in China and the WHO Headquarters found out about the pneumonia outbreak of suspicious origin in Wuhan and then sought confirmation from the Chinese government (IPPPR 2021: 22). The right of non-state actors to report disease outbreak events and for the WHO to use these reports—as permitted under the revised IHR—has progressed the norm of outbreak reporting (Davies 2019). Normatively, even the most reluctant states have recognized the value in detection because it is better to be in control of the news cycle than putting out infodemic rumours. Even in those instances when a state does not formally notify the WHO, the information rapidly reaches the organization. When PRO-Med Mail published a local government report on the outbreak of novel pneumonia cases of unknown origin in Wuhan on 30 December, this information paved the way for the WHO to request more information from the Chinese government on 31 December. As a result, all states were alerted to the outbreak via WHO internal communication channels by 5 January 2020. Throughout January 2020, Thailand, then Japan and South Korea, reported their first confirmed COVID-19 cases. More facts around the Wuhan pneumonia outbreak was ascertained, which led to the PHEIC declaration on 30 January.

The problem for most states is how to act upon surveillance information. The IPPPR has referred to problem as 'two worlds at different speeds': epidemic surveillance communicated the outbreak in rapid time, while states and the WHO were slow to react to the pace of information they were receiving (IPPPR 2021: 26). The result of the two-world pace was that February 2020 was a lost month for the world: 'when steps could and should have been taken to curtail the epidemic and forestall the pandemic' (IPPPR 2021: 29). The consequence was a failure by some states to detect early, with catastrophic consequences (i.e. Iran, Indonesia, and Russia). Inadequate early response was followed by a failure to scale up the necessary testing (i.e. Belorussia, Brazil, the United States).

At the onset of COVID-19, the greatest concern was the lack of adequate testing and the harm it would bring to citizens in low- and middle-income countries (LMIC) such Mexico, Pakistan, and Indonesia. However, high-income countries were revealed to be struggling with such tasks, irrespective of health system capacity. The problem in each site was different from the 'usual' LMIC resource gap problem of detection, access, and reporting. Surveillance is a political as much as a technical activity. Brazil and the United States both had the information available to adopt 'aggressive' containment procedures, but chose not to do so, while some states, such as Vietnam and Thailand, have, in 2021, experienced an upsurge in cases, despite being the *ones that rapidly detected and reported their first outbreaks early in 2020*. The lessons in surveillance are that no one state or organization has the answers, other than the need for open and transparent reporting: open access to non-state-provided event surveillance reports is vital. States may seek to report early, but they don't always confirm outbreak events early enough. Diversified sources for surveillance reports supports the precautionary principle: it provides all states with the information (if not the will) to act. With enhanced surveillance tools must then also come a more nuanced understanding of when and why detection 'failures' occur in each instance: assumptions are politically harmful and not impact-neutral.

The IHR were constructed to combat the systemic past failures to report the early growth of disease outbreaks. Despite it all the problems, COVID-19 revealed that the drafters of the IHR were right to shift underlying norms on surveillance and reporting: most states report more fulsomely and more quickly than they did before the adoption of the IHR in 2005. Most outbreaks can be detected by non-state surveillance systems and make their way into the WHO system. Of course, there are states that have failed to report; but they have generally paid a price in greater disease spread. There are also states, of various health system capacity and strength, that fail to act on reports.

In April 2021, the *Report of the Review Committee on the Functioning of the International Health Regulations (2005) during the COVID-19 response* found that:

> much of what is in the Regulations is well considered, appropriate and meaningful in any public health emergency of international concern. However, it was clear to us that in the context of a pandemic, countries that in 2005 approved the IHR, in 2020 only applied the Regulations in part, were not sufficiently aware of them, or deliberately ignored them.
>
> (WHA 2021: 7)

The COVID-19 pandemic revealed that the IHR was not wrong to promote detection and reporting under an international system of cooperation and trust, and its drafters were right to insist on Article 11 and permit non-state actors to report: political systems and leaders are fallible.

Human Rights

In 2014, there were many concerns—in real time—about the delayed response of the WHO Executive to the outbreak of Ebola in West Africa. The outbreak began in Guinea in December 2013, and then spread to Liberia and Sierra Leone in March 2014. An IHR Emergency Committee was not convened in response to this health emergency until 6 August 2014, which was then followed by a UN Security Council resolution one month later. As the months went by, there was an increased sense of urgency and desperation, communicated by individuals such as Dr Joanne Liu, then International President of Médecins Sans Frontières (MSF), for the WHO and other states to act. There were nearly 1,000 recorded deaths before a PHEIC was declared in August 2014. This outbreak would become the largest and most fatal Ebola outbreak ever recorded.

The affected states, the WHO, and the international community collectively failed to prioritize the right to health of the populations who were exposed to a deadly disease with a 50% fatality rate. The 2015 review of the WHO's response, led by Dame Barbara Stocking, noted that the IHR are meant to be implemented with full regard for the dignity, human rights, and fundamental freedoms of persons. This did not occur during the Ebola outbreak. The political response was heavily securitized: health-care workers were threatened with imprisonment if they did not turn up to work, and they were threatened if they spoke out against their government. Schools were closed, markets were shut, violence against women rose, and existing health morbidities increased (see Chapter 9 in this volume by Smith for an understanding of the gendered effects of pandemics). The realization that not every individual had agency and power in response to this outcome eventually led to improved health advice and risk communication, but the economic and social damage was immense and these communities are still healing five years later.

Compared to the West African Ebola outbreak in 2014, there has been more discussion and greater focus on particular groups at risk of neglect and discrimination during the COVID-19 pandemic from the outset. There is greater collective awareness and advocacy that individual human rights must not be compromised by the COVID-19 response (Sekalala et al. 2020). The United Nations (UN) has provided a series of factsheets and reports on groups at risk of discrimination during this outbreak, including the rights of individuals with disabilities, refugees, migrant workers, and women. There has been a consistent message from the UN and the World Bank that the economic recovery should focus not only on immediate relief, but should also support longer-term, sustainable development, including the creation of an international funding campaign to assist LMICs with preparedness to reach the Sustainable Development Goals 2030 Agenda.

Globally, there have been active advocacy campaigns to identify violations of economic, social, and civil rights during the COVID-19 outbreak: in the early stages of the outbreak, social media campaigns called out instances where ethnic Chinese were targeted for racist and xenophobic abuse (Human Rights Watch 2020), and media reported on women experiencing a higher volume of unpaid care duties and higher risk of job losses (Smith et al. 2021). There were calls for governments to address the higher risk of intimate and family violence during self-isolation or quarantine; the health risk to low-income workers and migrant workers living in cramped living conditions; the income vulnerability of casual workers now facing risk of wage loss and unemployment; and to aid the elderly and disabled, who were not prioritized for intubation and intensive care (Human Rights Watch 2020).

These examples of human rights advocacy during the COVID-19 pandemic have not overcome the silent, pernicious ways in which human rights have been abused. In many places, people—including frontline medical workers—who have challenged authority and spoken out against government messages that are dangerous, discriminatory, or neglectful have faced threats of violence, censorship, and even imprisonment. There are serious concerns about the use of emergency laws passed to implement lockdowns to also shut down political parties and civil society groups under 'spreading misinformation' laws that were introduced to support the public health response. Governments have also securitized the enforcement of various emergency laws.

A quick study of the Oxford COVID-19 Government Response Tracker, a composite measure [value 0–100] based on school closures, workplace closures, curfews, internal movement restrictions, and travel bans, reveals that in the first six months of the pandemic (declared 11 March 2020) the majority of countries adopted restrictions that sat well above the composite score 60 (100 is strictest) (Hale et al. 2021). Lockdown as a public health measure legitimated the power of the state to control the movement of people and the implications of this were quickly observed, with lockdowns being used to justify democratic 'backsliding' and tighter surveillance laws (e.g. in Hungary and the Philippines) (Billing 2020; Flinders 2021). Travel restrictions, mandatory quarantine, and biosecurity surveillance methods were not in accordance with the IHR or the recommendations of the WHO Director General. The *Report of the Review Committee on Function of the IHR during COVID-19 response* found 'no mechanism for monitoring the implementation of key provisions of the IHR, including those that cover human rights' (WHA 2021: 6).

The dilemma moving forward is how to progress the protest movement into distribution and reform. Those who have been most affected by COVID-19—in terms of health care, economic impact, social justice, and protection—are the populations who were already shouldering highest inequity burdens before the pandemic (Jensen et al. 2021). In terms of reform, a recent review of the IHR response to COVID-19 recommended that the 'WHO needs to collaborate with international human rights bodies to monitor States Parties' actions during health emergencies and to regularly reiterate the importance of respecting international human rights principles, including the protection of personal data and privacy, as agreed by States Parties in the IHR' (WHA 2021: 44).

The direct impact of COVID-19 policies on human rights, and the indirect impact of the COVID-19 regime on rights fulfilment, has been met with *global* protest movements on race relations, women's safety, the right to abortion, pro-democracy, workers' rights, anti-lockdowns, anti-vaccines, and climate change (Carothers and Wong 2020). Transnational networks collaborated in 2020 to fight for the right to peaceful protest during the pandemic and won this right under international law (Human Rights Law Centre 2020; UN News 2020). The right to peaceful protest challenges the legality of any government legislation that introduces public health regulations and laws during this pandemic that compromise the civil, political, economic, and social rights of individuals. The implementation, reform, and distribution obstacles remain high, but the activism to articulate a human-rights-centred response to COVID-19 has been unprecedented compared to recent health emergencies (Human Rights Watch 2020).

Scientific Cooperation

A third area where informal cooperation flourished was amongst civil society organizations, philanthropic agencies, and research institutions globally. Cooperation in areas of technical endeavour, such as science, mapping, weather, health, and digital are political, but they can also serve as functional pursuits that enhance international cooperation, in spite of the differences amongst the political actors. COVID-19 has revealed the best of collective scientific endeavours: it began when a group of scientists in China, then Thailand, released the virus genomic sequence on 10 and 14 January 2020, respectively (Corman et al. 2020).

The most obvious forms of effective cooperation outside formal international institutions were in the fields of vaccine discovery, diagnostics, and treatment. Progress in these fields was achieved through a combination of public (state and international government organizations) and private actors. It was the Group of 20 (G20), in March 2020 that called for the creation of an international initiative to fund and coordinate the delivery of vaccines, diagnostics, and treatments. This was the shared enterprise of France, the European Commission, and the World Health Organization, which led to the creation of the Access to COVID-19 Tools- Accelerator (ACT-A) in April 2020. The ACT-A created four pillars: promote diagnostics, treatment, vaccines, and health system strengthening.

The COVAX Facility (the vaccine pillar of ACT-A) has been the most innovative response since the H1N1 vaccine crisis, and it is not state managed or led. COVAX is led by GAVI (the Global Alliance for Vaccines and Immunisation), the Coalition for Epidemic Preparedness Innovations (CEPI) [two public–private partnerships], and the WHO. COVAX now has over 170 state signatories. The COVAX advanced market commitment is the ACT-A pillar most talked about: its ambition is to produce and distribute at least 2 billion vaccines by the end of 2021 (to approximately 20% of the world's population) in low-income countries. Despite its failures (and there are many), COVAX and the ACT-A is an innovative model of science diplomacy.

The leadership of ACT-A and COVAX is three-levelled: France (state); the European Commission (a regional organization); and the WHO (international); moreover, it is heavily dependent on non-state actors: financial and coordination commitments from two public–private initiatives (GAVI and CEPI), and a philanthropic agency, the Bill & Melinda Gates Foundation. The WHO is a co-convenor, like France and the European Commission, but not the leader in this arrangement. The absence of the United States was striking, albeit not surprising, given the Trump administration's position on COVID-19 and the WHO in 2020). In the past, the United States had been a strong leader in global health initiatives, including the joint UN Programme on HIV/AIDS (UNAIDS), the Global Fund to Fight AIDS, Malaria, and Tuberculosis, the President's Emergency Plan For AIDS Relief (PEPFAR), and the Global Health Security Agenda. The United States' interest in ACT-A and COVAX immediately changed with the election of President Biden. The United States joined COVAX and pledged support for ACT-A. Nonetheless, the structure of ACT-A and COVAX is novel, in that it does not permit one state to dominate the process. However, there are clearly some interests that dominate the process, to date, and this has been a significant problem.

The first caveat to the above is the serious funding shortfall in the ACT-A, including COVAX. Quite simply, states are investing in their own vaccine purchase agreements, rather than trusting COVAX and pooling resources into this facility. The principle of COVAX was that 20% of the world's population (mostly health-care workers and the most vulnerable) would be vaccinated first. To make matters worse, even if COVAX had the budget to purchase the vaccines needed, it is unable to access the supply, due to high-income countries hoarding both vaccines and the materials needed to make the vaccine (Samuel 2021). When countries, including the United States, the UK, and Israel arranged their own bilateral vaccine purchase agreements with pharmaceutical companies, all other countries (that could afford to do so) followed suit. In September 2020, there was a $300 million shortfall for the 2020 COVAX budget; and a $5 billion shortfall for 2021 (GAVI 2020). The 2021 vaccination target of 20% will not be reached, due to funding and vaccine shortfalls (Tooze 2020; Samuel 2021). Outside of vaccine discovery and production, the three other ACT-A pillars have been struggling to achieve operational funding. The Paris Peace Forum, held in November 2020, was arranged to secure more funding commitments to the ACT-A. At the Forum, it was announced that new contributions had brought the total commitment to US$ 5.1 billion. This was still US$ 4.2 billion short of the total funds needed in 2020; and short of a further US$ 23.9 billion required in 2021 to distribute vaccines, diagnostics, treatments, and basic health system support to deliver on the pillars of ACT. Italy, as chair of the G20 for 2021, with the European Commission, organized the first G20 global health summit to try to deliver a 'Rome Declaration' that would address the funding gaps and the vaccine shortfalls, and garner support for a 'pandemic treaty'. However, the event revealed deep divides between the members of the G20 with no statement on the pandemic treaty, no increased commitment to ACT-A, and no commitment to G20 members South Africa and India's call for a vaccine intellectual property waiver (Balmer and Guarascio 2021).

In addition to failure to invest in COVAX and ACT-A, support for the four-pillar programme is being seriously harmed by the vaccine waiver dispute. Since October 2020, India and South Africa have formed a political coalition calling for the World Trade Organization (WTO) to suspend all intellectual property (IP) rights related to COVID-19 vaccines, medicines, and other new technologies needed to control the pandemic (Usher 2020). Over 100 countries have joined this call (including China), with growing support from non-state actors, including public health associations, MSF, Amnesty International, and Oxfam International. In April 2021, US President Biden's administration announced their support for the waiver after months of opposition. However, a number of states, including Germany, France, Switzerland, and the UK, are holding out. These states are the headquarters for a number of big pharmaceutical companies that have led the COVID-19 vaccine production, including Pfizer and BioNTech. Until recently, one of the major contributors to COVID-19 vaccine discovery and production, the Bill and Melinda Gates Foundation, was not in favour of the waiver, but turned around its position after the US government announcement in May 2021. The alliance to block the vaccine waiver—which could effectively permit LMICs to produce their own COVID-19 vaccines—is causing growing rifts between states, private actors, and scientists. For example, it has led to a number of LMICs suggesting that they will block any reform to the IHR and a proposed pandemic treaty (to promote more international cooperation around early warning surveillance systems) until the vaccine waiver dispute is settled (Ramakrishnan et al. 2021).

Careful analysis of cooperation during the COVID-19 pandemic requires analysis of what failed, but also of what was attempted to unite global cooperation, to ensure that the right lessons are learned. States didn't 'go it alone' in the areas of disease detection and surveillance. However imperfect, there have been unprecedented calls for a human rights-centred response to COVID-19. The pace of international cooperation in the fields of science and technology—despite vaccine and intellectual property nationalism—has led to rapid research progress and state–private partnerships to develop responses to this pandemic. The backlash against the hoarding instincts of wealthy states and pharmaceutical companies was almost immediate and is growing in strength every day.

Conclusion: Future Diplomatic Entry Points for Global Health Security

The absence of a coordinated effort to address COVID-19 through formal institutions such as the UN Security Council pushed many analysts to consider this another example of a weakening international order. Yet in practice, global health governance—in science, rights, technology, and surveillance—has proven more complex and durable and has demonstrated its potential to facilitate cooperation that is diverse and inclusive. Appreciated this way, the avenues for global health security are expanding (see the Introduction to this volume by Ackerly et al.). This is not to diminish critical challenges relating to politics, financing, and participation, only that blockages within the two-level game of states and international organizations have not wholly inhibited the pursuit of knowledge sharing, advocacy, cooperation, and innovation by non-state actors, including civil society, scientists, and international non-government organizations across national, regional, and international boundaries.

Health security can be *both* a universalist public goods principle that required the international community to transcend the 'low-priority' political framing of health matters (Youde 2016) and a threat mitigation practice that identifies pathogenic risks in order to defend and protect the 'normal' political sovereign order. In the case of COVID-19, the language of health security used by states has often put national governments in competition for resources and undermined international cooperation.

The lack of state-level coordinated action in response to COVID-19 reveals the terms on which health issues, such as infectious diseases, are 'sold': international 'buy-in' is geared to protect states—through trade, travel, and now vaccines. Yet, calls for global cooperation have persisted—even thrived—in the face of traditional multilateralism stalling. States such as India and South Africa have called for an alternative vision of international cooperation. States were not the only actors who learned lessons from the failure of international cooperation in response to SARS and H1N1. Transnational networks across the sciences, civil society, philanthropic, and technology sectors were ready to detect COVID-19 and to respond to COVID-19. Existing global health governance networks were used to engage states and international organizations to secure participation in arrangements such as COVAX, which was thought impossible before the COVID-19 pandemic. International order may return to the status quo, but the global networks of cooperation and innovation exhibited during COVID-19 has been operational for some time. It is still possible to promote innovative and progressive tools in response to this pandemic and the next global health crisis.

References

Abbott, Kenneth W., Philipp Genschel, Duncan Snidal, and Bernhard Zangl. 2015. 'Orchestration'. In *International Organizations as Orchestrators*, edited by Kenneth W. Abbott, Philipp Genschel, Duncan Snidal, and Bernhard Zangl, pp. 3–36. Cambridge: Cambridge University Press.

Associated Press. 2020. 'China Delayed Releasing Coronavirus Info, Frustrating WHO'. 2 June. https://apnews.com/article/3c061794970661042b18d5aeaaed9fae.

Balmer, Crispian, and Francisco Guarascio. 2021. 'Failure for Humanity': Rich World Aims to End Vaccine Inequities', *Reuters*, 21 May. https://www.reuters.com/world/g20-health-summit-looks-boost-vaccine-access-drugmakers-offer-cut-price-shots-2021-05-21/.

Billing, Lynzy. 2020. Duterte's Response to the Coronavirus: 'Shoot Them Dead'. *Foreign Policy*, 16 April. https://foreignpolicy.com/2020/04/16/duterte-philippines-coronavirus-response-shoot-them-dead/

Borger, Julian. 2020. 'Caught in a Superpower Struggle: The Inside Story of the WHO's Response to Coronavirus'. *The Guardian*, 18 April. https://www.theguardian.com/world/2020/apr/18/caught-in-a-superpower-struggle-the-inside-story-of-the-whos-response-to-coronavirus.

Brown, Gordon. 2020. 'A Letter to the International Community'. *Project Syndicate*, 17 August. https://www.project-syndicate.org/commentary/save-our-future-education-funding-during-covid19-by-gordon-brown-2020-08?barrier=accesspaylog.

Carothers, Thomas and David Wong. 2020. 'Global Protests Start to Return'. *Carnegie Endowment for International Peace*. 30 June. https://carnegieendowment.org/2020/06/30/global-protests-start-to-return-pub-82225.

Centers for Disease Control and Prevention. 2019. '2009 H1N1 Pandemic (H1N1pdm09 virus)'. https://www.cdc.gov/flu/pandemic-resources/2009-h1n1-pandemic.html.

Clark, Helen. 2020. 'Missing In Action: The Lack of a Globally Co-ordinated Response to Covid-19'. *Sunday Star Times*. 12 April. https://www.g-l-f.org/who-we-are/glf-members-listed-by-region/helen-clark/missing-in-action-the-lack-of-a-globally-co-ordinated-response-to-covid-19/

Corman Victor M., Olfert Landt, Marco Kaiser, et al. 2020. 'Detection of 2019 Novel Coronavirus (2019-nCoV) by real-time RT-PCR'. *Euro Surveillance 25* (3): 2000045.

Davies, Sara E. 2017. 'Advocating Global Health Security'. In *Global Insecurity: Futures of Global Chaos and Governance*, edited by Anthony Burke and Rita Parker, pp. 253–72. London: Palgrave Macmillan.

Davies, Sara E. 2019. *Containing Contagion: The Politics of Disease Outbreaks in Southeast Asia*. Baltimore, MD: Johns Hopkins University Press.

Drezner, Daniel. 2020. 'The Song Remains the Same: International Relations after COVID-19'. *International Organization* 74 (supp): pp. E18–E35.

Duong, David, Helen E. Clark, Francesca Colombo, and Lucas Sherdel. 2020. 'More, Not Less, Multilateralism Is Needed to Fight the Coronavirus Pandemic'. World Economic Forum, 20 May. https://www.weforum.org/agenda/2020/05/more-multilateralism-needed-fight-coronavirus-pandemic.

Eccleston-Turner, Mark. 2020. 'COVID-19 Symposium: The Declaration of Public Health Emergency of International Concern'. *OpinioJuris*, 31 March. http://opiniojuris.org/2020/03/31/covid-19-symposium-the-declaration-of-a-public-health-emergency-of-international-concern-in-international-law.

Fidler, David P. 1999. *International Law and Infectious Diseases*. Oxford: Clarendon Press.

Fidler, David P. 2004. *SARS, Governance, and the Globalisation of Disease*. Basingstoke: Palgrave Macmillan.

Fidler, David P., and Lawrence O. Gostin. 2007. *Biosecurity in the Global Age: Biological Weapons, Public Health, and the Rule of Law*. Stanford, CA: Stanford University Press.

Fineberg, Harvey A. 2014. 'Pandemic Preparedness and Response—Lessons from the H1N1 Influenza of 2009'. *New England Journal of Medicine 370*: pp. 1335–42.

Flinders, Matthew (2021). 'Democracy and the Politics of Coronavirus: Trust, Blame and Understanding'. *Parliamentary Affairs 74* (2): pp 483–502.

Freedman, Lawrence. 2020. 'Coronavirus and the Language of War'. *New Statesman*, 14 April. https://www.newstatesman.com/science-tech/2020/04/coronavirus-and-language-war.

Global Alliance for Vaccines and Immunisation (GAVI). 2020. 'Countries Pledge Nearly US$ 1 Billion to Support Equitable Access to COVID-19 Vaccines'. 6 October. https://www.gavi.org/news/media-room/countries-pledge-nearly-us-1-billion-support-equitable-access-covid-19-vaccines.

Hale, Thomas, Noam Angrist, Rafeal Goldszmidt, Beatriz Kira, Anna Petherick , Toby Phillips, et al. 2021. 'A global panel database of pandemic policies (Oxford COVID-19 Government Response Tracker)', Nature Human Behaviour (5): pp. 529–538.

Harman, Sophie, and Clare Wenham. 2018. 'Governing Ebola: Between Global Health and Medical Humanitarianism'. *Globalizations 15* (3): pp. 362–76.

Human Rights Law Centre. 2020. 'Explainer: Protest Rights in the COVID-19 Pandemic'. https://www.hrlc.org.au/protest-rights-covid19.

Human Rights Watch. 2020. 'Progress Protecting Rights While Combatting COVID-19'. 27 October. https://www.hrw.org/news/2020/10/27/progress-protecting-rights-while-combatting-covid-19.

Independent Panel for Pandemic Preparedness and Response. 2021. 'Covid-19: Make It the Last Pandemic'. May. https://theindependentpanel.org/mainreport/.

International Health Regulations. 2005. 'Guidance Document for State Party Self-Assessment Annual Reporting Tool'. Geneva: World Health Organization.

Jensen, Nele, Ann H. Kelly and Mauricio Avendano. 2021. 'The COVID-19 pandemic underscores the need for an equity-focused global health agenda'. *Humanities and Social Sciences Communications* 8 (15): ppE1–E6.

Johnson, Tana. 2020. 'Ordinary Patterns in an Extraordinary Crisis: How International Relations Makes Sense of the COVID-19 Pandemic'. *International Organization 74* (supp): pp. E148–E168.

Kupferschmidt, Kai. 2020. 'Mission Impossible? WHO Director Fights to Prevent a Pandemic without Offending China'. *Science*, 10 February. https://www.sciencemag.org/news/2020/02/mission-impossible-who-director-fights-prevent-pandemic-without-offending-china.

Lee, Kelley, Suzanne Fustukian, and Kent Buse. 2002. 'An Introduction to Global Health Policy'. In *Health Policy in a Globalising World*, edited by Kelley Lee, Kent Buse, and Zuanne Fustukian, pp. 3–17. Cambridge: Cambridge University Press.

Pillinger, Mara. 2020. 'Virus Travel Bans Are Inevitable but Ineffective'. *Foreign Policy*, 23 February. https://foreignpolicy.com/2020/02/23/virus-travel-bans-are-inevitable-but-ineffective.

Price-Smith, Andrew. 2009. *Contagion and Chaos*. Cambridge, MA: Massachusetts Institute of Technology Press.

Ramakrishnan, Nithin, K. M. Gopakumar, and Sangeeta Shashikant. 2021. 'WHO: Should Members Pursue a Pandemic Treaty in the Midst of a Global Pandemic?' *Third World Network*. 12 May. www.twn.my/title2/health.info/2021/hi210507.htm.

Samuel, Segal. 2021. 'Why Covax, the Fund to Vaccinate the world, Is Struggling'. *Vox*. 20 May. https://www.vox.com/future-perfect/22440986/covax-challenges-covid-19-vaccines-global-inequity.

Sekalala Sharifah, Lisa Forman, Roojin Habibi, and Benjamin Mason-Meier. 2020. 'Health and Human Rights Are Inextricably Linked in the COVID-19 Response'. *BMJ Global Health 5*: e003359.

Smith, Julia, Sara E. Davies, Huiyun Feng, Connie C. R. Gan, Karen A. Grépin, Sophie Harman, et al. 2021. 'More than a public health crisis: A feminist political economic analysis of COVID-19', *Global Public Health 16*:8–9: pp.1364–1380.

Tooze, Adam. 2020. 'The World Is Winning—and Losing—the Vaccine Race'. *Foreign Policy*, 19 September. https://foreignpolicy.com/2020/09/19/the-world-is-losing-the-vaccine-race.

Tsai, Feng-Jen, and Rebecca Katz. 2018. 'Measuring Global Health Security: Comparison of Self- and External Evaluations for IHR Core Capacity'. *Health Security 16* (5): pp. 304–310.

UN News. 2020. 'How Do You Define Lawful Peaceful Protest? The UN Human Rights Committee Has a Clear Answer'. 29 July. https://news.un.org/en/story/2020/07/1069211.

Usher, Ann Danaiya. 2020. 'South Africa and India push for COVID-19 patents ban'. *Lancet 396* (10265): 1790–1791.

Whelan, Mary. 2008. 'Negotiating the International Health Regulations'. *Global Health Working Paper No. 1.* Geneva: The Graduate Institute. World Health Assembly. 2021. 'WHO's Work in Health Emergencies'. A74/9 Add.1, 5 May. https://cdn.who.int/media/docs/default-source/documents/emergencies/a74_9add1-en.pdf?sfvrsn=d5d22fdf_1&download=true.

WHO. 2018. International Health Regulations (2005) State Party Self-assessment Annual Reporting Tool. Geneva: World Health Organization. https://apps.who.int/iris/bitstream/handle/10665/272432/WHO-WHE-CPI-2018.16-eng.pdf?sequence=

WHO. 2020a. 'WHO Director-General's Statement on IHR Emergency Committee on Novel Coronavirus (2019-nCoV)'. 30 January. https://www.who.int/dg/speeches/detail/who-director-general-s-statement-on-ihr-emergency-committee-on-novel-coronavirus-(2019-ncov).

Youde, Jeremy. 2016. 'High Politics, Low Politics, and Global Health'. *Journal of Global Security Studies 1* (2): pp. 157–70.

13

How COVID-19 Is Shaking Up Pharmacy

Luc Bergeron and Martin Darveau

The SARS-CoV-2 (more commonly known as COVID-19) pandemic hit us with full force and without warning in 2020. We were presented with the unique challenge of a new pathogen (albeit one that is closely related to another previously encountered virus, the SARS-CoV-1) and a new clinical syndrome that we knew nothing about. This pandemic, in all likelihood, will not be an isolated event, and similar challenges might very well arise in the future. Because pharmacy is central to the acquisition and management of drugs worldwide, and also because the pharmacist is one of the most (if not the most) accessible of health-care professionals, the impacts of a global health calamity such as the COVID-19 pandemic are significant. These impacts on pharmacy and pharmacists are also present whether health infrastructures are developed or not. There are also many wider global issues, such as the limited number of countries sourcing active pharmaceutical ingredients (API) and the impact of a pandemic on their production or shipping capacity for the multitude of countries depending on API to manufacture drugs or the risk of major drug shortages if, for example, transportation is restricted by public health measures to contain the dissemination of the virus (Edwards et al. 2021). While the repercussions of a pandemic on pharmacy activities and pharmacy practice can be observed on many levels, as clinical practitioners we elected to address and reflect on some of the impacts COVID-19 has had on three important components of the practice of pharmacy: ethics and the use of drugs in a pandemic context, challenges regarding logistics (drug supplies), and the impact on pharmaceutical care.

Therapeutic and Ethical Challenges with COVID-19

With the emergence of COVID-19 in early 2020, we had to contend with an unexpected, widely spreading, and potentially fatal disease for which there was no established treatment. The short-lived epidemic of severe acute respiratory syndrome (SARS) (caused by coronavirus SARS-CoV-1) in 2003 prevented the clinical trials initiated from producing tangible results. Some clinical studies were also started to evaluate the clinical effectiveness of several antivirals during the

Luc Bergeron and Martin Darveau, *How COVID-19 Is Shaking Up Pharmacy.* In: *A Multidisciplinary Approach to Pandemics.* Edited by Philippe Bourbeau, Jean-Michel Marcoux, and Brooke A. Ackerly, Oxford University Press.
 DOI: 10.1093/oso/9780192897855.003.0014

recent Ebola outbreaks. However, more or less all of these studies were non-comparative (i.e. without a concurrent group in which patients did not receive an experimental drug), which led to no definitive conclusion about the efficacy or safety of the drug tested (Kalil 2020). A disease without a known treatment is particularly challenging because the development of new drugs typically takes a long time, often decades, to bring promising substances to market (Hay et al. 2014). Many of these drugs will never reach the market, either because of disappointing results in clinical trials or because of unexpected toxicity or poor tolerance. Time was not a resource we had at our disposal when COVID-19 hit, thus one of the first reactions of scientists was to take a look at the therapeutic arsenal already available to identify drugs that might have potentially useful antiviral activity against SARS-CoV-2. Some previous *in vitro* work had already been done with other related coronaviruses (SARS-CoV-1 and MERS-CoV) and with the Ebola virus, which pointed to a few drugs that showed promising antiviral activity. However, none of these drugs had been proven to be effective in the treatment of the disease.

A group of drugs which emerged rapidly as a possible viable treatment option for the coronavirus was the 4-aminoquinolines, and more specifically chloroquine and hydroxychloroquine. Hydroxychloroquine and chloroquine are used for the prevention and treatment of malaria, but also in the treatment of some autoimmune diseases such as rheumatoid arthritis and lupus. They are easily available worldwide, cheap, and considered safe for use. The apparently encouraging preliminary results of clinical trials, mainly from small or non-controlled trials, indicated a possible beneficial effect for the treatment of COVID-19 (Gautret et al. 2020). Initially, this looked like a potential 'game changer', to paraphrase a well-known politician. However, this seemingly good news raised a number of issues, in part triggered by the influence of social media.

The Impact of Social Media and 'Artificial Shortages'

Unbridled enthusiasm elicited by the public release of some of the results of early trials with chloroquine and hydroxychloroquine, amplified by social media and some political figures, led to a disproportionate increase in demand for these drugs. Liu and colleagues (2020) conducted a study of Google searches originating from the United States that included the terms 'buy', 'order', 'Amazon', 'eBay', or 'Walmart' in combination with 'chloroquine' or 'hydroxychloroquine' per 10 million total searches. They looked at fluctuations in the searches and found that Twitter posts by prominent individuals who have a vast number of followers (e.g. Elon Musk and Donald Trump) triggered a spectacular increase in searches on Google to obtain hydroxychloroquine and chloroquine (see Figure 13.1).

This disproportionate interest in hydroxychloroquine and chloroquine put significant pressure on pharmacists, who were inundated with requests from their

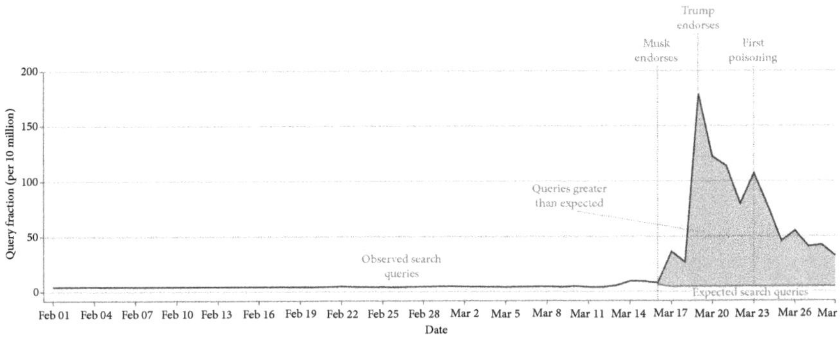

Fig. 13.1 Internet searches for purchasing hydroxychloroquine during the first weeks of the COVID-19 pandemic

Notes: Queries included the term « hydroxychloroquine » in combination with « buy », « order », « Amazon », « eBay », or « Walmart » (the latter being the top three e-commerce companies). The first dotted vertical line corresponds to entrepreneur Elon Musk's tweet on 16 March, the second corresponds to President Donald Trump's endorsement on 19 March, and the third corresponds to the first reported chloroquine poisoning on 23 March.
Source: reprinted with permission from Liu et al. (2020).

patients about these drugs and their availability. They also received several inappropriate prescriptions for hydroxychloroquine and chloroquine, clearly intended to prevent or treat COVID-19, from patients not known to have been diagnosed with inflammatory bowel disease, lupus, or malaria. All this unexpected (and urgent) interest in hydroxychloroquine and chloroquine led pharmacists and hospitals to request greater supplies of these drugs to constitute stockpiles, which in turn led to artificial shortages.

This pressure on pharmacies and drug wholesalers finally led to patients treated for established indications, such as lupus and rheumatoid arthritis, sometimes being denied their usual treatment. In March 2020 in Quebec, the Institut national d'excellence en santé et services sociaux (INESSS 2020), a provincial government agency whose mission is to promote clinical excellence and the efficient use of resources in the health and social services sector, issued a collective prescription that allowed pharmacists to limit the dispensing of hydroxychloroquine to patients known to have been diagnosed with lupus, juvenile rheumatoid arthritis, or to pregnant women. This practice ended after a few days, when it became clear that hydroxychloroquine would not be used on a large scale and the risk of a significant shortage became pointless.

Meanwhile, some caveats on the use of 4-aminoquinolines emerged. For instance, in the particular case of chloroquine, despite being effective against Chikungunya virus *in vitro*, French researchers observed that chloroquine was instead associated with a paradoxical effect (persistent arthralgia) when administered to patients for the treatment of this viral infection (Roques 2018; Guastalegname 2020). Moreover, most of the administration schedules advocated for hydroxychloroquine in the treatment of COVID-19 are derived from *in vitro* data and mathematical simulations (*in silico*) and have not been formally validated. In the end, groups of researchers and clinicians use different doses of the drug. For instance, while Didier Raoult's group suggests giving 200 mg of hydroxychloroquine 3 times a day for 10 days (Gautret et al. 2020), the Canadian CATCO research protocol (associated with the international Solidarity clinical trial conducted by the World Health Organization (WHO); US National Library of Medicine 2020) has proposed instead 800 mg twice daily for 1 day, followed by 400 mg twice daily for 9 days.

Concerns were also raised about the possible cardiac effects of hydroxychloroquine, as 4-aminoquinolines can cause arrhythmia problems. It was feared that the use of higher doses than those commonly used for the treatment of lupus in the treatment of COVID-19 would increase the risk of cardiac adverse effects (Fihn et al. 2020; Juurlink 2020). These fears explain in part the decision of the WHO, on 4 July 2020, to discontinue the hydroxychloroquine treatment arm of the WHO's SOLIDARITY trial. This randomized clinical trial was designed to compare different treatment approaches for COVID-19 (WHO 2020). This decision was made after close examination of the scientific basis (i.e. the clinical data supporting the drug's efficacy and safety) behind the choice of 4-aminoquinolines in the treatment of COVID-19.

The Ethics Angle

Many ethical challenges arise in a context where a proven effective treatment for a disease is lacking. For instance, if a drug is reputed to be safe for a given condition (e.g. lupus), can it be implied that it will remain as safe when it is administered to patients with a new disease of which we know very little about? As health professionals, are we required to offer any *potentially* beneficial drug to patients infected with coronavirus? Must one try unproven therapies at all costs when no treatment has been proven safe and effective, particularly when knowledge about the disease is evolving rapidly? What about the societal pressure put on clinicians by all the publicity and perhaps unrealistic expectations about certain drugs touted as 'miracle drugs'? What are the obligations of the pharmacist?

The patient's best interest must always be at the centre of a pharmacist's decisions and actions and is one of the cardinal principles of the profession's code of ethics. Pharmacists usually tend to err on the side of caution. However, in exceptional situations, such as pandemics caused by new pathogens, the right course of action is not always clear. We interact with physicians on a daily basis to ensure optimal use of drugs, and we use data from randomized clinical trials (RCTs) to convince them to change the nature of a drug therapy (agent, dosing, etc.) or modify the duration of treatment. However, the urgency brought upon us by the COVID-19 pandemic, with rapidly increasing numbers of sick patients needing hospitalization and a growing number of deaths, put pharmacists somewhat at odds with their science-based training (quality of evidence or RCTs) and the temptation to offer a possible cure for this deadly disease.

Some experts have formulated an ethical framework for the use of alternative medications with little or uncertain efficacy and safety data (Thompson 2020; Thompson et al. 2006; Leider et al. 2017). Beneficence (*primum non nocere*) is the common thread of this framework (see Table 13.1). Notably, the use of drugs within a research protocol (if access to research protocols is indeed available) is one of the components of the proposal and makes a lot of sense. The framework of a research project makes it possible to control several factors (efficacy measures, adverse effects) in a standardized and rigorous way that is impossible to achieve in the context of regular daily care of the patient. It also emphasizes the importance of the informed consent of the patient and the balance of risks and benefits. One should be aware of this balance because in a situation such as the one the pandemic put us in, we might emphasize the potential benefits of the drug at the expense of safety issues (Kalil 2020).

On the Importance of Doubt in Science

Doubt is at the heart of the scientific process. Health sciences, and infectious diseases in particular, are far from exact sciences. For instance, the optimal duration of antibiotic treatment for a significant number of everyday infections has not been clearly defined by rigorous studies (Llewelyn et al. 2017; Lambert 1999). Pharmacists and other health professionals have been trained in the past decades to rely on scientific facts (evidence-based medicine) in the decision-making process of

Table 13.1 Guidance for the use of drugs with little or uncertain efficacy and safety data

- Use of best available scientific evidence
- Consider the risk/benefit ratios, which may be different for patients who are critically ill
- Ensure that the patient or proxy is able to give informed consent
- Provision of drugs/treatment in the context of research (when accessible) is preferable
- Ensure that actions are not contributing to drug shortages for patients who are benefiting from medication for proven clinical indications
- Ensure equity of access

Adapted from Thompson 2020

selecting a treatment for a particular disease. Mishaps can occur over the course of drug development. Drugs that looked promising in early phases of development were abandoned because of unexpected problems or subsequently disappointing clinical results. In 2017, the US Federal Drug Administration (FDA) published a report describing examples of drugs for which phase 2 and phase 3 trials had divergent results (FDA 2017). In this regard, it seemed legitimate to have some degree of doubt or scepticism regarding the first presumably spectacular results reported with hydroxychloroquine. Hence the importance for pharmacists to take this step back to try to assess the issues, the balance of benefits and advantages, and the quality of the information available more objectively.

In addition, manuscripts presenting the results of several clinical trials as a prepublication also played a role in the frenzy surrounding hydroxychloroquine in the early months of the pandemic. Usually, when someone wants to publish the results of their work, the manuscript is submitted to the editors of a journal and generally peer-reviewed. This process acts as a sieve, to ascertain whether the work submitted is sound and whether the results and their interpretation by the authors are valid and objective. It is a form of quality assurance. Only a few of the immense quantity of manuscripts submitted every year will be chosen for publication. The dissemination of scientific data through preprint servers, such as *medRxiv.org*, represents a relatively new outlet for scientific data. Websites such as *medRxiv.org* allow free access to unpublished manuscripts on health sciences issues. In contrast with the conventional publication process, no subscription fee is required by the user to read the scientific work submitted. While preprint publication is allowing scientific work to be circulated to a wider audience, it is important to understand that the manuscripts have yet to undergo peer review. The website's home page notes that 'Preprints are preliminary reports of work that have not been certified by peer review. They should not be relied on to guide clinical practice or health-related behavior and should not be reported in news media as established information.' However, most of the users will not necessarily read the caution and will proceed directly to the manuscripts downloaded on the platform. There is thus a risk of providing unfiltered access to scientific results, without the appropriate interpretations and nuances that are often necessary, to people with limited or no scientific background. It might lead to misinterpretation and at times feed conspiracy theories and rumours that are posted and disseminated via social media (Islam et al. 2020). The hype around some drugs, such as hydroxychloroquine or ivermectin, was partly fed by the enthusiasm of readers who accessed preprint manuscripts but did not look at the methodology and analyses with a critical viewpoint, but rather disseminated the overly optimistic conclusions of the authors (Davey 2020b).

The standard publication process is not flawless, however, and can backfire on scientists. COVID-19 has provided us with a spectacular example of this with the publication and subsequent retraction of the results of an international study examining the effectiveness of chloroquine and hydroxychloroquine for the treatment of COVID-19 (Mehra et al. 2020). This study, published in the prestigious journal *The Lancet*, presented results that were supposed to originate from a vast multinational registry analysis of the use of hydroxychloroquine or chloroquine for COVID-19 treatment. However, some discrepancies in the number of patients taking hydroxychloroquine in Australia, when compared to official coronavirus data, were found and reported by a journalist at *The Guardian Australia* in the days following the publication of the study (Davey 2020a). This led to a wider investigation of the database provided by one of the investigators and ultimately resulted in the retraction of the study.

Knowledge about this new disease is accumulating at a phenomenal speed. Scientists and physicians published guidelines for the management of COVID-19 that became more or less obsolete within just a few weeks (Institute of Tropical Medicine, Antwerp, Universiteit Antwerpen, CHU Saint-Pierre, Agence fédérale des médicaments et produits de santé 2020)! Once again, one must remember to take a critical view regarding the information, its quality, and its interpretation. Clinical practice and science in medicine and pharmacy are seldom black and white.

The Unpredictable Impact of COVID-19 on the Drug Supply to Hospitals

The supply of drugs to hospitals is generally based on a well-regulated system where each component depends on another. In this chain, starting at the pharmaceutical industry, predictability is the key factor to ensuring a good drug supply to hospitals. From an individual perspective, one might think that predictability and the old concept of supply and demand cannot really be applied in health care because of the unpredictable nature of disease itself. However, this basic economic principle is rather well established when one considers a large-scale national health-care system. Indeed, it is based upon the historical consumption of each drug, which the pharmaceutical industry uses to anticipate the demand to come, and hence the amount to supply yearly, to each hospital. Thus, market predictability automatically regulates not only the production and availability of drugs nationally, but also drug inventories at distributors and in hospitals. Consequently, in a stable situation of supply and demand, a constant periodic turnover occurs between the pharmaceutical company, the distributor, and the hospital pharmacy.

At a certain level, the balance is precarious and can be quickly disrupted because of a supply disturbance, which is usually caused by an industrial production shutdown. Indeed, upstream in the supply chain, problems related to pharmaceutical ingredients or drug recalls can lead to a significant drop in production and, ultimately, to drug shortages. However, it will be relatively rare that the balance will be greatly and quickly affected because of a significant and unpredictable increase in drug demand. But this situation was observed worldwide during the COVID-19 pandemic (Ammar et al. 2020; Badreldin and Atallah 2020; Elbeddini et al. 2020; Shuman et al. 2020).

At first sight, there was no sign to suggest the extent of the spread that would occur, nor that the dissemination of SARS-CoV-2 would take an unusual path. This explains why medical teams and health system managers were in a very alert mode, but as observers rather than active players. Afterwards, the situation evolved too quickly, with the Wuhan outbreak taking just a few weeks to spread internationally. Despite the fact that health-care stakeholders promptly changed their perspective and formed strategic committees, most of them were still one step behind and found themselves in reaction mode instead of being fully in control of the situation. This weakened the precarious drug balance and exposed hospitals to the risk of not being able to meet the drug needs to treat intensive care unit (ICU) patients with COVID-19.

What should we remember from this period? How could the supply of drugs have been planned in a timely manner against a virus with flu-like symptoms for which no vaccine or effective treatment was available at the time of the outbreak? At the beginning, in terms of drug supply, actions were mainly limited to acquiring supportive drug therapies for the most threatening consequences of COVID-19, which were respiratory distress (Ammar et al. 2020) and secondary pulmonary infections (Dabestani et al. 2020). But because the COVID-19 pandemic was nothing but uncertain, numerous questions remained about adequate treatment of these consequences: How many patients would require such care? Which drugs would these patients need and for how long? To what extent should drug inventories in hospitals be increased rapidly without weakening the supply chain and leading to drug shortages? How much effort should be reasonably deployed before the virus is even present in the country? What is the status of drug inventories in hospitals? What would be the capacity of the industry to produce further drugs in a reasonable time? All these questions, and many others, are important during pathogen outbreaks and must be answered quickly.

Based on this experience, what emerged from the first wave of the COVID-19 pandemic is that the robustness of a national drug supply system depends mainly on four factors: (1) the centralization of information or, at the very least, the IT interconnection and harmonization of supply systems between hospitals at the regional level to make it possible to quickly obtain a reliable drug inventory status; (2) the ability of drug supply managers to act quickly and obtain a concerted drug supply plan in close collaboration with government authorities; (3) an effective and transparent communication strategy; and (4) the responsiveness of the industry as a partner. It appears that all these factors are necessary to the implementation of an action plan to be ready to face any new pandemic.

The Action Plan for Pharmacists in Times of Pandemics

Step 1: Estimating drug inventories at regional and national levels

During pandemics, the first step is to gather the status of drug inventories available in all hospitals at the regional and national level. It is essential to promptly obtain the opinion of clinicians to establish a list of the drugs most likely to be used. Then, drug supply managers must determine how many units of these drugs are available in each hospital. For example, pharmacists had to determine whether drug inventories were sufficient to treat ICU patients with COVID-19. However, if collecting information from all hospitals of a region is the easy part, it is far more complicated to collect and aggregate these data on a national level if there is no IT interconnection among hospital drug supply systems. Indeed, hospitals from different regions have different drugs suppliers, and therefore drug concentration and vial sizes differ.

Step 2: Estimating drug needs for a standardized patient

During pandemics, it is essential to estimate the drug requirements in milligrams (mg) for each patient affected by the virus. For each of the drugs on the list established by the clinicians, an average daily dose and a duration of treatment must be calculated. This standardized consumption, for example in mg/24 hours, must then be converted into the number of vials needed to treat a patient with this drug for 24 hours. For example, in the first wave of the COVID-19 pandemic, drug requirement calculations were based on the premise that ICU patients with COVID-19 would need more drugs, the proxy being an acute respiratory distress syndrome (Ammar et al. 2020), a well-known but infrequent clinical condition. One of the main challenges encountered during this pandemic was to provide enough drugs to treat a condition that was anticipated to require a large amount of drugs to support mechanical ventilation. Thus, once a critical drug list was established with an average daily dose for each drug, it was possible to calculate the autonomy of a hospital and a region to treat patients with COVID-19 in the ICU.

Step 3: Estimating the epidemiological curve

As all hospitals in the region are mobilized to face a pandemic, drug supply planning is completely disrupted. Indeed, some hospitals will significantly increase their bed capacity to add critically ill patients while others will discharge patients with no acute conditions and reduce their usual medical activities to deal with the pandemic. It is therefore impossible to plan medicine supply based on historical drug consumption data. In other words, predictability does not exist. There are important data to obtain to facilitate the implementation of a good action plan. For example, knowing the maximum capacity of ICU beds at regional and national levels is part of the data necessary to build up drug inventories in a pandemic situation. These data, coupled with epidemiology estimates, will help to establish how many patients are likely to occupy these beds regionally and nationally and to what extent these patients will need drugs.

Step 4: Reassessing the estimates daily

The centralization of data or the capacity of hospitals to exchange information related to drug inventories in each hospital at the regional and national levels is essential. Indeed, one of the main challenges during a crisis is to obtain accurate and real-time information so that concerted actions can be taken to avoid drug supply disruptions. It is essential for hospitals from the same region to share their drug data with others, which have to be updated daily according to drug consumption and the occupancy rate of beds by patients suffering from the virus. It is essential that drug supply managers know the following parameters in real time: (1) the number of vials of each drug available regionally and nationally; (2) how many patients could be treated with this amount of drug and for how many days; (3) the number of patients hospitalized daily; and (4) epidemiological estimates of the anticipated number of patients expected in the hospital over time. Lack of information on any of these parameters will compromise the ability of drug supply managers to act adequately.

Step 5: The responsiveness of the pharmaceutical industry

As previously stated, every part of the drug supply chain is important. Pharmaceutical industries must be quickly made aware of drug needs during a pandemic. They must act as partners in the action plan to ensure good responsiveness. Close discussions between stakeholders must be held, based on estimates of drug needs regionally and nationally.

The Communication Plan

One of the main challenges encountered during a pandemic concerns the communication of the status of hospital drug inventories by hospital pharmacists. While the importance of transmitting accurate and transparent information seems obvious, how to transmit this information, how much information to share, and to whom remains more complex. It appears that the communication plan should primarily aim to inform four categories of stakeholders: (1) government authorities; (2) those responsible for the supply of drugs in hospitals; (3) hospital care managers; and (4) clinical teams.

During a national crisis, government authorities must be informed daily about the status of drug inventories based on the parameters described above. Thus, government stakeholders have to know in real time the capacity to treat patients at the regional and national levels and the degree of information transmitted has to be limited to aggregated information. The same information has to be available to those responsible for the supply of drugs in hospitals—not only aggregated at the national level, but also granularly, detailed by hospital and by region.

Also, clinical teams in hospitals need to be involved to ensure the appropriate use of drugs that are at risk of shortages. They must use these drugs according to inventories and respect the measures put in place to reduce losses. Adequate information must be provided to clinical teams that takes into account the regional and national supply contexts. Indeed, during a pandemic, some regions are affected earlier, or more so than others. The uncertainty surrounding the rate and extent of spread, as well as the level of impact on hospitalizations by region, is a real challenge in planning drug needs in each hospital.

Add to this that, at any time, a less-affected hospital might be forced to share drugs with hospitals that are more affected, meaning that the less-affected hospital's drug inventory status can be rapidly reduced. This is an important factor to consider in the information to be transmitted to the clinical teams. With this information in hand, they are even more aware that drug inventories can decrease rapidly despite good planning. The main dilemma remains the following: who within the clinical teams should receive the information, and what level of information should be conveyed, as it must be properly interpreted in order to achieve the intended objectives?

Although it may seem obvious, it is important to remember that in a crisis situation, the right information must be sent to the right stakeholder. In other words, there is a need to control the message to some extent to achieve a balance between disseminating all data and withholding some information. The first situation will create a high risk of misinterpreting the data, causing the message to be distorted and running the risk of inappropriate use of drugs that could lead to drug shortages. The second situation will lead to inertia of the teams and a lack of confidence in drug supply managers. To overcome these situations, it is worthwhile to limit and identify the people who will receive all the information and act as message carriers; heads of medical departments could play this crucial role. They must be trained to fully understand all the data transmitted, the factors affecting drug inventories, and the uncertainty surrounding the context of the pandemic. At this level, charts, graphs, and colour codes could be useful to properly illustrate the status of drug inventories. Heads of medical departments must then convey clear guidelines to their clinical teams.

The most important thing is to maintain a clear, lean, and consistent message for clinicians throughout the crisis. Also, clinical tools indicating therapeutic alternatives must be shared to ensure adequate and uniform treatment of patients: for example, 'A low level of "*drug A*" is encountered, please use the proposed drug alternatives unless no option is clinically suitable for the patient.' Thus, in the context of COVID-19, the heads of emergency, intensive care, anaesthesia, and paediatrics departments were identified as message carriers and had to be well informed with frequent updates.

The Interpretation of Data

There are a few important factors to consider in the analysis and interpretation of drug inventories. First, some usual clinical activities are generally offloaded in a crisis. It is important to consider that drugs not used for these activities will cause a temporary increase in the inventories available to treat patients affected by the virus. However, at some point during a pandemic, these activities will have to be resumed. Those in charge of drug supply must be able to assess to what extent the inventories will allow a proportion of these usual activities to be resumed, depending on the evolution of the pandemic. The key element is to maintain enough drug inventories to treat possible patients suffering from the virus while maintaining the supply of drugs for other patients. This last element is a particularly important factor, since it significantly affects the status of drug inventories.

To overcome this uncertainty, drug inventory data must be translated into the number of days of autonomy to treat usual patients and to what extent these inventories are affected by the arrival of patients affected by the virus. For example, based on historical consumption data, the drug inventories available in a hospital for '*drug A*' would allow 80% of usual activities in addition to 10 ICU patients affected by the virus, while the arrival of additional ICU patients affected by the virus would reduce the drug availability for usual activities to '*x* %'. Again, charts and graphs could be useful to illustrate the links and the impact of each factor on drug inventories.

The Challenges for Pharmaceutical Care

The pharmacist is often the most accessible health professional to the population. Patients frequently consult their pharmacist before going to the doctor or the hospital. Pharmacies were also one of the few businesses that remained open during the lockdown instituted at the beginning of the COVID-19 pandemic. Pharmacists and pharmacy staff are, of course, not immune from developing the infection. Pharmacies everywhere in Canada had to implement new protocols—in just a few days—to limit access to the pharmacy to reduce the risk of transmission, install plexiglass panels, and provide personal protective equipment (PPE) for personnel.

Challenges in the maintenance of standards of care both in community and hospital practices were significant, with pharmacists and other staff members becoming infected. In small work teams, such as are frequently encountered in small community pharmacies, one infected member of the staff could have great repercussions. The infection of a pharmacist or technician could sometimes lead to a temporary closure of the pharmacy, since often a significant number of staff had to subsequently quarantine. Similar situations were encountered in hospital pharmacies. Furthermore, the hierarchy of pharmaceutical care activities had to be reassessed and resulted in the reallocation of personnel from their usual clinical tasks to other responsibilities because of COVID-19. Other challenges also loom. Now that there are safe and effective vaccines available, there is, there will be a need to administer this vaccine to most of the population on this planet. Pharmacists will most likely be called upon to help with mass vaccinations, and this will certainly put an additional strain on pharmacists and may even negatively affect access to pharmaceutical care by patients.

Furthermore, this pandemic has also led to the emergence of new technological approaches to alleviate staffing shortages or sick leaves associated with COVID-19. Teleworking, which up until 2020 had been rather marginal, is increasingly becoming a plausible solution to maintain pharmacy services. Many pharmacy tasks, such as the verification of prescriptions, can be done remotely. A pharmacist who must stay at home to care for a sick partner or child, for example, may very well be able to do at least part of their work from home. However, some problems remain with this approach, notably the need for secure networks to ensure that there is no breach in confidentiality. Also, there is great variability in the computer hardware available at home: Many employees do not have webcams, home computers that are compatible with pharmacy system requirements, and so on. Planning by health organizations (community and hospital pharmacies) for upgrades and improvements in home computer systems will be necessary in the near future. The COVID-19 pandemic will herald many changes in pharmacy practice.

However, one also has to recall that the practice of pharmacy is far from uniform worldwide. Access to pharmacy services (and to drugs) can rapidly become particularly challenging in regions where qualified personnel are scarce, and even more so in developing or emerging countries. COVID-19 should also be a reminder that there are still great variabilities in access to pharmaceutical care and pharmacy services.

Conclusion

The 2020 COVID-19 pandemic almost instantly took pharmacists out of their comfort zone and had vast repercussions on various aspects of pharmacy practice, particularly with regard to availability and access to therapeutic options, management of possible drug shortages and the drug supply chain, and impact on human resources. The unpredictability and speed of the spread, as well as the uncertainty surrounding the effects of SARS-CoV-2, had to be counterbalanced by a systematic, objective, and rigorous approach.

Above all, there is now a window of opportunity to review our practices, both in terms of supply chain logistics and clinical practice, to improve the response to the next pandemic, prevent future drug shortages, ensure access to therapeutics or vaccines, and offer a better quality of care to our patients.

References

Ammar Mahmoud A., Gretchen L. Sacha, Sarah C. Welch, et al. 2020. 'Sedation, Analgesia, and Paralysis in COVID-19 Patients in the Setting of Drug Shortages'. *Journal of Intensive Care Medicine*: 885066620951426. doi:10.1177/0885066620951426.

Badreldin Hisham A., and Bassam Atallah. 2020. 'Global Drug Shortages due to COVID-19: Impact on Patient Care and Mitigation Strategies'. *Research in Social and Administrative Pharmacy* 19 May: S1551-7411(20)30569-6. doi:10.1016/j.sapharm.2020.05.017.

Dabestani Arash, Dawn DeAngelo, Sophia R Chhay, Bayli J. Larson, and Michael C. Ganio. 2020. 'Medication Utilization in Patients in New York Hospitals during the COVID-19 Pandemic'. *American Journal of Health-System Pharmacy 77* (22): pp. 1885–1892. doi:10.1093/ajhp/zxaa251.

Davey Melissa. 2020a. 'Questions Raised over Hydroxychloroquine Study which Caused WHO to Halt Trials for COVID-19'. *The Guardian Australia*, 28 May. https://www.theguardian.com/science/2020/may/28/questions-raised-over-hydroxychloroquine-study-which-caused-who-to-halt-trials-for-covid-19.

Davey Melissa. 2020b. 'Unreliable Data: How Doubt Snowballed over COVID-19 Drug Research that Swept the World'. *The Guardian Australia*, 4 June. https://www.theguardian.com/world/2020/jun/04/unreliable-data-doubt-snowballed-covid-19-drug-research-surgisphere-coronavirus-hydroxychloroquine?CMP=share_btn_link.

Edwards Brian, Charles A. Gloor, Franck Toussaint, Chaofeng Guan, and Dominic Furniss. 2021. 'Human Factors: The Pharmaceutical Supply Chain as a Complex Sociotechnical System'. *International Journal for Quality in Health Care 33* (S1): pp. 56–9. doi:10.1093/intqhc/mzaa102.

Elbeddini Ali, Thulasika Prabaharan, Sarah Almasalkhi, and Cindy Tran. 2020. 'Pharmacists and COVID-19'. *Journal of Pharmaceutical Policy and Practice 13*: Article no. 36. doi:10.1186/s40545-020-00241-3.

Fihn Stephan D., Eli Perencevich, and Steven M. Bradley. 2020. 'Caution Needed on the Use of Chloroquine and Hydroxychloroquine for Coronavirus Disease 2019'. *JAMA Network Open 3* (4.23): e209035. doi:10.1001/jamanetworkopen.2020.9035.

Food and Drug Administration (FDA). 2017. '22 Case Studies Where Phase 2 and Phase 3 Trials Had Divergent Results'. 21 December. https://www.fda.gov/about-fda/reports/22-case-studies-where-phase-2-and-phase-3-trials-had-divergent-results.

Gautret Philippe, Jean-Christophe Lagier, Philippe. Parola, et al. 2020. 'Hydroxychloroquine and Azithromycin as a Treatment of COVID-19: Results of an Open-Label Non-Randomized Clinical Trial'. *International Journal of Antimicrobial Agents 56* (1): p. 1.

Guastalegname Maurizio, and Alfredo Vallone. 2020. 'Could Chloroquine/Hydroxychloroquine Be Harmful in Coronavirus Disease 2019 (COVID-19) Treatment?' *Clinical Infectious Diseases 71* (15): p. 887.

Hay Michael, David W. Thomas, John L. Craighead, Celia Economides, and Jesse Rosenthal. 2014. 'Clinical Development Success Rates for Investigational Drugs'. *Nature Biotechnology 32*: p. 40.

Institut national d'excellence en santé et services sociaux (INESSS). 2020. 'Ordonnance collective nationale d'interruption de l'hydroxychloroquine et de la chloroquine par les personnes atteintes de maladies chroniques dans le cadre d'une rupture d'inventaire'. https://www.inesss.qc.ca/fileadmin/doc/INESSS/COVID-19/COVID-19_OC-PMN_HCQ.pdf.

Institute of Tropical Medicine, Antwerp, Universiteit Antwerpen, CHU Saint-Pierre, Agence fédérale des médicaments et produits de santé. 2020. 'Interim Clinical Guidance for Patients Suspected of/Confirmed with COVID-19 in Belgium 16 mars 2020; Version 3'. http://www.biotech.ca/wp-content/uploads/2020/03/COVID-19_InterimGuidelines_Treatment_ENG.pdf.

Islam Md, Saiful, Tonmoy Sarkar, Sazzad Hossain Khan, et al. 2020. 'COVID-19–Related Infodemic and Its Impact on Public Health: A Global Social Media Analysis'. *American Journal of Tropical Medicine and Hygiene 103* (4): pp. 1621–9. doi:10.4269/ajtmh.20-0812.

Juurlink David N. 2020. 'Safety Considerations with Chloroquine, Hydroxychloroquine and Azithromycin in the Management of SARS-CoV-2 Infection'. *Canadian Medical Association Journal 192* (17): E450.

Kalil Andre C. 2020. 'Treating COVID-19—Off-Label Drug Use, Compassionate Use, and Randomized Clinical Trials During Pandemics'. *JAMA 323* (19): p. 1897.

Lambert H.P. 1999 'Don't Keep Taking the Tablets?' *The Lancet 354*: p. 943.

Leider Jonathan P., Debra DeBruin, Nicole Reynolds, Angelica Koch, and Judy Sieberg. 2017. 'Ethical Guidance for Disaster Response, Specifically around Crisis Standards of Care: A Systematic Review'. *American Journal of Public Health 107* (9): e1.

Liu, Michael, Theodore L. Caputi, Mark Dredze, Aaron S. Kesselheim, and John W. Ayers. 2020. 'Internet Searches for Unproven COVID-19 Therapies in the United States'. *JAMA Internal Medicine 180* (8): p. 1116.

Llewelyn Martin J., Jennifer M. Fitzpatrick, Elizabeth Darwin, et al. 2017. 'The Antibiotic Course Has Had Its Day'. *British Medical Journal 358*: j3418. doi:10.1136/bmj.j3418.

Mehra, Mandeep. R., Sapan S. Desai, Frank Ruschitzka, and Amit N. Patel. 2020. 'Hydroxychloroquine or Chloroquine with or without a Macrolide for Treatment of COVID-19: A Multinational Registry Analysis'. *The Lancet*. https://doi.org/10.1016/S0140-6736(20)31180-6.

Roques Pierre, Simon-Djamel Thiberville, Laurence Dupuis-Maguiraga, et al. 2018. 'Paradoxical Effect of Chloroquine Treatment in Enhancing Chikungunya Virus Infection'. *Viruses 10* (5): p. 268.

Shuman Andrew G., Erin Fox, and Yoram Unguru. 2020. 'Preparing for COVID-19-Related Drug Shortages'. *Annals of the American Thoracic Society 17* (8): pp. 928–31. doi:10.1513/AnnalsATS.202004-362VP.

Thompson, Alison K. 2020. 'Prescribing the Right Course of Action: Pharmacy Ethics in a Pandemic'. CSHP COVID-19 RX webinar. 7 May. https://cshp.ca/sites/default/files/Webinars/COVID-19%20Ethics%20and%20Pharmacy%20Practice%20May%202020.pdf.

Thompson, Alison K., Karen Faith, Jennifer L. Gibson, and Ross E. G. Upshur. 2006. 'Pandemic Influenza Preparedness: An Ethical Framework to Guide Decision-Making'. *BMC Medical Ethics 7* (12). https://doi.Org/10.1186/1472-6939-7-12.

US National Library of Medicine. 2020. 'Treatments for COVID-19: Canadian Arm of the SOLIDARITY Trial (CATCO)'. https://clinicaltrials.gov/ct2/show/NCT04330690.

World Health Organization (WHO). 2020. 'WHO Discontinues Hydroxychloroquine and Lopinavir/Ritonavir Treatment Arms for COVID-19'. 4 July. https://www.who.int/news-room/detail/04-07-2020-who-discontinues-hydroxychloroquine-and-lopinavir-ritonavir-treatment-arms-for-covid-19.

14

COVID-19 and the Economics of Population Health

Analysing Direct and Indirect Effects

Markus Herrmann and Maripier Isabelle

Pandemics, from the Spanish flu 100 years ago to the more recent coronavirus disease 2019 (COVID-19) can bring private and public health-care systems to the brink of collapse. Developing vaccines, finding cures, and securing personal protective equipment mobilize considerable resources, time, and energy. Governments and individuals alike face a new set of costs and heightened uncertainty about the consequences of their decisions (see Chapter 3 in this volume by Goldstone). Drawing on evidence from the COVID-19 pandemic, this chapter addresses the economic determinants on which public policy can help preserve population health via mitigation strategies, but also on how individuals can (re)act as pandemics unfold beyond the early detection and containment phases. It also describes how income and employment losses incurred on the labour market as a result of public health mitigation strategies may affect population health in the long run, once the pandemic is over. While we focus our attention on diseases for which, like the recent COVID-19, a path to eradication is difficult[1] as the associated pandemic unfolds, we also draw occasionally on lessons from the eradication of others.

In the short run, contagion of communicable diseases, as well as their containment, bear epidemiological and socio-economic components. Indeed, the rate at which the disease spreads heavily depends on the social acceptance of the sanitary measures[2] established by public health authorities, but also on how individuals perceive the disease and their opportunity cost of secluding from public life, including possibly having to stop working. Public health authorities, relying on

[1] For example, in the absence of vaccines providing long-term immunity, in the presence of non-human carriers of the disease, etc.

[2] Sanitary measures include social distancing (also called physical distancing), hand hygiene and respiratory etiquette, use of masks, environmental cleaning and ventilation, and lockdowns of non-essential businesses. Social acceptance is important, as the compliance by individuals and businesses cannot always be easily enforced.

Markus Herrmann and Maripier Isabelle, *COVID-19 and the Economics of Population Health.* In: *A Multidisciplinary Approach to Pandemics.* Edited by Philippe Bourbeau, Jean-Michel Marcoux, and Brooke A. Ackerly, Oxford University Press. © Oxford University Press (2022). DOI: 10.1093/oso/9780192897855.003.0015

simulations of epidemiological models, have a broader view and can account for the current and future spread of an infectious disease in terms of morbidity, mortality, and congestion within the health-care system. Their goal is to preserve the public good of population health. Individuals, however, are less likely, and possibly even unable, to account for the indirect consequences, or external effects, of their own actions during a pandemic. Rather, and unless public authorities move forward with compulsory policies such as lockdowns and bans on public gatherings, individuals will consciously (and sometimes unconsciously) abide by the sanitary measures or, independently, develop their own protection strategy if they judge that they are not forgoing too much well-being (happiness, income, etc.) by doing so.

We argue that governments should account for both the social benefits and costs of containing the pandemic, even if they do not necessarily have complete knowledge of the future health and economic costs. Indeed, uniform sanitary measures, such as social distancing and lockdowns, may translate into different private economic costs for individuals, which, in turn, may not be neutral in terms of long-term health outcomes for certain segments of the population (see also the Introduction in this volume by Ackerly et al.). Accounting for these complex, indirect, and potentially lasting effects in a context riddled with uncertainty thus becomes a challenge for public authorities seeking to take action in the early days of a pandemic and to define, if possible, an initial lockdown strategy.

While any strategy chosen by governments to address the risks of contagion will have consequences that percolate through numerous spheres of individuals' lives, the costs associated with labour market transformations and shifts in income distributions are generally among the first ones to materialize and to be measured. As policymakers seek to sequentially adjust their responses to pandemics using updated flows of data, understanding the nature, magnitude, and distribution of private costs associated with these labour market changes is crucial. Moreover, historical experience, economics, and public health shed light on the private health costs that may result from the impact of social distancing measures on labour markets. Understanding these dynamics can also help to shape policy responses that are complementary to the initial sanitary measures and define a broader optimal strategy in the face of pandemics.

Figure 14.1 illustrates the dynamics explored in this chapter, which is structured as follows. Section 2 addresses how a health crisis initially unfolds and discusses from an economic perspective the drivers of the related costs for society as a whole, as well as for the individual. Section 3 then focuses on the likely aggregate costs that the public health measures put in place by governments might impose on the economy and discusses how such costs are distributed among individuals. It also investigates how this distribution of private costs, stemming from a disrupted labour market and the impact on absolute and relative incomes, may translate into

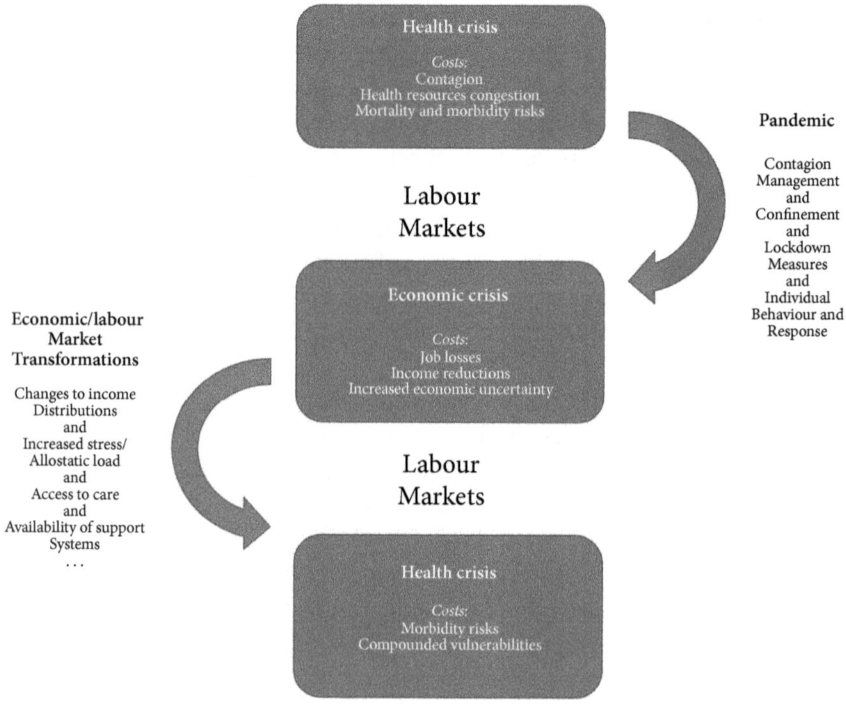

Fig. 14.1 Pandemics, labour markets, and health outcomes

longer-term health burdens for some individuals. Finally, Section 4 concludes and reflects on long-term policymaking, including eradication strategies, as societies navigate the threats and uncertainties associated with pandemics.

The Initial Crisis

Preserving public health is a valuable public good. It is well understood in economics that the provision of a public good may be suboptimal from a societal point of view because individuals mostly account for their own benefit but not for the aggregate, social benefit.[3] Transposed to the context of a pandemic, an individual incorporates ('internalizes') their private benefit of preventing infection, but does

[3] The same type of 'underprovision' of a public good in economics is often studied in the context of environmental crises, where the lack of investment from parties involved threatens our capacity to reach climate goals. Similarities can indeed be identified in the structure of and problems underlying environmental crises (current and future) and pandemics. Why policy response and governance systems are different is discussed in Chapter 6 in this volume by Morin et al. In the same vein, Davies (Chapter 12 in this volume) addresses the failure of international health cooperation and discusses how cooperation at this level has become intertwined with other domains of international cooperation.

not account for the 'external' benefits possibly provided to others (through mask-wearing, for instance). These non-realized social benefits turn into social costs that a governmental authority may be particularly concerned with at the beginning of the crisis.

Contagion and Congestion Externalities and the Social Health Costs of a Pandemic

Not avoiding contagion within society implies a social cost in terms of increased morbidity and mortality imposed on others. It can also lead to congestion within the health-care system. This last scenario becomes more likely when the elderly constitute the majority of infected individuals because they tend to suffer more from respiratory complications (as was seen in northern Italy, Paris, and the Alsace region in eastern France during the first wave of the COVID-19 pandemic).

So far, many economic studies on population health have concentrated on the mortality of pandemics by putting a value on the lives (to be) lost to determine the direct social health cost, and thus have abstracted from the morbidity and congestion cost.[4] Determining the social cost of mortality raises many legitimate ethical questions. Should the life of a rich person be valued more highly than the life of a poor person? How does one account for age?

Economics circumvents these issues by assigning the value of a *statistical* life (VSL), possibly accounting for the expected remaining life-years. This value relies on methods considering either revealed or stated preferences of economic agents for life-threatening health risks.[5] Its calculation depends on the population or data sample, such that 'substantial heterogeneity in the VSL [is observed] both within and across countries' (Kniesner and Viscusi 2019: 5). While richer countries have higher VSLs, the evidence on the relationship between VSL and age is less clear, as reported in Kniesner and Viscusi (2019), who review the economic theory behind VSL and provide a guide to the literature. The US Department of Transportation guideline establishes US$9.6 million for the US VSL in 2016 (Department of Transportation (DOT) 2016). In Quebec (Canada), the value is much lower at C$3.4 million (Ministère des Transports du Québec 2016).

An alternative approach to the VSL that is used in the health domain is based on determining a quality-adjusted life-year (QALY) to which a value is then attributed. Stated-preference techniques in a population sample can be used to

[4] In the context of the COVID-19 pandemic, work by Kniesner and Sullivan (2020) on the social cost attributed to morbidity is a notable exception and is discussed later.

[5] Economic theory and evidence suggest that, in equilibrium, riskier jobs imply higher wages while neighbourhoods with lower health hazards imply higher house prices, both of which can reveal the individual's 'taste' and thus willingness-to-pay for risk reduction. Stated preferences methods, such as conducting surveys on the valuation of risk reduction, are also used in the literature (Kniesner and Viscusi 2019).

attribute utility weights to the quality of a year of life, which allows researchers to reduce two dimensions (health status and time) into a one-dimensional health index. A year of life in perfect health is given the weight of 1, while death corresponds to zero. QALY measures can then be combined with VSL measures. Another possibility consists in observing the revealed choice made by public health agencies to recommend (or not) a costly new treatment or technology. In Canada, Griffiths and Vadlamudi (2016) find evidence of a threshold value of C$50,000 per QALY up to which the Canadian Agency for Drugs and Technologies in Health (CADTH) recommends treatment. The UK Department of Health values a QALY in 2009 at £60,000 (Griffiths and Vadlamudi 2016).

As discussed below, the use of the VSL approach tends to attribute a higher social cost to mortality as compared to the QALY approach, even as both methods correct for age. Depending on the approach used, some researchers, public authorities, and stakeholders may consider an analysis built on the VSL approach to have a favourable bias towards stricter policy actions aimed at preventing more deaths, especially if it does not account for age. Economics does not claim to provide the just value of life to public authorities: Even economists disagree. Rather, it renders the different values and possible choices, whether they are taken more on efficiency or equity grounds, transparent. The public authority's own preference of avoiding the spread of infection is revealed through the approach and planning horizon chosen, which ultimately becomes a political question.

Barla and Herrmann (2020) contrast both methodological approaches when calculating the benefits of avoided deaths of early COVID-19 sanitary measures in Quebec. In their analysis, the VSL and QALY (valued at the benchmark value provided by the CADTH) are adjusted by age group and the remaining life expectancy (properly discounted), assuming that the above-cited values from the Ministère des Transports du Québec and CADTH apply for an individual of average age. The values are shown in current-value terms (2020) in Figure 14.2. The VSL approach leads to values up to three times higher than those obtained with the QALY approach. They range from C$5.1 million for individuals between 0 and 9 years of age for the VSL to C$0.3 million for individuals who are 80 years or older for the QALY approach.

The VSL approach has been used to value avoided fatalities in the COVID-19 pandemic by Thunström and colleagues (2020), Fischer (2020), and many others. It can be criticized on the grounds that pandemics may affect too many people and that the risk is not hypothetical, violating its economic foundations, which are built on marginal evaluations and variations of risk. Pindyck (2020) points out that during the pandemic, COVID-19 is not a potential but a real threat to life, and VSL 'overstate[s] the benefit from lives saved, even if we base that benefit on individual preferences toward mortality risk' (2020: 20); he mentions the use of the QALY methodology as an alternative. Vaillancourt (2020) also favours QALY, as 'it can be used in shifting health resources between various types of activities such as

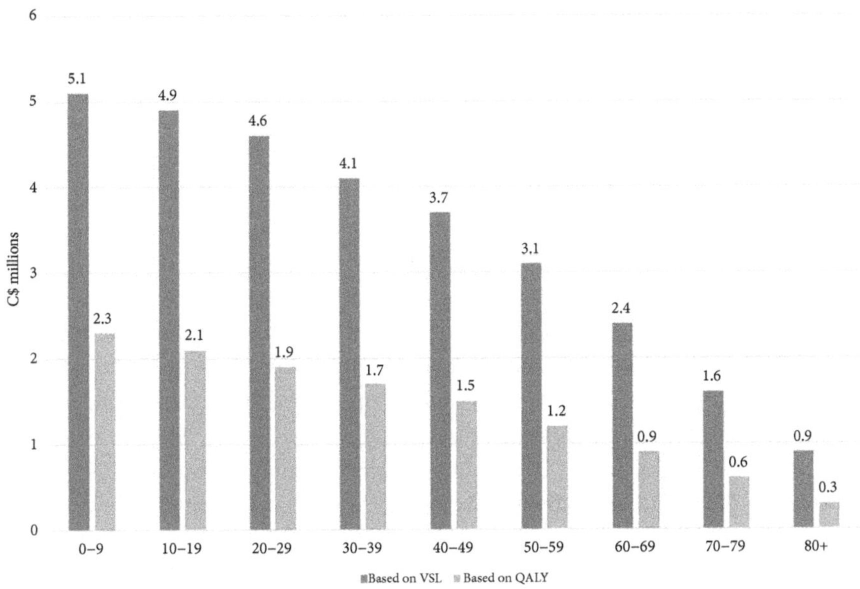

Fig. 14.2 VSL and QALY adjustment for Quebec (in C$millions)

allocating resources for COVID-19 patients and thus removing them from other patients (cancer ...) although this is a less common use' (2020: 2).

However, this is precisely what happened in Quebec as the COVID-19 pandemic unfolded: to prepare for an outbreak, 6,000 hospital beds were freed up in April 2020 by postponing other 'non-urgent' medical treatments. While the cost of such a policy (e.g. postponed surgeries, cancelled appointments and treatments, which may lead to complications or heightened anxiety for the patients) is mostly privately incurred, it provides a social benefit of avoiding congestion in the health-care system. It is the social benefit net of private costs due to the avoided congestion that should be accounted for when evaluating the social desirability of such a policy. To our knowledge, no economic analysis has estimated the congestion cost, or the benefit of avoiding it, in the context of the COVID-19 pandemic so far.

Kniesner and Sullivan (2020) evaluate the morbidity cost of COVID-19. Based on the six injury categories described in a report from the US Department of Transportation (DOT 2016), the authors define and value (QALY-adjusted VSL) four severity categories for symptomatic individuals suffering from COVID-19: no hospitalization (US$32,700), general hospital admission (US$512,300), intensive care unit without mechanical ventilation (US$1,144,500), intensive care unit with mechanical ventilation (US$2,899,400). Asymptotic individuals are valued at US$11,000. The study calculates an overall morbidity cost of approximately US$2.2 trillion as of July 27 (US$46,000 per case), which, to avoid double accounting, needs to be adjusted for possible fatalities that occur in the different severity categories (lowering the cost by 0.2 to 20%). Comparing this figure to the social cost of mortality of US$1.6 trillion (attributable to the 147,000 COVID-19 fatalities as of 27 July 2020), the study points to the importance of accounting for the morbidity cost, which will otherwise greatly underestimate the social health cost of pandemics.[6]

So far, we have only dealt with the contagion and congestion cost of the disease that may translate into a social health cost. But what are the direct costs of treating a pandemic patient? An early estimate of treatment cost of a 'representative patient' during the COVID-19 pandemic comes from the model presented by Lee (2020), who calculates the *median* cost of hospitalization in the United States, which is equal to US$14,400. A representative patient that does not require hospitalization but has symptoms is attributed a median cost of US$3,000, which is four times higher than the cost associated with common, symptomatic influenza (Lee 2020). These direct treatment costs do not necessarily add to the social cost insofar as individuals account for them. A wealthy individual (or one with health insurance) may be ready to pay (or get reimbursed) the sum that is due. Poorer (and uninsured) individuals may be unable to incur the full direct treatment cost such that the uncovered part becomes a social cost.

Vaccination Campaigns and Their Social Health Benefit

Infectious diseases, especially viruses, are effectively fought with vaccination campaigns, if a vaccine is available. By vaccinating a sufficient number of individuals, herd immunity can be reached (at least theoretically) within the population.[7] A population that is characterized by herd immunity conveys immunity to those individuals that have not become infected yet because the virus has stopped spreading (i.e. the infection starts to die out because each new infection case causes less than one further infection[8]).[9] Clearly, an effective vaccine procures a private benefit for the person that gets vaccinated, but it also creates a social benefit by

[6] Building on Kniesner and Sullivan's estimate for the morbidity cost, Dave and colleagues (2021) find evidence that public gatherings at a motorcycle rally held in South Dakota in August 2020 may have turned that event into a super-spreader, generating a public health cost of US$12.2 billion.

[7] Following Kim and colleagues (2011), herd immunity conveyed by a worldwide vaccination programme of the World Health Organization (WHO) has played a major role in eradicating smallpox at a global scale. Following Thompson and Tebbens, '[t]he prerequisites for global eradication include the ability to eradicate [the] disease from all countries contemporaneously and a global commitment to coordinate efforts' (Thompson and Duintjer Tebbens, 2011: 120). As an example of such a commitment, the authors refer to Global Polio Eradication Initiative. Types 2 and 3 were declared successfully eradicated in 2015 and 2019 (Centers for Disease Control and Prevention (CDC) 2021).

[8] It may also arise naturally if people become perfectly immune to the virus due to antibodies of the disease.

[9] Currently available vaccines against COVID-19 do not necessarily provide sterilizing immunity in the long run, that is, prevent vaccinated people from reinfection, and hence, communication

protecting those who are still susceptible to becoming ill (Boulier et al. 2007). Gersovitz and Hammer (2003) address this externality and propose economic instruments (notably a tax and subsidy policy) for preventative or therapeutic measures. Of course, the value of the benefits of a vaccine relative to its costs also depends on whether the immunity it provides lasts for extended periods (such as the vaccine that contributed to the eradication of smallpox in the 1970s) or not (such as the ones developed in 2020 to protect against COVID-19).

In the case of the COVID-19 pandemic, these social benefits, and eventually the avoided costs associated with other sanitary measures, should be accounted for when deciding how much to spend on the development and distribution of new vaccines. Vaccination against COVID-19 provides an additional health policy tool, but it won't substitute, neither immediately nor completely, for the portfolio of sanitary measures put in place at the beginning of the pandemic. Indeed, capacity constraints for administering the vaccine has slowed down building up immunity, while new variants of COVID-19 may circumvent vaccination efforts and negatively affect the population's willingness to get vaccinated in the future.[10]

The Individuals' Behavioural Responses to Disease Prevalence, Vaccine, and Treatment Availability

So far, we have dealt with how economics allows us to determine contagion and congestion externalities (that are not accounted for by individuals) but which should be accounted for in the evaluation of public health policies. However, individuals do adapt to risky environments and may try to control, as much as possible, the risk of contagion themselves, whether this is complementary to an existing public health policy or not. Philipson (2000) presents a survey of models integrating epidemiology and economics, creating the term 'rational epidemics'. Concentrating only on the private benefits that one gets from being healthy, the theoretical model presents individuals' behavioural changes as a response to disease prevalence. This determines a private demand for prevention that is prevalence-elastic—that is, it implies a rate at which individuals will seek out more protection from the disease as 1% more people in their environment become infected. Evidence for such prevalence-related behaviour is found by Wise et al. (2020),

of the disease. Vaccines clearly have a positive impact by attenuating the pathology of the disease, and may lower the rate of transmission, as have other vaccines to corona diseases (Lavine et al. 2021).

[10] Some people have argued in favour of letting herd immunity build up naturally (by enough people getting infected and recovering from the disease) in the case of COVID-19, stating that it is economically too damaging to preserve public health through lockdowns. Because of the high number of fatalities associated with COVID-19, however, such a policy may be considered unethical. Nor does it necessarily represent an economically efficient policy. Without public intervention, it is only hypothetical that younger individuals (who have lower morbidity and mortality risk) contract the disease and help build up herd immunity for the whole society, while senior citizens remain perfectly, and voluntarily, sheltered.

who show that people in the United States at the beginning of the COVID-19 pandemic adopted more stringent sanitary measures when perceiving a higher risk of infection. Following Bauch and Galvani (2013), risk perceptions can indeed be fundamental drivers of behavioural shifts within the population that faces an infection outbreak. A link can be established here to the disease that has probably got the most attention from researchers analysing the private demand for preventing contagion: the human immunodeficiency virus (HIV) (and associated acquired immune deficiency syndrome, AIDS).[11] Early evidence by Ahituv and colleagues (1996) suggests that individuals' propensity to avoid contracting HIV (use of condoms) increases by 50% as the AIDS prevalence increases by 1%. Auld (2003) shows that an anticipated treatment of AIDS tends to lower the prevalence of infection even before the treatment arrives because individuals may self-discipline. Once treatment is available and has proven effective, individuals may lower their guards and disengage from social distancing (or other preventative measures). This is supported by evidence in the context of HIV, where successful antiretroviral (ART) therapy (allowing doctors to control the virus load in an HIV patient) may make individuals behave in riskier ways. A study by Mei and colleagues (2011) in Amsterdam shows that this effect may even outweigh the beneficial effects of ART therapy. This result implies that it is not only prevalence but also the perceived lethality of the disease that individuals account for.

Given this interdependency between individual behaviour and disease prevalence, Bauch and Galvani (2013) argue in favour of imbedding social networks into models of biological contagion. Such models could also account for 'social contagion', when 'highly connected nodes suggest that the vaccine carries risks, … fueling vaccine scare and a drop in vaccine coverage'. As an example, the authors refer to the fear by parents that their child may suffer from autism due to a measles–mumps–rubella vaccine.

Not accounting for the individuals' behaviour when designing public health policies can negatively affect their efficiency, especially if they abstract from the health status of individuals. Fenichel (2013) highlights the importance of accounting for individuals that have recovered and become immune to the disease. Non-discriminate public policies implying social distancing ignore the fact that immune individuals contribute to less contagious contacts for those that are uninfected, which possibly decreases welfare. Clearly, the results rely on the hypothesis that individuals know their own health status. Regarding COVID-19, it must be noted that recovery does not necessarily convey lasting immunity, and knowledge about the approximate time during which an individual is immune after being infected was lacking for most of the first wave of the pandemic. Hence, even if a

[11] Chapter 1 in this volume by Jacobsen discusses from an epidemiological perspective whether HIV/AIDS classifies as an epidemic or a pandemic. The chapter also delivers insights on how governments have responded at an international scale to this disease in order to treat, prevent, and eventually eradicate it.

uniform health policy may not be the 'first-best' solution (i.e. the one among several alternatives that maximizes net benefits), it can still be preferred to no policy at all, given the information constraints.

New models of disease transmission include 'learning dynamics derived from evolutionary game theory' to account for the impact of individual adherence to sanitary measures (see Jentsch et al. 2021; on the evolutionary approach, the interested reader may also refer to Chapter 2 in this volume by Johnson).[12] In the context of a pandemic, like COVID-19, where vaccination does not provide immediate, nor possibly lasting immunity, the vaccination rollout must be accompanied with ongoing sanitary measures with which individuals should comply. Jentsch and colleagues (2021) use mobility and health data for Ontario, Canada, to calibrate adherence of the population in this type of model and analyse different strategies of vaccination rollout minimizing COVID-19 fatalities. More deaths can generally be avoided by targeting the eldest first with the available vaccine. However, a higher perceived cost of vaccination incurred by individuals may invalidate this result and make administering the vaccine independently of age or prioritizing those individuals with the highest contact rates the optimal strategy.

To Confine or Not Confine? The Efficiency of Governments' Initial Sanitary Measures

If social distancing can be an effective measure to limit the spread of a pandemic in the absence of an effective vaccine or treatment (both directly and by facilitating contact tracing when infections occur), it comes at the cost of further slowing down an already fragile economy.[13] This trade-off is analysed nicely in Pindyck (2020), who shows, with the help of a stylized epidemiological model, that a second wave of infection is possible once social distancing measures are relaxed and contact rates among individuals rise sufficiently. Historical evidence for multiple waves is provided, for example, by Caley and colleagues (2008) in the context of the Spanish flu in Sydney, Australia, in 1919. Such dynamics also became evident as the COVID-19 pandemic unfolded in 2020 and 2021.

In the context of COVID-19, social distancing during the initial phase of the pandemic was used more or less intensively, depending on jurisdictions; this variation can be used statistically to determine the relative effectiveness of these measures (for European countries, see the report by the COVID-19 response team

[12] These models bear resemblance with economic models, but do not rely on the same microfoundations for the individuals' objective functions, which underly their decision-making processes.

[13] Following Thompson and Duintjer Tebbens (2011), an example of a newly emerging disease that could successfully be stopped before it became endemic is the severe acute respiratory syndrome (SARS). The containment of this new disease, which originated in 2002 in China and led to transmission chains in six countries around the world, was achieved through sanitary and quarantine measures as 'a result of globally coordinated activities' (Thompson and Duintjer Tebbens 2011: 118).

at Imperial College London (2020), and for Quebec in particular see Lacroix (2020)). The key parameter to be estimated in these analyses is the basic reproduction number (known as R0), which relates to the contact rate among individuals.

What exactly has been driving governments' reactions to the COVID-19 pandemic is a question too early to answer on scientific grounds. It appears that many health authorities and governments were mainly concerned about mortality, tracing the disease, and possible congestion of the health-care system.[14] From an economic point of view, any project or policy put in place by public decision-makers should undergo a test of whether its benefits outweigh its costs—that is, whether it is efficient.

Economists have started to analyse the efficiency of social distancing measures in the context of COVID-19 by concentrating on the immediate, direct health costs. At an early stage in the pandemic, Thunström and colleagues (2020) relied on hypothetical scenarios of social distancing (based on a reduction of 38% of the contact rate obtained in the Caley et al. (2008) study and on a highly stylized epidemiological model) and informed conjectures on the related economic recovery to test the economic efficiency of social distancing. Sensitivity checks show that the benefits of social distancing, measured as the value of lives saved (based on VSL), outweigh the costs (in terms of a slower gross domestic product recovery) by US$1.1–7.8 trillion, and US$5.2 trillion, as compared to the baseline scenario where no reduction in the contact rate occurs. Some parameters were close to their break-even values, meaning that the benefits and costs were close to equal, such that small variations in any of them (or in any of the hypotheses underlying the calculations) may reverse the result.

Fischer (2020) proposes a more sophisticated bio-economic model that accounts for the population's age structure (which affects the mortality rate of COVID-19) and job-dependent social distancing measures (affecting, to a different degree, schoolchildren, the vulnerable, and people that can work from home or not). The analysis accounts for wage loss, childcare expenses, and the cost of the disease, as well as morbidity and mortality. Among the policies analysed, the least-cost one is keeping the vulnerable, people who can work from home, as well as all schoolchildren at home while the remainder of society practices social distancing. Fischer also calculates the private costs incurred by an additional non-essential worker who is working from home to stop doing so, as well as the external cost imposed on society as a whole. The private cost for the first worker to 'leave' the lockdown scenario is about US$350, while the external cost amounts to US$4,500. The cost tends to increase tenfold for scenarios in which more people are circulating freely.

[14] Some public health authorities and governments seem to have argued in favour of building up herd immunity, such as Sweden or the UK (Jones and Helmreich 2020).

Barla and Herrmann (2020) carry out a cost–benefit analysis of Quebec's stringent measures of shutting down non-essential economic sectors for two months (from 17 March 2020 to 17 May 2020) as compared to a softer approach of pursuing more voluntary social distancing, as in Sweden (based on a study by Britton (2020), who found a distancing of 37% for the Stockholm region). Their research is also built on a bio-economic model like Fischer's (2020) and controls for the time when a vaccine arrives. If a vaccine had been available by the end of March 2021, up to 8,900 lives could have been saved, which declines to 2,600 if no vaccine had arrived before the end of the pandemic (i.e. herd immunity would then be achieved naturally). Based on the QALY method presented above, results show that Quebec's stringent policy is efficient, leading to a net benefit of C$2.1 billion in a scenario where the vaccine would have arrived at the end of March 2021. The result is reversed, leading to a potential cost of C$2.7 billion if no vaccine had become available.[15]

The rationale for public health action in the context of pandemics is therefore often rooted in the disproportionate health externalities coming from individual behaviour, given the communicable nature of the illness at play: individuals make their decisions based on a comparison of the private costs and benefits that they expect to incur with each possible action. In doing so, they often fail to factor in the consequences that emanate from these actions and that affect those around them. This paves the way for the imposition of *some* form of social distancing measures by governments.[16] To decide which (if any) actions to take to limit the spread of infection, governments therefore should estimate and weigh the costs of inaction (in terms of direct fatalities and morbidity, but also in terms of the collateral damage that could result from the congestion of health-care systems, and so on) against the different measures they can implement (most importantly focusing on forgone gross domestic product (GDP) and a rise in unemployment associated with stay-at-home orders, social distancing measures, the shutdown of certain sectors of activity, etc.).

Hence, selecting an efficient policy response to pandemics (such as to confine or not confine, and if so, to what extent) in the short run heavily relies on whether social costs and social benefits associated with different options have been correctly accounted for.[17] The uncertainty that arises with the share of asymptomatic carriers further increases the complexity associated with policy decision-making in pandemic times, as would suggest a comparison between the mitigation of

[15] Using a VSL approach adjusted for life expectancy, their results show that the stringent policy remains efficient even in that case. Note that the benefit for both approaches is underestimated, as the authors abstract from the morbidity cost of being infected.

[16] It is important to note here that such individual actions are not necessarily driven by a lack of altruism or consideration for others, but may originate from a lack of information on the nature or extent of these consequences to others (externalities).

[17] Adda (2016) provides evidence that, historically, the measures implemented may not have proven to be cost-effective in hindsight.

COVID-19 and endeavours such as the eradication of smallpox (with only symptomatic cases) and the elimination of severe acute respiratory syndrome (SARS) (with mainly symptomatic cases).[18]

A Contaminated Economy

An early key feature of most pandemics is a lack of knowledge on ways to either immunize people or treat the virus. As such, measures limiting social interactions often present themselves as primary candidates when seeking to take immediate action to protect populations. History indeed presents numerous occurrences in which viral outbreaks have led to the adoption of such measures: from orders to close pubs in seventeenth-century England during the plague epidemic to the shutdown of schools and public meeting spaces in several nations during the 1918 influenza pandemic.[19] Such measures are even more likely to be adopted when a virus is characterized by a high rate of asymptomatic carriers, which would limit the efficiency with which more targeted mitigation strategies could be deployed.

Overall, social distancing behaviours inevitably affect the economy and labour markets. At the start of the second wave of the COVID-19 pandemic, a 4.5% decline in global GDP was projected for the year 2020, and a number of economies were expected to have not fully recovered by the end of 2021 (Organisation for Economic Co-operation and Development (OECD) 2020). This impact can be linked to the rather uniform shutdown measures implemented by governments and to individuals' behavioural changes to limit their exposure to the virus.

Rare are public authorities' decisions that have a symmetrical impact on all individuals within the targeted population. While this is true in general, a rich literature that draws on both contemporary and historical evidence suggests a substantial degree of heterogeneity in the labour market impacts of responses to health crises borne by individuals.[20] An important question thus becomes: who are the most likely to bear the costs of social distancing behaviour, either imposed or driven by individuals' own fear of the virus? As illustrated in Figure 14.1, these

[18] As of March 2021, the CDC estimated that 30% of COVID-19 cases were asymptomatic ones, with an infectiousness level at 75% that of symptomatic cases (CDC 2021a). Interestingly, smallpox was eradicated with vaccines and contact tracing as primary tools, in the absence of known treatment for the disease (CDC 2018). This eradication effort was facilitated by, among other things, the absence of non-human carriers and the existence of a vaccine offering long-term immunity, characteristics not shared by the viruses at the heart of more recent pandemics and epidemics (Nelson 1999). In parallel, the opportunity cost of non-eradication was extremely high for smallpox, given the lethality of the disease and the absence of a cure.

[19] See Arthi and Parman (2020) for a review of historical responses to pandemics, Adda (2016) for evidence from France, and Markel et al. (2007) for a more detailed account of actions taken during the 1918 influenza pandemic. Chapter 1 in this volume by Jacobson addresses the health regulations tackling historic and more recent pandemics.

[20] Chapter 9 in this volume by Smith highlights the important gender dynamics associated with pandemics on labour markets.

different economic costs may translate into health inequities in the long run—a second-order impact of the virus, looping from a health crisis to an economic one, and to another health crisis for some.

Focusing on the perhaps most stringent measures adopted in the first wave of the COVID-19 pandemic, the economic burden borne by some may be accentuated by constraints that limit their options to adapt to—and avoid the income losses associated with—measures such as social distancing, lockdowns, and shutting down economic sectors. These costs may pave the way to a new challenge in terms of population health.[21]

The Labour Market Costs of Social Distancing

The relative importance of the economic drag imposed by social distancing measures compared to the labour market impacts of the lethal nature of the virus itself varies across pandemics (Arthi and Parman 2020). Historically, the relative aggregate cost of lockdown measures would often be dwarfed by the potential economic consequences of inaction. For example, the 1918 and 2009 influenza epidemics were particularly lethal among working-age people (World Health Organization 2010).[22] Accordingly, while several social distancing measures were implemented during the 1918 pandemic, the most important shock to the economy was attributable to a reduction in the labour force and a deceleration in aggregate production caused by the direct health impacts of the influenza virus (Velde 2020). On the other hand, the recent COVID-19 crisis hit the elderly more aggressively than working-age people in most jurisdictions. Thus, except in a few sectors, the economic turmoil observed in the initial wave of this pandemic was not caused by a negative labour supply shock from mortality and morbidity. Rather, it came from the decline in consumption, which led to the closure of small businesses and the resulting temporary and permanent loss of employment, mostly attributable to shutdown measures and to individuals' behavioural changes to limit their exposure to the virus.

Official survey data also finds that almost one-fifth of the civilian non-institutional population in the United States had been unable to work at some point in the month of May 2020 because their employer had either lost some of their business or completely shut down due to the pandemic. Of the 12% who were still unable to work two months later, one-third were unemployed and one-sixth had left the labour force altogether (US Bureau of Labor Statistics 2020). In Canada,

[21] As mentioned in Goldstone (Chapter 3 in this volume), the distribution of these costs may also raise challenges in terms of political stability.

[22] Prior exposure to different strains of viruses and related immune system responses are one of the explanations put forward for this phenomenon (Gostic et al. 2016).

employment dropped by nearly 16% in the two months following stay-at-home orders and the shutdown of several sectors of the economy (Statistics Canada 2020). Lockdown measures implemented in the initial wave of the pandemic in Europe were estimated to be responsible for up to 5% of labour force participants losing their job permanently, and for another 23% becoming temporarily unemployed (Eurofound 2020).

The sectors hardest hit through the first wave of the COVID-19 pandemic were those most likely to be directly impacted by shutdown measures and by voluntary or mandatory reduction in social contacts. Reports looking at real-time microdata from US consumers and firms highlight such dynamics. Between March and May of 2020, social distancing and shutdowns had an important impact on consumer spending at bricks-and-mortar establishments and smaller businesses, regardless of local demographic or geographic characteristics. Alexander and Karger (2020) estimate a *causal* impact of governments' stay-at-home orders corresponding to a 19% reduction in smaller businesses' revenues, or half the total loss of income observed for those firms during the period. Looking at foot traffic, Goolsbee and Syverson (2020) find important impacts of measures taken to limit contagion in terms of reduction of activity in physical businesses, which they mostly attribute to voluntary social distancing behaviours.

One phenomenon that exacerbates not only health implications but also economic symptoms of modern-day pandemics is globalization. Of course, individuals' geographic mobility facilitates viral spreads.[23] The routes of propagation of historical epidemics would often coincide with trade routes (Alfani and Murphy 2017; Adda 2016). In addition, the integration of economies, starting with global supply chains, plays an important role in the rapid cross-border spread of the economic consequences associated with governments' and individuals' responses to viral outbreaks. Confinement in one nation will influence labour markets and production processes in several others, in addition to the direct economic impact of the public health measures taken locally. History therefore doesn't always offer a complete portrait of the extent to which modern-day pandemics can contaminate economies and individuals' economic outcomes. The availability of e-commerce can, of course, attenuate the impact of lockdowns or social distancing measures on consumer spending and economic activity. However, dematerialized commerce can concentrate power in companies with global distribution networks, which are

[23] Outbreaks of other infectious diseases in the twenty-first century could be contained at a much smaller geographic scale. Among these, the WHO has considered SARS as the 'first severe and readily transmissible new disease to emerge in the 21st century [showing] a clear capacity to spread along the routes of international air travel'. Originating in southern China in 2002, the disease found its way via Hong Kong to Toronto, Canada, in early 2003, causing more than 40 deaths. Other examples are the Ebola virus, known for its outbreak in West Africa between 2014 and 2016, as well as Middle East respiratory syndrome (MERS), which originated in 2012 on the Arabian Peninsula, but also caused an outbreak in South Korea in 2015. Note that these diseases can only be considered eliminated, and not eradicated, as the pathogen still may exist in some non-human reservoir.

also less likely to have a local labour force presence. While potentially mitigating some economic impacts of confinement, it might therefore enhance the heterogeneity in the distribution of costs among individual economic players, both firms and workers.

An Unequal Burden: Who Can Adjust, and How?

Lack of detailed or comprehensive data has, for most of the twentieth century, limited economists' and other scientists' capacity to estimate the extent and the distribution of health and economic impacts from global waves of infectious diseases. Importantly, this has affected their capacity to assess the impact of social distancing measures on these distributions. However, given recent advances in data collection methods and computing capacity, the COVID-19 pandemic offers a unique opportunity to do so. Moreover, constant flows of information coming from administrative or private sources make it possible for changes in health and socio-economic status, as well as changes in behaviour, to be observed in real time. These data flows are valuable to track mechanisms and anticipate the long-run impacts of pandemics on individuals.

A first observation stemming from such data is that vulnerable groups tend to be disproportionately hit by the virus.[24] Contagion and mortality rates, as in most other pandemics, have been significantly worse among visible minorities and low-income individuals in the United States (CDC 2020), the UK (White and Nafilyan 2020), Canada (Toronto Public Health 2020), Sweden (Drefahl et al. 2020), and Belgium (Decoster et al. 2020), to name just a few. An important income gradient also characterizes early COVID-19 statistics, as is true with most global influenza outbreaks.[25]

While lockdown-type measures can reduce such pandemic-specific health inequities by limiting the rate of contamination, they can also have a disproportionate economic impact on more vulnerable individuals. Just as it affects morbidity risks, occupational segregation is associated with variations in the individual economic burden imposed by widespread social distancing. First, the direct impact of shutting down certain economic sectors, as was done by numerous governments in the control and mitigation phase of COVID-19, leads to a mechanical increase in unemployment concentrated in sectors often characterized by a higher degree of precarity and lower wages, like the services or tourism industries. Baylis and colleagues (forthcoming) found that these direct impacts of shutdown measures during the first wave of the COVID-19 pandemic were an important factor in a

[24] The impact of pandemics on gender inequality and vulnerability of women is addressed in Chapter 9 in this volume by Smith.
[25] See, e.g. Hadler et al. (2016) for recent epidemics in the United States or Mamelund (2006) for a discussion relating to the 1918 Spanish flu pandemic in Norway.

pandemic-induced gender gap in the labour market in Canada. They document that work-from-home arrangements were the least likely to be implemented in occupations and industries based on interactions and contact with the public, in which women and low-income individuals are overrepresented. These groups thus disproportionately suffer from layoffs as governments move forward with shutdown or stay-at-home orders, or as individuals voluntarily choose to reduce their contacts.

Such a relationship between the economic burden of the pandemic and the high-contact and low-flexibility nature of certain occupations is found in a variety of contexts (see, e.g. Leibovici et al. (2020) and Mongey et al. (2020) for the United States; Joyce and Xu [2020] for the UK; and Adams-Prassl et al. (2020) for Germany, the UK, and the United States).[26] Further, the family and living arrangements of an important proportion of women and lower-income people in the context of a lockdown are often barriers to working from home. Finally, even after the relaxing of social distancing rules and the reopening of some sectors of the economy, these workers are more likely to experience a slower job recovery, partially because of weaker links with their former employers.[27] Zabai (2020) also highlights a negative relationship between COVID-19-induced unemployment and households' initial degree of financial resilience. Long-term inequities could thus stem from short-term imbalances in the pandemic risks and in the costs of distancing borne by individuals.

Overall, individuals who are most likely to be able to avoid the private economic costs of imposed or generalized social distancing measures are often those who are the most likely to be able to adjust their behaviour to avoid contagion risks. As this greater capacity to avoid pandemic risk is often derived from their lower level of ex-ante economic vulnerability, this evidence suggests that pandemics exacerbate socio-economic inequalities[28] in a way that could pose a new wave of health consequences for those at the bottom of the income distribution.

Economic Vulnerability, Relative Income, and Health

Low income is generally found to be a strong predictor of poor health outcomes (Marmot and Wilkinson 2005; Commission on Social Determinants of

[26] Adams-Prassl et al. (2020) also present evidence that factors beyond experience, the type of industries or occupation, and the proportion of tasks that individuals can achieve from their home environment seem to be a driving part of the gap in the economic impact of confinement measures between genders in certain jurisdictions (United States, UK). They suggest that part of the remaining difference may be driven by the predominant role of women in caring for children (especially in the case of school and day-care closures).

[27] The same sectors are also more likely to suffer from reductions in discretionary savings stemming from an increase in uncertainty and a reduction in income at the global level.

[28] See, e.g. Papageorge et al. (2020).

Health 2008). Although reverse causality[29] is a challenge when trying to interpret this association, growing evidence in economics suggests that a causal channel from income to health may be at play,[30] even where health-care coverage is offered universally. Such findings offer interesting insights on the potential long-term health consequences that can arise from the impact of social distancing on labour market outcomes and income distributions.

A key channel through which low income could harm individuals' health, the allostatic load, finds its roots far beyond economics (McEwen and Stellar 1993). This phenomenon is described as a physical 'wear and tear' experienced by individuals and caused by important, repeated, or lasting stress. Exposed to important economic challenges over a certain period of time, individuals could experience physiological reactions that can weaken their cardiovascular, endocrine, and immune systems, leaving them more vulnerable to several diseases and health problems (Schneiderman et al. 2005).[31] In addition to these responses to economic stress, changes in individuals' behaviour as they experience income and employment losses could also have longer-run health impacts. Work by economists looking at exogenous job losses or exogenous shocks to people's incomes provides causal evidence in line with these mechanisms (see, e.g. Adda and Fawaz 2020; Browning and Heinesen 2012) and with a channel linked to mental health also documented extensively in psychology.

But beyond the relationship between one's own income and health, an additional phenomenon increases the potential health consequences of the skewed distribution of the economic costs associated with actions taken to contain a pandemic. Experimental and clinical studies have provided evidence that one's position on the socio-economic ladder—or one's social status—can have an impact on physical and mental health trajectories.[32] These findings echo predictions stemming from the relative income hypothesis (Veblen 1899; Duesenberry 1949), which suggests that an individual's income relative to others' might affect their well-being. Economics also provides some evidence that relative income matters for individuals' health and well-being (Marmot 2004; Luttmer 2005; Daly and Wilson 2009; Daly et al. 2013).[33]

[29] Income may influence people's health, but their health also influences their earning capacity and their income.

[30] Lleras-Muney (2018) presents a review of important work investigating this question.

[31] Schneiderman et al. (2005) consider exposure to a stressor to be persistent exposure that lasts over a month. Others employ more stringent thresholds. Overall, most periods of exposure are coherent with the lasting economic impacts of pandemics on vulnerable individuals.

[32] For example, Marmot (1999) found changes in high-density lipoprotein (HDL) cholesterol levels for British civil servants who experience a change in their status within the hierarchy. Important work on this question has also been conducted on animal models (Sapolsky 1993, 2004; Snyder-Mackler et al. 2016), although their bearings on human populations are less clear.

[33] Some studies, however, yield equivocal conclusions. For example, Ifcher et al. (2018) suggest that the association between one's own well-being and relative income depends on the level of geography over which the reference group is defined.

Existing evidence on the health impacts of changes to absolute and relative incomes is helpful to understand how pandemics may impose long-term health costs beyond the direct impact of the virus at its origins. For example, using high-frequency private-sector data for the United States, Chetty and colleagues (2020) show that the negative impact of social distancing measures on employment during the first wave of the COVID-19 pandemic was concentrated among low-income workers in affluent areas. This finding differs from the patterns observed in most recessions, where job losses are generally concentrated among low-income workers living in low-income areas. The distribution of economic costs stemming from social distancing in response to COVID-19 is therefore likely to generate more important changes in the relative income of those who suffer from these costs. Such patterns could translate into additional negative health consequences for the most vulnerable, potentially generating a new health crisis for this group.[34] Understanding the full health impacts of pandemics, therefore, implies considering the dynamic process between health and income and the amplifying role of inequality in this loop.

Conclusion

From health risks to job losses and economic struggles, pandemics come with an array of costs that few individuals and communities can avoid. This chapter has identified important externalities associated with individual behaviours in the context of a serious threat of viral contagion and which command that public authorities take action to reconcile the overall costs and benefits of social interactions. Individuals themselves may also adjust some of their behaviours to limit their exposure to the virus, beyond what authorities suggest. While limiting the mortality and morbidity toll of a pandemic, these actions will lead to additional costs, importantly economic costs, which are often distributed in a way that exacerbates initial inequities within a society. This chapter has concentrated on the pandemic-disrupted labour market as a major driving mechanism that leads to additional indirect costs at the individual level. Our analysis clearly shows explains how such dynamics, from health threats to economic woes, can circle back to long-run health concerns that go beyond the initial viral threat.

The labour market is clearly not the only possible driving mechanism that merits investigation: the stock market and housing market can also be heavily impacted by pandemics, affecting income (and hence health outcomes, as our argument goes) in the short and long run. Access to schooling and higher education have

[34] Long-term consequences of pandemics can come from a variety of other causes that go beyond the scope of this chapter. For example, the fetal origins hypothesis suggests that cohorts of children *in utero* during the COVID-19 pandemic may do worse in terms of health and economic outcomes without adequate compensatory measures (Almond and Currie 2011).

become more complicated for those who are less well off, impacting their income in the long run. Interestingly, higher mortality among the rich elderly should lead to more inheritance and further foster the initial endowment gap in society.

Our assessment of the private and social costs of the pandemic, in the short and long run, raises questions about the portfolio of economic policies governmental authorities use during a pandemic and what criteria should be applied to navigate the subsequent health crises. We have argued that cost–benefit analysis of sanitary measures provides important information to the government in the short run; indeed, 'the cure must not be worse than the problem itself'; however, from an economic point of view, not only private but all social benefits and costs of the cure must be accounted for correctly.

Furthermore, our assessment has demonstrated that even when they are efficient from a society's perspective, social distancing policies come with indirect effects on income and health that can be tackled better with a richer portfolio of redistributional policies.

In the long run, a healthy economy is inseparable from a healthy population. In a context of new infectious diseases, like COVID-19, this assertion holds even for the world population. Increased population health obtained through social distancing policies and vaccination accomplishments in one country can easily be undone when new, more aggressive variants surface somewhere on the planet and start travelling. Experts and scientists have started to analyse under which circumstances the COVID-19 pandemic may transition to an endemic state, that is, a situation in which the disease may only have sporadic outbreaks, like other pandemics did in the past (Lavine et al. 2021).

What we can learn from the mitigation and eradication of other infectious diseases, like tuberculosis and smallpox, respectively, is that it is only an international, collective effort that may lead the way. Currently, available vaccines for COVID-19 do not necessarily prevent people from communicating the disease. This, combined with a lack of production capacity at the global scale and evolving variants, leaves an open question of whether highly contagious diseases like COVID-19 may be eradicated in the near future. More scientific insight is necessary in order to mitigate such pandemics in the long run. Whether such scientific insight finds the support of a majority of countries, and whether their citizens adhere to the proposed health policies, including continuous vaccination programmes, is a question several social sciences can help to answer.

References

Adams-Prassl, Abigail, Teodora Boneva, Marta Golin, and Christopher Rauh. 2020. 'Inequality in the Impact of the Coronavirus Shock: Evidence from Real Time Surveys'. IZA Institute of Labor Economics Discussion Paper No. 13183.

Adda, Jerome. 2016. 'Economic Activity and the Spread of Viral Diseases: Evidence from High Frequency Data'. *Quarterly Journal of Economics 131* (2): pp. 891–941.

Adda, Jerome, and Yarine Fawaz. 2020. 'The Health Toll of Import Competition'. *The Economic Journal* 130(630): pp. 1501–1540.

Ahituv, Avner, V. Joseph Hotz, and Thomas Philipson. 1996. 'The Responsiveness of the Demand for Condoms to the Local Prevalance of AIDS'. *Journal of Human Resources 31* (4): pp. 869–98.

Alexander, Diane, and Ezra Karger. 2020. 'Do Stay-at-Home Orders Cause People to Stay at Home? Effects of Stay-at-Home Orders on Consumer Behavior'. Federal Reserve Bank of Chicago Working Paper No. 2020–12.

Alfani, Guido, and Tommy E. Murphy. 2017. 'Plague and Lethal Epidemics in the Pre-Industrial World'. *Journal of Economic History 77* (1): 314–43.

Almond, Douglas, and Janet Currie. 2011. 'Killing Me Softly: The Fetal Origins Hypothesis'. *Journal of Economic Perspective 25* (3): pp. 153–72.

Arthi, Vellore, and John Parman. 2020. 'Disease, Downturns, and Wellbeing: Economic History and the Long-Run Impacts of COVID-19'. *Explorations in Economic History* 79: 101381.

Auld, M Christopher. 2003. 'Choices, Beliefs, and Infectious Disease Dynamics'. *Journal of Health Economics 22* (3): pp. 361–77.

Barla, Philippe, and Markus Herrmann. 2020. 'COVID-19: Fallait-il mettre sur pause l'économie québécoise? Une analyse avantage-coûts'. CREATE Working Paper Series, No. 2020–21.

Bauch, Chris T, and Alison P. Galvani. 2013. 'Social Factors in Epidemiology'. *Science 342* (6154): pp. 47–9.

Baylis, Patrick, Pierre-Loup Beauregard, Marie Connolly, et al. Forthcoming. 'The Distribution of COVID-19 Related Risks'. *Canadian Journal of Economics.*

Boulier, Bryan, Datta Tejwant S., and Robert Goldfarb. 2007. 'Vaccination Externalities'. *B.E. Journal of Economic Analysis & Policy 7* (1): 1–27.

Britton, Tom. 2020. 'Basic Estimation-Prediction Techniques for COVID-19, and a Prediction for Stockholm'. *MedRxiv*. 14 May. https://www.medrxiv.org/content/early/2020/05/14/2020.04.15.20066050.

Browning, Martin, and Eskil Heinesen. 2012. 'Effect of Job Loss Due to Plant Closure on Mortality and Hospitalization'. *Journal of Health Economics 31* (4): pp. 599–616.

Caley, Peter, David J. Philp, and Kevin McCracken. 2008. 'Quantifying Social Distancing Arising from Pandemic Influenza'. *Journal of the Royal Society, Interface 5* (23): pp. 631–9.

CDC. 2018. 'Prevention and Treatment—Smallpox'. https://www.cdc.gov/smallpox/prevention-treatment/index.html.

CDC. 2020. 'COVID-19 Hospitalization and Death by Race/Ethnicity'. Updated 9 September 2021. https://www.cdc.gov/coronavirus/2019-ncov/covid-data/investigations-discovery/hospitalization-death-by-race-ethnicity.html.

CDC. 2021a. 'COVID-19 Pandemic Planning Scenarios'. Updated 19 March 221. https://www.cdc.gov/coronavirus/2019-ncov/hcp/planning-scenarios.html.

CDC. 2021b. 'Polio Disease and Poliovirus'. https://www.cdc.gov/cpr/polioviruscontainment/diseaseandvirus.htm.

Chetty, Raj, John N. Friedman, Nathaniel Hendren, Michael Stepner, and Opportunity Insight Team. 2020. 'How Did COVID-19 and Stabilization Policies Affect Spending and Employment? A New Real-Time Economic Tracker Based on Private Sector Data'. National Bureau of Economic Research Working Paper No. 27431.

Commission on Social Determinants of Health. 2008. *Closing the Gap in a Generation: Health Equity through Action on the Social Determinants of Health*. Geneva: World Health Organization.

Daly, Mary, and Daniel J. Wilson. 2009. 'Happiness, Unhappiness, and Suicide: An Empirical Assessment'. *Journal of the European Economic Association 7* (2–3): pp. 539–49.

Daly, Mary, Daniel J. Wilson, and Norman J. Johnson. 2013. 'Relative Status and Well-Being: Evidence from US Suicide Deaths'. *Review of Economics and Statistics 95* (5): pp. 1480–500.

Dave, Dhaval., Drew McNichols, and Joseph J. Sabia. 2021. 'The Contagion Externality of a Superspreading Event: The Sturgis Motorcycle Rally and COVID-19'. *Southern Economic Journal* 87(3): pp. 769–807.

Decoster, André, Thomas Minten, and Johannes Spinnewijn. 2020. 'The Income Gradient in Mortality during the Covid-19 Crisis: Evidence from Belgium'. *Covid Economics 50*: pp. 74–105.

Department of Transportation (DOT). 2016. 'Revised Department Guidance 2016: Treatment of the Value of Preventing Fatalities and Injuries in Preparing Economic Analyses'. https://www7.transportation.gov/office-policy/transportation-policy/revised-departmental-guidance-on-valuation-of-a-statistical-life-in-economic-analysis.

Drefahl, Sven, Matthew Wallace, Eleonora Mussino, et al. 2020. 'Socio-Demographic Risk Factors of COVID-19 Deaths in Sweden: A Nationwide Register Study'. Stockholm Research Reports in Demography.

Duesenberry, James S. 1949. *Income, Saving, and the Theory of Consumer Behavior*. Cambridge, MA: Harvard University Press.

Eurofound. 2020. 'Living, Working and COVID-19: First Findings—April 2020'. Technical report, Luxembourg. Updated 6 November 2020. https://www.eurofound.europa.eu/publications/report/2020/living-working-and-covid-19.

Fenichel, Eli P. 2013. 'Economic Considerations for Social Distancing and Behavioral Based Policies during an Epidemic'. *Journal of Health Economics 32*: pp. 440–51.

Fischer, Carolyn. 2020. 'Six Degrees of Separation for Covid-19: The External Costs and Benefits of Extended Distancing for Different Social Groups'. *Covid Economics 25*: pp. 1–22.

Gersovitz, Mark, and Jeffrey S. Hammer. 2003. 'The Economical Control of Infectious Diseases'. *Economic Journal 114* (492): pp. 1–27.

Goolsbee, Austan, and Chad Syverson. 2020. 'Fear, Lockdown, and Diversion: Comparing Drivers of Pandemic Economic Decline 2020'. Becker Friedman Institute, University of Chicago Working Paper No. 2020–80. Chicago, IL: University of Chicago.

Gostic, Katelyn M., Monique Ambrose, Michael Worobey, and James O. Lloyd-Smith. 2016. 'Potent Protection against H5N1 and H7N9 Influenza via Childhood Hemagglutinin Imprinting'. *Science 354* (6313): pp. 722–6.

Griffiths, Elizabeth A., and Naga Vadlamudi. 2016. 'CADTH's $50,000 Cost-Effectiveness Threshold: Fact or Fiction?' *Value in Health 19*: A488–9.

Hadler, James L., Kimberly Yousey-Hindes, Alejandro Perez, et al. 2016. 'Influenza-Related Hospitalizations and Poverty Levels—United States, 2010–2012'. Technical Report 05, CDC. 12 February. https://www.cdc.gov/mmwr/volumes/65/wr/mm6505a1.htm.

Ifcher, John, Homa Zarghamee, and Carol Lee Graham. 2018. 'Local Neighbors as Positives, Regional Neighbors as Negatives: Competing Channels in the Relationship between Others' Income, Health, and Happiness'. *Journal of Health Economics 57*: 263–76.

Imperial College London. 2020. 'Report 13—Estimating the Number of Infections and the Impact of Non-Pharmaceutical Interventions on COVID-19 in 11 European Countries'. 6 August. https://www.imperial.ac.uk/mrc-global-infectious-disease-analysis/covid-19/report-13-europe-npi-impact.

Jentsch, Peter C., Madhur Anand, and Chris T. Bauch. 2021. 'Prioritising COVID-19 Vaccination in Changing Social and Epidemiological Landscapes: A Mathematical Modelling Study'. *The Lancet Infectious Diseases 21* (8): pp. 1097–1106.

Jones, David, and Stefan Helmreich. 2020. 'A History of Herd Immunity'. *The Lancet 396* (10254): pp. 810–11.

Joyce, Robert, and Xiaowei Xu. 2020. 'Sector Shutdowns during the Coronavirus Crisis: Which Workers Are Most Exposed?' Institute for Fiscal Studies Briefing Note BN278.

Kim, Tae Hyong, Jennie Johnstone, and Mark Loeb. 2011. 'Vaccine Herd Effect'. *Scandinavian Journal of Infectious Diseases 43* (9), 683–9.

Kniesner, Thomas J., and Ryan Sullivan. 2020. 'The Forgotten Numbers: A Closer Look at COVID-19 Non-Fatal Valuations'. *SSRN* 28 August. https://ssrn.com/abstract=3680348.

Kniesner, Thomas J., and W. Kip Viscusi. 2019. 'The Value of a Statistical Life'. In *Oxford Research Encyclopedia of Economics and Finance*. doi:10.1093/acrefore/9780190625979.013.138.

Lacroix, Guy. 2020. 'Les mesures de confinement sont-elles efficaces?' *CIRANO*, Perspectives/insights series, no 2020PE-11. https://cirano.qc.ca/fr/sommaires/2020PE-11.

Lavine, Jennie S., Ottar N. Bjornstad, and Rustom Anita. 2021. 'Immunological Characteristics Govern the Transition of COVID-19 to Endemicity'. *Science 371* (6530): 741–5.

Lee, Bruce Y. 2020. 'Coronavirus Medical Costs Could Soar into Hundreds of Billions as More Americans Become Infected'. *The Conversation*, 4 May. https://theconversation.com/coronavirus-medical-costs-could-soar-into-hundreds-of-billions-as-more-americans-become-infected-137479.

Leibovici, Fernando, Ana Maria Santacreu, and Matthew Famiglietti. 2020. 'Social Distancing and Contact-Intensive Occupations'. Federal Reserve Bank of St Louis technical report. 24 March. https://www.stlouisfed.org/on-the-economy/2020/march/social-distancing-contact-intensive-occupations.

Lleras-Muney, Adriana. 2018. 'Mind the Gap: A Review of the Health Gap'. *Journal of Economic Literature 56* (3): pp. 1080–111.

Luttmer, Erzo F. P. 2005. 'Neighbors as Negatives: Relative Earnings and Well-Being'. *Quarterly Journal of Economics 102* (3): pp. 963–1002.

Mamelund, Svenn-Erik. 2006. 'A Socially Neutral Disease? Individual Social Class, Household Wealth and Mortality from Spanish Influenza in Two Socially Contrasting Parishes in Kristiania 1918–19'. *Social Science and Medicine 62* (4): pp. 923–40.

Markel, Howard, Harvey B. Lipman, J. Alexander Navarro, et al. 2007. 'Nonpharmaceutical Interventions Implemented by U.S. Cities during the 1918–1919 Influenza Pandemic'. *JAMA 298* (6): 644–54.

Marmot, Michael. 1999. 'Multi-Level Approaches to Understanding Social Determinants'. In *Social Epidemiology*, edited by L. Berkman and I. Kawachi, pp. 349–367. Oxford: Oxford University Press.

Marmot, Michael. 2004. *The Status Syndrome: How Social Standing Affects Our Health and Longevity*. New York: Times Books.

Marmot, Michael., and Richard Wilkinson. 2005. *Social Determinants of Health*. Oxford: Oxford University Press.

McEwen, Bruce S., and Eliot Stellar. 1993. 'Stress and the Individual: Mechanisms Leading to Disease'. *Archives of Internal Medicine 153* (18): pp. 2093–101.

Mei, Shan, Rirck Quax, David van de Vijver, et al. 2011. 'Increasing Risk Behaviour Can Outweigh the Benefits of Antiretroviral Drug Treatment on the HIV Incidence among Men-Having-Sex-with-Men in Amsterdam'. *BMC Infectious Diseases* 11 (118).

Ministère des Transports du Québec. 2016. 'Guide de l'analyse avantages-coûts des projets publics en transport routier—paramètres (valeurs de 2015)'. https://www.transports.gouv.qc.ca/fr/entreprises-partenaires/entreprises-reseaux-routier/guides-formulaires/documents-gestionprojetsroutiers/guide-avantages-couts-projets-publics.pdf.

Mongey, Simon, Laura Pilossoph, and Alex Weinberg. 2020. 'Which Workers Bear the Burden of Social Distancing Policies?' National Bureau of Economic Research Working Paper No. 27085.

Nelson, Ann Marie. 1999. 'The Cost of Disease Eradication: Smallpox and Bovine Tuberculosis'. *Annal New York Academy of Science 894*: pp. 83–91.

Organisation for Economic Co-operation and Development (OECD). 2020. 'OECD Economic Outlook, Interim Report September 2020'. 16 September. https://www.oecd-ilibrary.org/economics/oecd-economic-outlook/volume-2020/issue-1_34ffc900-en.

Papageorge, Nicholas W., Matthew V. Zahn, Michèle Belot, et al. 2020. 'Socio-Demographic Factors Associated with Self-Protecting Behavior during the COVID-19 Pandemic'. National Bureau of Economic Research Working Paper No. 27378.

Philipson, Tomas 2000. 'Economic Epidemiology and Infectious Diseases'. In *Handbook of Health Economics*, Vol. 1, part B, edited by Antory Culyer and Joseph Newhouse, pp. 1761–99. London: Elsevier.

Pindyck, Robert S. 2020. 'COVID-19 and the Welfare Effects of Reducing Contagion'. National Bureau of Economic Research Working Paper No. 27378.

Sapolsky, Robert M. 1993. 'Endocrinology Alfresco: Psychoendocrine Studies of Wild Baboons'. *Recent Progress in Hormone Research 48*: pp. 437–68.

Sapolsky, Robert M. 2004. *Why Zebras Don't Get Ulcers: The Acclaimed Guide to Stress, Stress-Related Disorders and Coping*. New York: Henry Holt and Company.

Schneiderman, Neil, Gail Ironson, and Scott D. Siegel. 2005. 'Stress and Health: Psychological, Behavioural and Biological Determinants'. *Annual Review of Clinical Psychology 1*: pp. 607–28.

Snyder-Mackler, Noah, Joaquin Sanz, Jordan Kohn, et al. 2016. 'Social Status Alters Immune Regulation and Response to Infection in Macaques'. *Science 354* (6315): 1041–45.

Statistics Canada. 2020. 'Labour Force Survey, July 2020'. *The Daily*, 7 August. https://www150.statcan.gc.ca/n1/daily-quotidien/200807/dq200807a-eng.htm.

Thompson, Kimberly M., and Radboud J. Duintjer Tebbens. 2011. 'Economic Evaluation of the Benefits and Costs of Disease Elimination and Eradication Initiatives'.

In *Disease Eradication in the 21st Century: Implications for Global Health*, edited by Stephen L. Cochi and Walter R. Dowdle, pp. 115–30. Series Strüngmann forum reports. Cambridge, CA: MIT Press.

Thunström, Linda, Stephen C. Newbold, David Finnoff, Madison Ashworth, and Jason F. Shogren. 2020. 'The Benefits and Costs of Using Social Distancing to Flatten the Curve for COVID-19'. *Journal of Benefit-Cost Analysis 11* (2): pp. 179–95.

Toronto Public Health. 2020. 'COVID-19 Infection in Toronto: Ethno-Racial Identity and Income'. Updated 1 June 2021. https://www.toronto.ca/home/covid-19/covid-19-latest-city-of-toronto-news/covid-19-status-of-cases-in-toronto.

US Bureau of Labor Statistics. 2020. 'Labour Force Statistics from the Current Population Survey: Supplemental Data Measuring the Effects of the Coronavirus (Covid-19) Pandemic on the Labor Market'. Technical report. https://www.bls.gov/cps/effects-of-the-coronavirus-covid-19-pandemic.htm#data.

Vaillancourt, Francois. 2020. 'COVID-19 and the Health Policy Recession: Whatever It Takes, Grandma, or the Economy, or What Makes Sense?' *CIRANO*, Perspectives/insights series, No. 2020PE-01. 17 April. https://cirano.qc.ca/files/publications/2020PE-01.pdf.

Velde, Francois. 2020. 'What Happened to the U.S. Economy during the 1918 Influenza Pandemic? A View through High-Frequency Data'. Federal Reserve Bank of Chicago Working Paper No. 2020–11.

Veblen, Thorstein. 1899. *The Theory of the Leisure Class*. New York: MacMillan.

White, Chris, and Vahe Nafilyan. 2020. 'Coronavirus (COVID-19) Related Deaths by Ethnic Group, England and Wales: 2 March 2020 to 10 April 2020'. London: Office for National Statistics.

Wise, Toby, Tomislav D. Zbozinek, Giorgia Michelini, Cindy C. Hagan, and Dean Mobbs. 2020. 'Changes in Risk Perception and Self-Reported Protective Behaviour during the First Week of the COVID-19 Pandemic in the United States'. *Royal Society Open Science 7*: 200742.

World Health Organization (WHO). 2010. 'Emergency Preparedness Response: What Is a Pandemic?' Technical report. https://www.who.int/csr/disease/swineflu/frequently_asked_questions/pandemic/en.

Zabai, Anna. 2020. 'How Are Household Finances Holding Up against the Covid-19 Shock?' Bank for International Settlements Bulletin 22.

15

COVID-19

A Wake-Up Call for Sustainable Food Systems

*Geneviève Parent**

The COVID-19 pandemic, which continues to spread globally as we write this chapter, is having major negative impacts on food security and nutrition all over the world. This pandemic can certainly be described as an external shock on food systems that renders difficult, or even impossible, equitable access to healthy food (Food and Agriculture Organization (FAO) et al. 2020; High Level Panel of Experts (HLPE) 2020a).

As dramatic as this pandemic is for humanity, its importance should not overshadow the fact that other pandemics have had, and will have, similar impacts on food systems. Furthermore, other kinds of external shocks can also limit or prevent access to healthy food, such as climate change, locust invasions, storms, and financial crises (FAO et al. 2017; HLPE 2020a). For instance, above and beyond the problem of the financialization of markets in staple foods, the 2008 financial crisis revealed the risks associated with entrusting national food security to the global food system. The food riots that occurred clearly exposed the problems encountered by countries that rely primarily on the importation of staple foods to feed their citizens to the detriment of developing their own agriculture. For the first time, middle-class households in Egypt, Algeria, Senegal, Cameroon, and Burkina Faso, which do not generally experience food insecurity, found it difficult to provide for themselves and their families because they were no longer able to rely on low-cost food imports (Janin 2009).

However, unlike the 2008 financial crisis, the COVID-19 pandemic affected all countries regardless of their level of economic development, which is bringing the international community together around the idea of a necessary reform to food systems through the United Nations' Food Systems Summit held in 2021. The willingness expressed by several governments for achieving greater food self-sufficiency because of the pandemic also underlines the need for such a transformation.

* The author would like to thank Josiane Jean, research professional at the Legal Research Chair in Food Diversity and Security.

Geneviève Parent, *COVID-19.* In: *A Multidisciplinary Approach to Pandemics.*
Edited by Philippe Bourbeau, Jean-Michel Marcoux, and Brooke A. Ackerly, Oxford University Press.
 DOI: 10.1093/oso/9780192897855.003.0016

Indeed, as stated on several occasions by the UN Secretary General António Guterres, one of the main challenges facing humanity is to build sustainable food systems that are resilient to any shock. This will ensure food security and nutrition for all in such a way that the economic, social, and environmental bases needed to generate the food security and nutrition of future generations are not compromised (HLPE 2014).

Food system resilience relates to a combination of three capacities: adaptative, absorptive, and transformative (FAO et al. 2017). These capacities determine how and to what extent individuals, households, communities, and states are able to cope with and adapt to external shocks such as pandemics.

This chapter is structured to address the two sets of ethical imperatives presented in the introduction of this book. We highlight the shortcomings of the current food system, addressing its lack of resilience and sustainability as well as the vulnerabilities and the injustice associated with these flaws, while also considering the reform of food systems as one of the ways to be better prepared for future pandemics (see the Introduction to this volume by Ackerly et al.).

We argue that the reflection launched by United Nations' Food Systems Summit in 2021 is an opportunity to move beyond the traditional rhetoric opposing the global food system and more territorialized food systems to trigger an effective reform of all food systems so that they become powerful drivers for planetary health[1] in accordance with the UN Sustainable Development Goals set up in 2015.

The Impacts of Pandemics on Food Systems: Learning from COVID-19

There are many different food systems. Some of them are interconnected and their sum constitutes the 'global food system' (HLPE 2014). A food system can be defined as the way in which people organize themselves, in space and time, to obtain and consume their food (Malassis 1979). For the HLPE, 'a food system gathers all the elements (environment, people, inputs, processes, infrastructures, institutions, etc.) and activities that relate to the production, processing, distribution, preparation and consumption of food, and the output of these activities, including socio-economic and environmental outcomes' (HLPE 2014, 2017).

As the coronavirus (COVID-19) pandemic continues to spread around the world, scientists from different fields are still trying to understand the complex impacts of pandemics on food security and nutrition. Moreover, according to international organizations such as the World Health Organization (WHO), the

[1] 'Planetary health' is described as 'the achievement of the highest attainable standard of health, wellbeing, and equity worldwide through judicious attention to the human systems—political, economic, and social—that shape the future of humanity and the Earth's natural systems that define the safe environmental limits within which humanity can flourish' (Whitmee et al. 2015).

World Food Programme (WFP), and the FAO, the worst effects will be long lasting (HLPE 2020b; WFP 2020). However, research derived from a variety of disciplines identifies some of the pandemic's negative effects on food systems. We are already able to assert that COVID-19 (the virus on its own, but also the set of measures put in place to limit its spread) and the economic slowdown that it has generated have set in motion a series of reactions impacting almost all elements of the food system and all stakeholders, from agricultural producers to consumers (HLPE 2020b; Petetin 2020).

It is not possible or necessary in the context of this chapter to present all those impacts. However, from the following non-exhaustive list we can conclude that the global food system and the current individual food systems in general are not resilient enough. They have shown little capacity to adapt and avoid disruption and difficulty to accommodate change. In short, they are not capable of providing sufficient, adequate, and accessible food to all, over time, while coping with unpredictable disruptions (Hendrickson 2015; HLPE 2020a; Petetin 2020).

Major Disruption in the Global Food Supply Chain

The movement of food through international trade is especially affected by the COVID-19 pandemic, as well as by the means to limit its spread (HLPE 2020b; Petetin 2020). The global supply chain is long, involved, depends on many actors from farm to fork, and is driven by a small number of multinationals (Cheriet and Lubello 2017; Hendrickson 2015). It works on a 'just-in-time' model, where supply varies according to the standard of demand (e.g. holidays, seasons, events; Hobbs 2020; Petetin 2020). The current global food system works in a way that the actors in the chain must coordinate among themselves and be efficient because when one actor is disturbed, all actors are equally affected. Therefore, there can be long ramifications to disruptions or delays (Gaupp 2020; International Panel of Experts on Sustainable Food Systems (IPES–Food) 2020; Petetin 2020).

The global supply chain is divided into two main parts: retail consumption (grocery stores) and food-service markets. The two lines operate differently. One requires predetermined packaging and quantities based on expected consumer demand, and the other provides large quantities in barrels or tank trucks planned for the needs of different institutions. Many difficulties have been encountered throughout both parts of the global chain due to the COVID-19 pandemic, such as difficulty in adapting to demand disruptions caused both shortages in the retail market (e.g. empty supermarket shelves) and food losses in large-scale production (Barrett 2020).

Furthermore, the COVID-19 pandemic has led many countries to impose export restrictions that have had damaging effects on import-dependent countries, such as a shortage of food and an increase in the prices of food (HLPE

2020b; IPES-Food 2020). Some export-dependent countries have lost a significant amount of perishable food due to lockdowns (HLPE 2020a).

Production systems and farmers have been particularly affected by the crisis. The pandemic has highlighted the importance of farmers' contributions to food systems and their damaging dependence on other actors to ensure the delivery of fresh products to consumers (Petetin 2020). The pandemic has also shown the high value of migrant farmworkers to the economy and the food security of many developed countries (HLPE 2020b; Larue 2020). As a result of movement restrictions, many crops were lost because they were not harvested, and farmers all over the world have been impacted. Many of these farmworkers were forced to choose between farming work that is profitable for their family but risky and remaining with their family to protect the health of its members (IPES-Food 2020).

Indeed, the closure of food plants because workers contracted the virus is another example of disruptions in the food supply chain (HLPE 2020a). More than 30,000 workers in food-processing plants in the United States and Europe contracted COVID-19 (as of April 2020), leading to plant closures or slowdowns (Laborde et al. 2020). This has resulted in delays in international transport (HLPE 2020b; Larue 2020).

There is still little formal analysis of the impact of COVID-19 on more local food supply chains and their actors (Béné 2020). However, it is clear that the major impact of COVID-19 on farmers, through the difficulties encountered by migrant farmworkers and the outbreaks on farms and in workplaces such as slaughterhouses, have also impacted local supply chains.

Impacts on Consumers and Food Environments

Food security and nutrition is closely correlated with household income. The closure of the economy to slow the spread of the virus means that low-income households may no longer have access to healthy and sufficient food (HLPE 2020a; IPES-Food 2020). Although the pandemic does not affect all countries in the same way, COVID-19 generally results in a decrease in household income throughout the world. And chain disruptions not only prevent food from reaching consumers, but also increase the prices of some products, putting food out of reach for many consumers (HLPE 2020b; Klassen and Murphy 2020). The WFP predicts that an additional 71 to 100 million people will fall into extreme poverty as a direct consequence of the pandemic (WFP 2020).

The COVID-19 pandemic and the measures put in place to limit its spread have exacerbated social inequities (HLPE 2020b; Klassen and Murphy 2020; WFP 2020). They have also highlighted the precarity and inadequate remuneration experienced by many of the most important stakeholders of food systems, such as migrant farmworkers (Klassen and Murphy 2020). In addition, food banks in many countries are struggling to keep up with demand as more middle-income households require their help. The demand for food aid has increased by 50–140% in the United States since February 2020 and increased by 20% in Canada between March and May 2020 (Leddy et al. 2020). In Latin America, the number of people requiring food assistance almost tripled in 2020 (HLPE 2020b).

The negative effects of COVID-19 on children are not distributed equally either. For instance, school closures impacted 300 million children around the world, who were deprived of school meals, which are an important part of their diet (FAO et al. 2020; Gaupp 2020; HLPE 2020a).

The pandemic also highlights health inequities. For instance, and as demonstrated by Smith in Chapter 9 of this book, the health impacts of a pandemic are often gendered. COVID-19 also emphasised the increase of diet-related non-communicable diseases (NCDs), another facet of food insecurity (Willett et al. 2019). According to recent studies, NCDs have been associated with a greater risk of contracting COVID-19 and, when contracted, with a higher death rate (Leddy et al. 2020; Yang et al. 2020).

As mentioned in the introduction to this book, the injustices that the pandemic reveals have been latent, which is particularly true in relation to food security and nutrition. The COVID-19 pandemic has forced the entire world to confront itself with a basic fact: the most important activities of our society, including feeding ourselves and future generations, rely on a generally poorly paid workforce who experience precarious employment and whose incomes are severely affected by the smallest economic perturbations and labour shortages.

Shortcomings of Food Systems beyond Pandemics

While the COVID-19 pandemic highlights the lack of adaptative capacities of food systems to external shocks, it also reveals their limited absorptive capacity. Indeed, the pandemic reveals that food systems have not been able to effectively take into account scientific evidence that demonstrates their negative impact on food security and nutrition in order to initiate significant change.

Yet long before COVID-19, the scientific community and international organizations concerned with food security, health, climate, the environment (see Chapter 6 in this volume by Morin et al.), and the right to food were urging states to reform food systems to make them true vectors of sustainability, food security and nutrition, and implementation of human rights (Committee on World Food Security (CFS) 2020; De Schutter 2014; FAO et al. 2017; FAO and WHO 2014; HLPE 2012; Intergovernmental Panel on Climate Change (IPCC) 2019). Even the United Nations called in 2015 for the transition to sustainable food systems in the 2030 Agenda for Sustainable Development. Under Sustainable Development Goal 2, which is to end hunger, achieve food security and improved nutrition, and promote sustainable agriculture, Objective 2.4 directly calls for the transition to sustainable food systems, calling on states to 'ensure sustainable food production systems and implement resilient agricultural practices that increase productivity and production, that help maintain ecosystems, that strengthen capacity for adaptation to climate change, extreme weather, drought, flooding and other disasters and that progressively improve land and soil quality' (UN 2015).

To better achieve Objective 2.4, just before the COVID-19 outbreak the UN Secretary General, António Guterres, announced the Food Systems Summit held in 2021. In doing so, he set forth the crucial importance of transforming food systems as part of the Decade of Action to deliver the Sustainable Development Goals, while condemning food waste and advocating for a world where nutritious food is available to all.

Nevertheless, the COVID-19 pandemic exacerbates a long-standing food and nutrition crisis that underpins the long-known negative impacts of current food systems.

Food Insecurity

Despite these clear recommendations and goals, after years of decline in the number of undernourished persons around the world it is on the rise again (FAO et al. 2020). In 2020, just before COVID-19 struck, 690 million people were undernourished, with an estimated 2 billion people experiencing moderate or severe food insecurity (FAO et al. 2020; IPES–Food 2020).

The international organizations expect these numbers to increase substantially because of COVID-19 and containment measures. The pandemic may add between 83 and 132 million people to the total number of undernourished in 2020, and an additional 71–100 million people are expected to fall into extreme poverty (WFP 2020; FAO et al. 2020). Recent estimates suggest that the rate of child wasting (i.e. children who are underweight for their height—an important predictor of under-five child mortality) could also increase, affecting an additional 6.7 million children (WFP 2020).

The sad fact is that there is enough food produced to feed the world population, but one-third of the food produced for human consumption is lost or wasted. It is estimated that 1.3 billion tons of food per year are being wasted all along the food chain, from agricultural production to consumption (FAO 2019a).

Health Impacts and Food Diversity Loss

The dramatic loss of agricultural and food diversity, the homogenization of food products and ways of producing them, and the simplification of diets are generally associated with the inadequacies of the global food system (Rastoin and

Ghersi 2010; Rastoin 2018; Willett et al. 2019). We are indeed witnessing a homogenization and simplification of diets towards a North American-style diet, which is rich in calories, animal protein, fat, and sugar (Khoury et al. 2014; Willett et al. 2019), with profound negative effects on agricultural diversity and human health. Agricultural and food multinationals depend directly on this homogenization of consumer habits for financial growth, so they aim to standardize products using a mass consumption model (Hendrickson 2015).

The past few decades have also seen notable increased in NCDs: cardiovascular disease, obesity, type 2 diabetes, hypertension, dyslipidemia, and cancer (FAO and WHO 2014). The principal cause of NCDs is overnutrition (i.e. excessive consumption of sugar, salt, and processed foods to the detriment of whole grains, fruits, and vegetables; Global Burden of Disease (GBD) 2017; Leddy et al. 2020; Whitmee et al. 2015).

Contrary to popular belief, obesity and undernutrition can coexist in the same population—even within the same household—in both developed and developing countries (FAO et al. 2020). Food insecurity, malnutrition, and obesity are in fact the three components of a global syndemic. A 'syndemic' can be understood as '[a] synergy of epidemics, because they co-occur in time and place, interact with each other to produce complex sequelae, and share common underlying societal drivers' (Swinburn et al. 2019). The cost associated with obesity and undernutrition is estimated at US$3,000–4,000 billion per year, or 5–6% of global gross domestic product (FAO et al. 2020; Swinburn et al. 2019).

Moreover, the intensive agriculture and livestock practices—a typical component of the global food system—generate significant negative externalities, such as soil degradation, pollution by pesticides and other chemical inputs, and groundwater contamination, while also contributing to climate variability through significant global greenhouse gas emissions (FAO et al. 2018; HLPE 2017).

Those practices also lead to an alarming loss of agricultural and food diversity, which includes seeds, farm animals, and plant and fish species, but also extends to the diversity of food heritage, traditional agricultural and processing practices, local and Indigenous knowledge, and rural landscapes. Such biodiversity brings many benefits to humanity, including a greater resilience to external shocks (FAO et al. 2017). For instance, of the 382,000 species of existing vascular plants, only about 6,000 are grown for food. As of 2014, only nine species accounted for 66% of all crop production in the world (sugar cane, maize, rice, wheat, potatoes, soybeans, oil-palm fruit, sugar beet, and cassava; FAO, 2019b).

Intensive livestock production (large numbers of animals in a limited space) also creates conditions for the emergence of infectious diseases, which are sometimes transmissible to humans (e.g. Ebola, swine flu (H1N1), COVID-19 (SARS-CoV-2); IPES–Food 2020). The risk of infectious disease is enhanced when ecosystems are destroyed by humans, thus dismantling the natural protective barriers and increasing close contact between humans and wildlife (Everard et al. 2020).

As mentioned by IPES–Food, 'The "efficiencies" of global trade have paved the way for increasingly uniform farming systems and removed the firebreaks of biodiversity' (IPES–Food 2020). In addition, diseases of animal origin account for two-thirds of human infectious diseases, causing millions of deaths each year, and research has found a significant link between poverty, livestock, and zoonotic diseases (Machalaba et al. 2015; FAO et al. 2017). Though the origins of COVID-19 are as yet unconfirmed, it is assumed they are zoonotic and linked to these dynamics.

The risk of pandemics has increased significantly in recent decades due to urbanization, worldwide movement, modification of land use, and intensive exploitation of natural resources (Galanakis 2020). As these trends increase, the threat is expected to continue to intensify.

Climate Change

The FAO, HLPE, and IPCC have all reached the same conclusion: climate change is severely impacting all aspects of food security and nutrition, particularly agricultural and food production, food availability, food utilization, and food price stability (FAO et al. 2018; HLPE 2012). The level of climate change we are experiencing today, including rising average temperatures, heavy rains, and intensifying extreme weather, is unprecedented (IPCC 2019). While the past decade was the warmest on record, the year 2019 breaks all records (World Meteorological Organization (WMO) 2020). Climate is the most important environmental factor influencing agricultural and food production and thus agricultural and food diversity (FAO et al. 2018).

The increase in climatic events caused by global warming exposes and exacerbates the lack of resilience of current food systems. For instance, in 2020 locust swarm invasions were the worst the East African region has experienced in 70 years (HLPE 2020a). This event, in conjunction with the COVID-19 pandemic, has many implications for food security.

The IPCC judges that the global food system, with its long supply chains and large-scale intensive production, is responsible for 21–37% of greenhouse gas (GHG) emissions worldwide. Of this estimate, 9–14% of GHGs are generated by agricultural production alone, and 8–10% by food losses and waste (IPCC 2019).

Clearly, current food systems are stretching our natural resources without meeting our nutritional needs, while global food insecurity continues to rise (FAO and WHO 2014). Unless an evidence-based food systems reform is made, this already dramatic state of planetary health will worsen and will provide a propitious environment for the emergence of new pandemics (HLPE 2020b; IPCC 2019; Rastoin 2018; Swinburn et al. 2019; Whitmee et al. 2015; Willett et al. 2019).

Towards Resilient and Sustainable Food Systems

As shown above, the COVID-19 pandemic has highlighted the lack of resilience of already unsustainable food systems. The Food Systems Summit held in 2021 will hopefully address ways to meet these challenges in order for food systems to become true vectors of food security and nutrition and planetary health.

The global awareness raised by COVID-19 has led to several states becoming committed to achieving greater food self-sufficiency through local food systems that are more resilient, in particular through greater sustainability (Hendrickson 2015; Rastoin 2018). However, this strategy can also be related to the hegemonic position of the global food system and underlies an important change in the international legal framework.

Global Food System in the Dock

Although the global food system contributes to global food security and nutrition, through international trade creating higher levels of food availability and accessibility and advanced knowledge in food safety, the scientific literature and most international organizations have identified the negative impacts of the global food system as the main causes of the crisis we have described above (IPCC 2019; Hendrickson 2015; Rastoin 2018; Swinburn et al. 2019; Whitmee et al. 2015).

This can be explained to a large extent by the fact that, since the mid-1990s, we have witnessed the rise of an intensive, concentrated, and financialized agro-industrial food system of mass production and consumption (Rastoin and Ghersi 2010). This agro-industrial food system is in the hands of a few multinational corporations (Cheriet and Lubello 2017; Fakhri 2020; FAO et al. 2020; Hendrickson 2015;). In 2009, the 15 largest agri-food multinationals accounted for 46% of sales in the agri-food sector worldwide (Cheriet and Lubello 2017). For instance, nearly three-fifths of the seed companies are controlled by four multinationals, three of which are also agro-chemical transnationals (Hendrickson 2015). Still driven by the promises of the Green Revolution and empowered by trade agreements, which have seen the liberalization of trade in agricultural products since 1995 in an almost identical way to other goods, the agro-industrial food system took over the global food system. The latest State of Food Security and Nutrition in the World report points out that '[f]ood systems have become more globalized, industrialized and dominated by large actors capable of economies of scale and of maintaining long supply chains' (FAO et al. 2020).

Under this agro-industrial food system, food is becoming a commodity like any other. This paradigm leaves little room for considerations such as the right to food and the fight against climate change or NCDs. (Fakhri 2020; GBD 2017;

De Schutter 2011), causing ever-increasing food insecurity and putting unprecedented stress on our ecosystem (Hendrickson 2015). Morin and colleagues in Chapter 6 of this text show that health and the environment also have a tense and ambiguous relationship with trade liberalization.

Following an important reflection emerging from the Food Systems Summit in 2021, we must avoid mistaking the global food system with the agro-industrial food system. Although the latter takes a hegemonic position in the global food system and has negative impacts on food security and nutrition, it should not be forgotten that nations have always traded food. These exchanges have contributed, and still contribute, to the development of food cultures around the world. It is therefore necessary to resolve the unproductive conflict that has been raging for several years between the global food system and local food systems to finally address the root causes of the hegemonic place the agro-industrial food system occupies in the global food system.

The Root Causes

It is incumbent on all of us to request a legal framework in which the global food trade operates to ensure that it supports agricultural and food practices that are sustainable and resilient and that safeguard planetary health, instead of simply enabling the development of an agro-industrial food system that negatively impacts food security and nutrition.

Trade agreements, the basis of the development of the agro-industrial food system, are characterized by their high efficiency. They are general, binding, and founded on reciprocal commitments. The dispute settlement mechanisms specific to those agreements are mandatory and highly effective. However, this legal regime leaves little room for food security and nutrition considerations and neglects the broader human rights perspective (Brodeur et al. 2010; De Schutter 2011; Fakhri 2020; Parent 2003; Parent and Modou 2019).

Adding to this already problematic situation is the fact that there are no universal, general, and binding agreements on sustainable food security and nutrition outside of international economic law under which states can declare they must be able to adopt measures to ensure food security and nutrition for their own population (Brodeur et al. 2010; Parent and Modou 2019).

The kind of market liberalization, launched within the World Trade Organization (WTO) by the Agreement on Agriculture and coupled with the increased deregulation and disinvestment of states in the agricultural sector, has created conditions ripe for the development of the agro-industrial food system. As the UN Special Rapporteur on the Right to Food points out, this agreement 'has privileged those States and corporations that already have access to resources, infrastructure, credit and foreign markets. More specifically, trade liberalization and domestic policies in the wealthiest countries increased the market power of transnational commodity traders and processors' (Fakhri 2020). We now know that the hegemonic position of the agro-industrial food system over local or regional ones has negative impacts on food security and nutrition, especially in lower- and middle-income countries and on vulnerable consumers worldwide (Willett et al. 2019).

The way in which international economic law is shaped combined with the legal vacuum regarding food security outside trade law explains why states, in spite of their willingness, are now limited in what they can achieve regarding more local and sustainable food systems and moving towards greater food self-compliance. Indeed, national laws must be elaborated in compliance with the states' international commitments. As a result, since the mid-1990s, national policies and legal measures affecting food security and nutrition have essentially been developed around economic considerations, with all the attendant negative impacts on human and planetary health that we see today. In this context, states lack the elbow room to move towards greater food security and nutrition.

As discussed in relation to health security by Davies in Chapter 12 of this text, in the face of the challenges posed by COVID-19 some states may also be tempted to return to protectionist food policies. However, studies show that a return to protectionism would magnify the initial shock caused by the pandemic on food security and nutrition (Espitia et al. 2020). This could be as detrimental to global food security and nutrition as continuing along the path we have taken so far (Kerr 2020; Espitia et al. 2020).

Michael Fakhri, the UN Special Rapporteur on the Right to Food in 2020, as well as his predecessor, have argued that an in-depth reform is needed within and outside the WTO (Fakhri 2020; De Schutter 2014). On the one hand, the vacuum outside trade agreements should be filled by an international binding instrument to restore balance between economic, food security, nutrition, environmental, and social concerns. On the other hand, the few references to food security and environmental protection in the WTO agreements, including the Agreement on Agriculture, need to be developed and strengthened in new international commitments (De Schutter 2014; Parent 2003). Fakhri goes even further by inviting states to advance trade policies based on winding down the WTO Agreement on Agriculture and negotiating new international food agreements based on a right-to-adequate-food perspective (Fakhri 2020).

In either case, the paradigm must be reversed: trade liberalization is not an end, but one of the means by which we can achieve better food security and nutrition. Such a reform would support greater coherence in international law that is based on fundamental rights, including the right to adequate food. This reform would provide a legal framework supportive of more resilient and sustainable food systems. Therefore, the Food Systems Summit has launched a constructive reflection on the reform of the international legal order relating to food security and nutrition to achieve the Sustainable Development Goals, with the aim of enabling states to support their local food systems while remaining open to international trade.

International Cooperation for More Inclusive Sustainable Food Systems

Addressing the root causes of the hegemonic place the agro-industrial food system enjoys and reforming the international legal framework to initiate a real transition towards resilient and sustainable food systems relies on vigorous international co-operation in which not only all states but also all stakeholders have a voice. This cooperation is a key element of the food systems' transformative capacity, which is an important component of the concept of the resilience of food systems (FAO et al. 2017).

As clearly expressed by the Chief of Cabinet of the Director General of the UN David Chikvaidze, 'we no longer live in a bipolar or unipolar world; and not yet in a multipolar one, but, rather, in an unsettled world with multiple actors of different caliber with clashing interests and often isolationist politics of fear and resentment' (Chikvaidze 2020). Thus, if strong multilateralism and effective mechanisms ensuring stakeholders' participation are essential for a successful food systems' transition, achieving those constitutes a significant challenge in current geopolitics.

Strengthening International Cooperation through Enhanced Multilateralism

As the world struggles with the COVID-19 pandemic, which is one of the most acute challenges to international cooperation, multilateralism is also undergoing an unprecedented crisis that threatens to wipe out all the coordination efforts since the Second World War (Chikvaidze 2020). The US policies and decisions under the presidency of Donald Trump have been identified as one of the main factors of this crisis: their nationalist policies, withdrawal from several international agreements, trade war on China, and cutting off US funding to the WHO in the middle of the COVID-19 pandemic are eloquent examples (Sachs 2020).

More specifically in the area of food security and nutrition, the multilateralism crisis can be felt in the lack of a coordinated response to the COVID-19 pandemic, the decline in efforts by several states to improve the Agreement on Agriculture at the WTO, the Trump administration's refusal to appoint new members to the WTO Appellate Body, and the withdrawal of the United States from the Paris Agreement on climate change (HLPE 2020a). In this context, the intention of a number of governments to achieve greater national food self-sufficiency may further affect multilateralism and global food security and nutrition (Kerr 2020).

The foundations of the international order are at such risk that the International Day of Multilateralism and Diplomacy for Peace was established by the UN General Assembly in 2018 and was first observed on 24 April 2019. France, Germany, and other partners then launched the Alliance for Multilateralism based on the conviction that a rules-based multilateralism is the only reliable guarantee for international stability and peace. The 'Declaration on the Commemoration of the Seventy-Fifth Anniversary of the United Nations' adopted by the General Assembly on 21 September 2020, also reiterates that 'multilateralism is not an option but a necessity as we build back better and greener for a more equal, more resilient and more sustainable world' (UN 2020).

However, we cannot ignore that the generalized mistrust on the part of citizens of the world towards global governance institutions is also an important contributing factor (Chikvaidze 2020; Petetin 2020). Petetin's recent work on food democracy demonstrates that in the COVID-19 context and beyond, 'citizens do not feel in control of the international food supply chain or food provenance and feel like food choice is imposed by the supply chain' (Petetin 2020). Therefore, future food systems agendas, like the 2021 Food Systems Summit, should aim to find solutions for a more inclusive, networked multilateralism without a hegemonic leader and not limited to states alone (Chikvaidze 2020; HLPE 2020a; Sachs 2020).

More Inclusive Governance

To this end, the 2030 UN Agenda for Sustainable Development encourages states to work towards a new 'networked and inclusive' governance (UN 2015). This means more intense cooperation between the different international organizations and effective participation of multiple stakeholders. This type of governance also underlies multisectoral coordination at local, national, regional, and international levels. It must give a voice to women, who are central to global food security, and to young people. It must also be a governance informed by reliable and independent scientific data.

Fortunately, unlike in the fields of health and the environment (see Chapters 6 by Morin et al. and 11 by Dufort and Clément in this text), inclusive governance is championed by the Committee on World Food Security (CFS) to ensure food security and nutrition for all (Golay 2010; CFS 2017). The CFS is a one-of-a-kind intergovernmental body that provides a platform of discussion and coordination to strengthen collaborative action among several constituents: governments, regional and international organizations and agencies (e.g. the FAO, International Fund for Agricultural Development, the WFP, the WHO, UNICEF, the UNDP, the Standing Committee on Nutrition, and the Special Rapporteur on the Right to Food), civil society and non-governmental organizations (e.g. family food producers, fishermen, women, youth, and consumers), the private sector, philanthropic foundations, financial institutions (e.g. the World Bank, the International Monetary Fund, regional development banks, the WTO), and international agricultural research institutions. The CFS reports to the UN General Assembly through the Economic and Social Council and to the FAO and institutionalizes the role of the HLPE in evidence-based decisions.

Although voting and decision-making is ultimately limited to member states, these stakeholders are actively involved in the work of the CFS. They have the right to speak in plenary sessions and in small-group discussions, where they contribute to the drafting of documents and make formal proposals. They then have a tangible impact on the policy products developed and adopted by the CFS (CFS 2017).

Even if the guidelines resulting from this colossal collective work are non-binding (meaning that it is up to each member state to choose to implement them at the national level), they have an important impact in the quest for better food security and nutrition (CFS 2017). They are the result of networked and inclusive governance, which facilitates their social acceptability and favours their application across many countries and regions.

The CFS is currently working on voluntary guidelines on food systems and nutrition (CFS 2020). The Food Systems Summit and the future food systems agendas could therefore be an opportunity to discuss the issues based on these guidelines.

The CFS has launched a real revolution in international governance, which could be pushed even further and emulated to be useful in times of pandemics. It is a beacon of hope for a renewed multilateralism towards achieving the Sustainable Development Goals. Since a recent evaluation of the CFS's work reveals that it is largely unknown outside of its headquarters in Rome (CFS 2017), the Food Systems Summit should be used as an opportunity to shed light on its unique experience.

Conclusion

The focus of this chapter was on demonstrating that the COVID-19 pandemic, as would any pandemic, has exacerbated the lack of resilience and sustainability of the agro-industrial food system and its negative impact on global food security and nutrition, while also considering how food systems might become more resilient in the face of external shocks such as pandemics.

Food systems are extremely complex. Interventions in one part of the system can have severe positive or negative impacts on other parts and stakeholders (CFS 2020). The complexity of the interrelationships within a food system, as well as the intricacy of the interactions and feedback between different systems, needs to be addressed to achieve a reform that tends towards greater resilience and sustainability. To do so, additional research in every discipline, as well as interdisciplinary research, are still needed.

Mistaking the global food system with the agro-industrial food system is an error. The global food system is the sum of several individual food systems that can contribute to global food security and nutrition. However, as documented above, the agro-industrial food system takes a hegemonic place in the global food system, while being simultaneously described as having the most negative impact on planetary health. Research should tackle this hegemonic position to initiate an effective and sustainable transition. A return to protectionist food policies could have devastating impacts on global food security and nutrition.

We have demonstrated that the current international legal framework supports, and even promotes, the agro-industrial food system instead of fostering the development of resilient and sustainable food systems. This legal framework explains in large part why an ever-increasing number of people go hungry or lack nutritionally adequate food. A global evidence-based reflection is needed on how to coordinate the global food system so that it is more supportive of sustainable and resilient food systems.

It is clear that the COVID-19 pandemic and its impacts will continue to exacerbate global food insecurity, but there is hope that the Food Systems Summit—and the international reflection that will continue afterwards—will stimulate discussion and scientific research on the root causes of the lack of resilience and sustainability of food systems to prepare an adequate response to other pandemics or external shocks. However, several concerns expressed by the non-governmental agencies are questioning the value of the results of this reflection in view of the central role that the dominant agricultural and food corporations already play. Past and present UN Special Rapporteurs on the Right to Food have expressed their concerns about the danger of bringing back business-led solutions imposed by the multinationals.

The success of this international discussion beyond the UN Summit and, more broadly, the ability of food systems reform to enhance global food security and nutrition are, therefore, dependent on a constructive discussion involving not only states but all stakeholders. There is a pressing need for an inclusive international cooperation to address food systems transition. This confirms the essential role the CFS could play in the transition of food systems towards greater resilience and sustainability as an essential forum for constructive discussion among all stakeholders.

UN-initiated thinking on food systems reform coupled with the glaring lack of resilience and adaptability of food systems to pandemics and other external shocks is creating unprecedented momentum that allows us to envision that lasting changes will be made.

References

Barrett Christopher B. 2020. 'Actions Now Can Curb Food Systems Fallout from COVID-19'. *Nature Food 1*: 319–20. https://doi.org/10.1038/s43016-020-0085-y.

Béné Christophe. 2020. 'Resilience of Local Food Systems and Links to Food Security: A Review of Some Important Concepts in the Context of COVID-19 and Other Shocks'. *Food Security 12*: 805–22. https://doi.org/10.1007/s12571-020-01076-1.

Brodeur Johanne, Catherine Del Cont, Bernard Colas, and Michel Jacquot. 2010. Pour une meilleure cohérence des normes internationales: Reconnaître la spécificité agricole et alimentaire pour le respect des droits humains. Cowansville, PA: Yvon Blais.

Cheriet Foued, and Pasquale Lubello. 2017. 'Concentration des grandes firmes et nouvelle division multinationale du travail: La révolution du système agroalimentaire mondial'. In *Systèmes agroalimentaires en transition*, edited by Pasquale Lubello, Alain Falque, and Leila Temri, pp. 115–58. Versailles: Editions Quæ. https://doi.org/10.3917/quae.lubel.2017.01.0115.

Chikvaidze David A. 2020. 'Multilateralism: Its Past, Present and Future'. *Cadmus 4*: pp. 127–33.

Committee on World Food Security (CFS). 2017. 'Evaluation of the Committee on World Food Security—Final Report'. 14 April. www.fao.org/fileadmin/templates/cfs/Docs1617/Evaluation/CFS_Evaluation_Final_Report__14_April_2017.pdf.

CFS. 2020. *CFS Voluntary Guidelines on Food Systems for Nutrition*. Rome: CFS.

De Schutter Olivier. 2011. 'The World Trade Organization and the Post-Global Food Crisis Agenda: Putting Food Security First in the International Trade System'. UN Special Rapporteur on the Right to Food.

De Schutter Olivier. 2014. 'Final Report: The Transformative Potential of the Right to Food'. UN Special Rapporteur on the Right to Food. A/HRC/25/57.

Espitia Alvaro, Rocha Nadia, and Michele Ruta. 2020. 'COVID-19 and Food Protectionism: The Impact of the Pandemic and Export Restrictions on World Food Markets'. Policy Research Working Papers, World Bank. https://doi.org/10.1596/1813-9450-9253.

Everard Mark, Paul Johnston, David Santillo, and Chad Staddon. 2020. 'The Role of Ecosystems in Mitigation and Management of COVID-19 and Other Zoonoses'. *Environmental Science and Policy 111*: pp. 7–17.

Fakhri Michael. 2020. 'The Right to Food in the Context of International Trade Law and Policy'. UN Special Rapporteur on the Right to Food. A//75/2019.

Food and Agriculture Organization (FAO). 2019a. *The State of Food and Agriculture 2019: Moving Forward on Food Loss and Waste Reduction*. Rome: FAO.

FAO. 2019b. 'The State of the World's Biodiversity for Food and Agriculture'. FAO Commission on Genetic Resources for Food and Agriculture Assessments. Rome: FAO.

FAO, International Fund for Agricultural Development (IFAD), United Nations International Children's Emergency Fund (UNICEF), World Food Programme (WFP), and World Health Organization (WHO). 2017. *The State of Food Security and Nutrition in the World 2017: Building Resilience for Peace and Food Security*. Rome: FAO.

FAO and WHO. 2014. 'Rome Declaration on Nutrition'. Second International Conference on Nutrition, Rome: FAO.

FAO, IFAD, UNICEF, WFP, and WHO. 2018. *The State of Food Security and Nutrition in the World: Building Climate Resilience for Food Security and Nutrition*. Rome: FAO.

FAO, IFAD, UNICEF, WFP, and WHO. 2020. *The State of Food Security and Nutrition in the World 2020: Transforming Food Systems for Affordable Healthy Diets*. Rome: FAO.

Galanakis Charis M. 2020. 'The Food Systems in the Era of the Coronavirus (COVID-19) Pandemic Crisis'. *Foods 9*: p. 523. https://doi.org/10.3390/foods9040523.

Gaupp Franziska. 2020. 'Extreme Events in a Globalized Food System'. *One Earth 2*: pp. 518–21. https://doi.org/10.1016/j.oneear.2020.06.001.

Global Burden of Disease (GBD) 2017. 'Diet Collaborators. 2019. "Health Effects of Dietary Risks in 195 Countries, 1990–2017: A Systematic Analysis for the Global Burden of Disease Study 2017"'. *The Lancet 393*: pp. 1958–72.

Golay Christophe. 2010. 'Crise et sécurité alimentaires: vers un nouvel ordre alimentaire mondial?' *International Development Policy 1*: pp. 229–48.

Hendrickson Mary K. 2015. 'Resilience in a Concentrated and Consolidated Food System'. *Journal of Environmental Studies and Sciences 5*: pp. 418–31. https://doi.org/10.1007/s13412-015-0292-2.

High Level Panel of Experts (HLPE). 2012. 'Food Security and Climate Change. Report #3'. Rome: HLPE.

HLPE. 2014. 'Food Losses and Waste in the Context of Sustainable Food Systems. Report #8'. Rome: HLPE.

HLPE. 2017. 'Nutrition and Food Systems. Report #12'. Rome: HLPE.

HLPE. 2020a. 'Food Security and Nutrition: Building a Global Narrative towards 2030. Report #15'. Rome: HLPE.

HLPE. 2020b. 'Impacts of COVID-19 on Food Security and Nutrition: Developing Effective Policy Responses to Address the Hunger and Malnutrition Pandemic'. September 2020. Rome: HLPE.

Hobbs Jill E. 2020. 'Food Supply Chains during the COVID-19 Pandemic'. *Canadian Journal of Agricultural Economics 68*: pp. 171–6. https://doi.org/10.1111/cjag.12237.

Intergovernmental Panel on Climate Change (IPCC). 2019. 'Special Report: Climate Change and Land'. https://www.ipcc.ch/srccl.

International Panel of Experts on Sustainable Food Systems (IPES–Food). 2020. 'COVID-19 and the Crisis in Food Systems: Symptoms, Causes, and Potential Solutions'. April. www.ipes-food.org/_img/upload/files/COVID-19_CommuniqueEN.pdf.

Janin Pierre. 2009. 'Les "émeutes de la faim": Une lecture (géo-politique) du changement (social)'. *Politique étrangère 2* (Summer): pp. 251–63.

Kerr William A. 2020. 'The COVID-19 Pandemic and Agriculture: Short- and Long-Run Implications for International Trade Relations'. *Canadian Journal of Agricultural Economics 68*: pp. 225–9.

Khoury Colin K., Anne D. Bjorkman, Hannes Dempewolf, et al. 2014. 'Increasing Homogeneity in Global Food Supplies and the Implications for Food Security'. *Proceedings of the National Academy of Sciences 111*: 4001–6.

Klassen Susanna, and Sophia Murphy. 2020. 'Equity as Both a Means and an End: Lessons for Resilient Food Systems from COVID-19'. *World Development 136*: 105104.

Laborde David, Will Martin, Johan Swinnen, and Rob Vos. 2020. 'COVID-19 Risks to Global Food Security'. *Science 369*: 500–2.

Larue Bruno. 2020. 'Labor Issues and COVID-19'. *Canadian Journal of Agricultural Economics 68*: pp. 231–7.

Leddy Anna M., Sheri D. Weiser, Kartika Palar, and Hilary Seligman, 2020. 'A Conceptual Model for Understanding the Rapid COVID-19-Related Increase in Food Insecurity and Its Impact on Health and Healthcare'. *American Journal of Clinical Nutrition 112* (5): 1162–9.

Machalaba Catherine C., Elizabeth H. Loh, Peter Daszak, and William B. Karesh. 2015. 'Emerging Diseases from Animals'. *State of the World*: pp. 105–16.

Malassis Louis. 1979. *Économie agroalimentaire, tome 1. Économie de la consommation et de la production agroalimentaire*. Paris: Cujas.

Parent Geneviève. 2003. 'La reconnaissance du caractère spécifique du commerce agricole à travers la prise en compte des considérations liées à la sécurité alimentaire dans l'accord sur l'agriculture'. *Les Cahiers de droit 44* (3): pp. 471–517.

Parent Geneviève, and Kader L. Modou. 2019. 'Les expressions de la spécificité agricole'. *Revue de droit d'Ottawa 50* (1): 101–29.

Petetin Ludivine. 2020. 'The COVID-19 Crisis: An Opportunity to Integrate Food Democracy into Post-Pandemic Food Systems'. *European Journal of Risk Regulation 11* (2): pp. 326–36.

Rastoin Jean-Louis. 2018. 'Éditorial Accélérer la transition vers une alimentation durable par un changement de paradigme scientifique et économique et des politiques publiques innovantes'. *Food Systems 3*: p. 17.

Rastoin Jean-Louis, and Gérard Ghersi. 2010. *Le système alimentaire mondial*. Versailles: Editions Quæ.

Sachs Jeffrey D. 2020. 'COVID-19 and Multilateralism'. *Consilience 22*: pp. 1–5.

Swinburn Boyd A., Vivica I. Kraak, Steven Allender, et al. 2019. 'The Global Syndemic of Obesity, Undernutrition, and Climate Change: The Lancet Commission Report'. *The Lancet 393*: pp. 791–846.

United Nations (UN). 2015. 'Transforming Our World: The 2030 Agenda for Sustainable Development'. A/RES/70/1.

UN. 2020. 'Declaration on the Commemoration of the Seventy-Fifth Anniversary of the United Nations'. https://www.un.org/pga/74/wp-content/uploads/sites/99/2020/07/UN75-FINAL-DRAFT-DECLARATION.pdf.

Willett Walter, Johan Rockström, Brent Loken, et al. 2019. 'Food in the Anthropocene: The EAT–Lancet Commission on Healthy Diets from Sustainable Food Systems'. *The Lancet 393*: pp. 447–92.

Whitmee Sarah, Andy Haines, Chris Beyrer, et al. 2015. 'Safeguarding Human Health in the Anthropocene Epoch: Report of the Rockefeller Foundation–Lancet Commission on Planetary Health'. *The Lancet 386*: 1973–2028.

World Food Programme (WFP). 2020. 'Global Report on Food Crises Update: In Times of COVID-19'. September.

World Meteorological Organization (WMO). 2020. *WMO Statement on the State of the Global Climate in 2019. WMO-No. 1248*. Geneva: WMO.

Yang Jing, Ya Zheng, Xi Gou, et al. 2020. 'Prevalence of Comorbidities and Its Effects in Patients Infected with SARS-CoV-2: A Systematic Review and Meta-Analysis'. *International Journal of Infectious Diseases 94*: pp. 91–5.

16

Force Majeure in International Law during a Pandemic

Lessons from the COVID-19 Crisis

Andrea K. Bjorklund

Immediately the COVID-19 crisis hit, questions about its effect on the performance of contractual obligations arose. One of the potential defences to the performance of contractual obligations is force majeure, a doctrine found in most municipal laws that excuses or arrests contractual obligations due to an external event—the 'Act of God' that is the force majeure event—or follow-on effects, whether factual or legal, that render performance impossible. Force majeure is also known in public international law; a state can raise force majeure as a circumstance precluding wrongfulness that obviates its obligation for the duration of the event. There are other defences that respondents seeking to escape liability might raise. A few of those will be touched on below, largely in contradistinction to force majeure, but the bulk of the chapter will concentrate on the ways that this particular pandemic illustrates the possibilities, and shortcomings, of a force majeure defence.

A quintessential force majeure event would be a hurricane, or tidal wave, or other natural phenomenon that is no person's fault but that prevents a specific event from occurring. Yet these examples, while of illustrative use, do not really explore fully all of the ramifications of a force majeure event. If, for example, a wedding had been planned to take place at a seaside hotel that was flattened by a tidal wave, force majeure suggests that the hotel would not be responsible for being unable to host the wedding, and that the bridal couple would not be responsible for paying any rental for the hotel, at least if there was a force majeure clause in the contract. But what about the deposit? Should the hotel refund it, or would the hotel get to keep it? If the hotel manager had already purchased thousands of dollars' worth of flowers on behalf of the couple, would the bridal couple at least have to pay for those flowers? One can spin this out in various ways, of course, but the principle should be clear—while a force majeure event might be viewed as excusing the performance of contractual obligations, significant questions about liability for

Andrea K. Bjorklund, *Force Majeure in International Law during a Pandemic.* In: *A Multidisciplinary Approach to Pandemics.* Edited by Philippe Bourbeau, Jean-Michel Marcoux, and Brooke A. Ackerly, Oxford University Press.
 DOI: 10.1093/oso/9780192897855.003.0017

expenses that have already been incurred or services that have already been given might still remain, particularly when there is a contract whose performance lasts over time.

A global pandemic such as the COVID-19 coronavirus fits somewhat uneasily under the force majeure umbrella. The examples set out above are events that occur all at once, whereas the spread of the COVID-19 coronavirus and its attainment of 'pandemic' status took some time—at the end of January 2020, the World Health Organization (WHO) noted it as a 'Public Health Emergency of International Concern', but it was not declared a pandemic until 11 March 2020 (Paddeu and Jephcott 2020: 1). Its severity, its practical consequences, and the governmental responses to it have varied significantly (and continue to vary significantly) across jurisdictions and, indeed, have changed frequently, even within individual jurisdictions, as infection rates have waxed and waned.

A pandemic itself is an overarching event, with multiple and often variable government measures implemented under it that themselves make the performance of a party's contractual obligations impossible, or at least exceptionally difficult. Thus, even if a pandemic qualifies as force majeure for only a limited period of time, government actions forbidding large gatherings might themselves suffice to excuse parties from contractual liability—force majeure on top of force majeure, as it were. China, for example, issued force majeure certificates to local exporters to exempt them from their obligation to fulfil contractual agreements with overseas trading partners, and other countries considered following suit (Paddeu and Jephcott 2020).

The example above involves a contract between private parties. If the parties come from different legal jurisdictions, their interaction would be governed by principles of private international law, which would dictate which particular contract law applies to their relationship. It would also direct which particular governmental dictates (e.g. the Chinese certificates mentioned above) might be invoked to excuse performance.

Force majeure can also affect the obligations between states, a matter of public international law. At public international law, a force majeure event involves an unforeseen and unavoidable external occurrence and constitutes a circumstance precluding wrongfulness when a state is simply incapable of complying with an obligation or is excused from having failed to prevent a problem from occurring (Bjorklund 2008: 465). A successful force majeure claim might involve a state arguing that it was not responsible for harm done by looters to another state's vessel sailing near an unfrequented part of the coast because 'the raid was one of those occasional and unexpected outbreaks against which ordinary and reasonable foresight could not provide' (International Law Commission (ILC) 2001b: para. 28 (internal quotation omitted)). The result would be to preclude the wrongfulness of a state's failure to fulfil its obligations whilst the force majeure event is still operative. After the event is over, however, the obligation returns (ILC 2001a).

Force majeure is only one of myriad ways in which a pandemic could intersect with public international law (Bradley and Helfer 2020: 572). This project is multidisciplinary in approach; one might say that the law itself is multidisciplinary, although the usual nomenclature is 'fragmented'. Different legal disciplines are sometimes described as siloed—there is trade law, and investment law, and human rights law, and international humanitarian law, and international criminal law, etc. All are different from each other, and all have their share of specialists. Polymathic lawyers attempt to learn from other disciplines within the law, as well as from disciplines outside the law. As the introduction to this volume states, '[w]ithout seeking to challenge the weaknesses of each discipline, a multidisciplinary approach thus builds on their strengths to prove a broader understanding of the phenomenon at hand' (Introduction by Ackerly et al.).

Force majeure crosses legal silos. It is a doctrine found in both municipal law and in public international law. In the public international law sphere in particular, it is applicable across disciplines, and might be invoked to excuse misconduct in the human rights, trade, or investment contexts—and in other contexts as well. A pandemic offers the opportunity to assess force majeure as it might appear in different factual scenarios. Nonetheless, the doctrine of force majeure plays only a small role in the pantheon of ways that a pandemic affects our world.

Force Majeure in Private International Law

Private international law regulates the relationships between private entities from different legal jurisdictions. Force majeure is known in the contract law of most countries and is recognized in the Convention on the International Sale of Goods and in the International Institute for the Unification of Private Law (UNIDROIT) Principles on International Commercial Contracts. (United Nations Convention on Contracts for the International Sale of Goods (CISG) Article 79; UNIDROIT 2016: Principle 6.2.2). In private international law, a force majeure event might be the aforementioned natural cause, yet it might also extend to the government's response to a particular phenomenon. Returning to our wedding example, what if the couple were from China, with the wedding to take place in Quebec? And what if there were no tidal wave, but rather an epidemiological disaster called COVID-19, which prompted the Canadian government to close its borders to foreign travellers and to forbid hotels from hosting guests? Is either the existence of the disease itself or the governmental response, or both, a force majeure event that excuses contractual performance? What if the government had not intervened formally, but had merely cautioned against travel? What if the prospective bridegroom had a medical condition making him especially vulnerable should he contract COVID-19, and thus he chose not to travel, even though most others in his situation would make a different decision? Would the couple be relieved of their contractual obligations, assuming the hotel had been able and willing to host the nuptials?

One of the reasons that answering these questions is so difficult is that the notion of excusing contractual performance goes against the fundamental reason that society recognizes contracts as binding—the point of entering into a contract is to solidify the agreement between the parties. This foundational idea will be explored below, before a short comparative analysis of the different approaches to the notion of binding contracts in the civil and common law traditions and different notions of the role judges should play in amending existing contracts, which lead to somewhat different approaches to doctrines such as force majeure. Those different approaches have an effect on risk allocation as parties enter into contractual relationships, and also have some impact on likely remedies if the contract is terminated.

Pacta sunt servanda

The foundation of contract law is the doctrine of *pacta sunt servanda*, or sanctity of contract—contracts are binding obligations that are not subject to unilateral rescission or alteration. The default rule is that a contract must be honoured, and that if one party decides to breach a contract, the other party is entitled to damages or, in appropriate circumstances, to specific performance.

One noted European commentator, who is sometimes regarded as the father of the *Principles of European Contract Law*, noted that *pacta sunt servanda*:

> is a basic principle in the laws of all countries. Many laws and courts stick to it with rigor. It is stated in the famous article 1134(1) of the French Civil Code. 'The agreements validly concluded are regarded as law for the parties,' the [UNIDROIT Principles] state [...] in art. 1.3. 'A contract validly entered into is binding upon the parties. It can only be modified or terminated in accordance with its terms or by agreement or as otherwise provided in these Principles.' A contracting party must be able to rely on the contract and exercise the rights granted to him or her under the contract. As the draftsmen of the CISG, the [Commission on European Contract Law] considered the principle to be so obvious that it was not stated in a special rule. It is, however, implied in several articles, including CISG art. 79 ... It is also implied in art. 6.111 (l) of the [Principles of European Contract Law] on change of circumstances, which provides that a party is bound to fulfil its obligations even if performance becomes more onerous.
>
> (Lando 2005: 388)

Particularly in common law jurisdictions, the reason for the breach is immaterial. A person who decides not to buy a house because a cancer diagnosis makes it imprudent to do so has no more right to seek rescission of a contract than the person who changes their mind because a different house that attracted them more became available. In one of his judicial opinions, US Supreme Court Justice Oliver Wendell Holmes, Jr emphasized that damages should remain the same whether the breach was innocent or wilful: 'If a contract is broken the measure of damages generally is the same, whatever the cause of the breach' (Holmes 1897: 544).

The conclusion that damages would be the same, regardless of the reason for the breach, is premised on the 'bad man theory of contract'—what kind of contract law do you need if you have a 'bad man' who would not abide by his legal duty out of a sense of moral obligation, but only because he would face adverse consequences in the event he failed to keep his word? Again, the classic reference is to Justice Holmes: 'The duty to keep a contract at common law means a prediction that you must pay damages if you do not keep it—and nothing else.' (Holmes 1897: 462)

The civil law tradition is more apt to recognize the moral underpinnings of a contractual obligation:

> [j]ust as in matters of mistake and of *réticence dolosive* [misleading silence] French law takes a moral stance while English law emphasizes the security of transactions and economic efficiency, so also French law treats breach of contract as a form of moral wrongdoing, while the Common law looks more to commercial considerations.
>
> (Nicholas 1992: 212)

Thus, in part because of this reliance on morality, the civil law tends to try to preserve a contract. This emphasis has several consequences. One is that parties are often limited in their ability to 'avoid' the contract—to treat it as no longer operative—without giving the injured party another chance to perform. This principle is known in German as '*Nachfrist*'. Another is that the law tends to approach remedies differently. The matter of fault on the part of the breaching party has an effect on the available remedy. Under French law, an injured party seeking money damages can get only foreseeable damages if the breaching party breached inadvertently, but can recover all damages proximately caused in the event of an intentional breach (Hyland 1994: 428). Fault also plays a role in German law, as there, it is also a prerequisite to bringing a cause of action in damages (Heldrich and Rehm 2005: 131).

In civil law systems, the remedy of specific performance (that the parties are ordered to perform the contract, rather than to pay damages in lieu of performing) is generally preferred, subject to certain exceptions. While specific performance is not necessarily sought, even when it could be, the fact that it is available can have an effect on the alacrity with which a party breaches, and also on settlement (Lando and Rose 2004: 473). Parties cannot simply breach and assume they will pay some sort of damages; the spectre of being ordered to perform the contract affects decisions they might make about breaching it.

In both the common law and the civil law, then, one sees a great deal of emphasis on guarding the sanctity of the contract, albeit in different ways. Yet in practice, even in common law systems, approaches might be different. Parties also have the right to renegotiate, or even to terminate, their contracts, and to agree that no negative consequences should ensue for either party. In particular, a non-lawyer might not take such a strictly commercial view of a contractual obligation, and might even be quite shocked at the suggestion that a contractual promise is not also subject to moral considerations, both with respect to abiding by the promise and conceivably with respect to being permitted to break it. A house seller confronted with a tragic story might not hold the buyer to his bargain. Even without a hard luck story, if the request to rescind the contract comes early such that the seller can easily find another buyer, the seller might let the buyer walk away. The default rule that the contract is enforceable might affect those negotiations, but the cost of enforcing the contract might also influence a seller. If the cost of enforcing the contract is relatively large, and obtaining substitute performance is relatively easy, the seller might not bother to try to enforce the contract.

Thus, although the law itself is relatively strict, in practice it might be less amoral than would seem to be the case. Nonetheless, the notion that contracts should be honoured means that excuses for contractual non performance are disfavoured, and there is a high bar to invoking them successfully.

The Force Majeure Doctrine

In the private law context, the doctrine of force majeure typically arises as a defence to the performance of a contract. Even in English, the French phrase 'force majeure' (superior force) is usually employed, though sometimes it is referred to as an 'Act of God'. The English phraseology is especially evocative—a force majeure event is beyond the control of the other party, and its occurrence renders performance impossible. Note that in addition to the requirement that neither party be responsible for the event and the requirement that they could not have avoided it, the event must also not have been foreseeable. To put it differently, the parties must not be expected to have allocated between themselves the risk of the event happening.

The doctrine is known in both the civil law and the common law, although there are important differences in applicability. It is part of the civil law, and applies regardless of whether the parties have included it in their contract or not. It is in Article 1218 of the French civil code, for example:

> In contractual matters, there is force majeure where an event beyond the control of the debtor, which could not reasonably have been foreseen at the time of the conclusion of the contract and whose effects could not be avoided by appropriate measures, prevents performance of the obligation of the debtor.

In the common law, on the other hand, a force majeure clause has to be included in the contract to be invoked as a reason for non-performance. It is not available in the absence of specification by the parties that it should apply. This difference reflects the greater deference to party autonomy that the common law holds. The presumption is that if the parties want a force majeure clause in their contract, they will include it; if they do not, then they do not want force majeure to provide an excuse for non-performance. The presumption in French law is the opposite—that the parties would want to have that ground for non-performance.

The breadth of a common law force majeure clause might also affect the outcome of any particular case. The so-called Spanish flu pandemic of 1918, the last great pandemic before the COVID-19 crisis, spawned its share of claims related to the pandemic, including some raising the doctrine of force majeure (Wajs 2020). In one Californian case, quarantine protocols delayed the ability of a soap manufacturer to deliver its wares; the court permitted a delay in performance because of a contractual provision suspending delivery in the event of outside interference (*Citrus Soap Co. v. Peet Bros* Mfg. Co. (1920) 194 P. 715). In one of the only force majeure cases resulting from the COVID-19 epidemic to have yet been decided, the court dismissed the claim for breach on the basis of the force majeure clause. While not enumerating epidemics on the list of excused events, it included 'circumstances beyond our or your reasonable control, including, without limitation, as a result of natural disaster, fire, flood, general strike, war, armed conflict, terrorist attack or nuclear or chemical contamination, we may terminate this Agreement with immediate effect' (*JN Contemporary Art LLC v. Phillips Auctioneers LLC* (2020) WL 7405262, S.D. N.Y., 16 December 2020). The pandemic fell within the rubric of natural disaster; the clause also had a introductory language suggesting that it extended to any language beyond the parties' control.

Each case is going to be highly fact-specific; less-broad clauses might lead to different results (Wajs 2020). The identity of the interpreter might also affect the outcome: 'Force majeure clauses are usually quite vague in their terminology and leave therefore ample room for the interpreter to superimpose the applicable law on the agreed terms. Therefore, depending on the applicable law, clauses with identical wording may be given different effects' (Cordero-Moss 2020: 50).

These differences in part stem from differences in terms of remedies. Civil law tribunals tend to be more comfortable ordering performance, revising contracts for the parties in order to maintain equilibrium, or otherwise adjusting them to ensure the continuing validity of the contract (Berger and Behn 2020: 39). This difference in approach is linked to the aforementioned differences in ideas about the moral underpinnings of contracts—if the contract is based in morality, then preserving it is imperative, whereas if it is based in the common will of the parties, and the will of one of them changes, then requiring that party to perform violates their will. Requiring that the party pay damages but not requiring actual performance is the unsurprising outcome. Relatedly, common law courts tend to regard court intervention with contract drafting or redrafting as a violation of party autonomy—it is for the parties to determine the terms of their contracts. If the parties want to continue to be bound contractually, they can renegotiate their contracts, but if they do not want to renegotiate, then it is not for the court to impose a new contract on them. These differences also explain the civil law's more ready embrace of doctrines related to force majeure, such as hardship—the idea that contractual performance should be excused or amended because it causes hardship for one of the parties (Cordero-Moss 2020: 52). The common law analogue—frustration of purpose—is much harder to trigger, and an English court, for example, does not regard itself as having the power to redraft the contract in light of the changed circumstances (Berger and Behn 2020: 39).

One should not, however, overstate the differences in the force majeure doctrine. Several elements are remarkably similar between the civil and the common law. First is the notion that the event must be beyond the control of the party (or parties) seeking to avoid the obligation. Second is the requirement that that party not have been able to avoid the effects of the event. Third is the idea that the parties could not have been expected to foresee the event at the time of the conclusion of the contract. This criterion is generally modified by the idea that the event be 'reasonably' foreseeable. Virtually anything is 'foreseeable' in that, if the parties employ their imaginations, they could likely come up with a long slate of theoretically foreseeable events. Yet we do not think it worthwhile for parties to a contract to put that much time, effort, and cost into hypothesizing about events that are not likely to occur. Thus, we look at events that the parties, at the time of contracting, might have been expected to consider as they concluded their contract, given the factual circumstances known to them at the time. The more an event was foreseeable, the more we expect that the parties could have, or should have, allocated the risk of its occurring in the contractual terms. The final requirement is that the obligation not be capable of performance—that it be impossible, or very nearly impossible. This is a deliberately high bar.

Let us return to the introductory hypothetical and amend the scenario from a tidal wave destroying the wedding hotel to the emergence of a global pandemic, such as COVID-19. In the first instance, there are some potential factual difficulties with establishing force majeure related to a pandemic. Unlike a tidal wave, which occurs at a time certain, the pandemic took several weeks to circulate around the globe. What might have been force majeure for a February wedding in Wuhan would not necessarily have been force majeure for a February wedding in Quebec. More difficult factual scenarios arise if we assume that either the bride and groom or some of the wedding guests were travelling across an international border (or even internally, given some governmental restrictions) to arrive at the hotel where the wedding was to be held. If the parents of the bride and groom resided in Wuhan and could not travel because they were locked down in China and unable to travel to Canada, would the bride and groom be able to invoke force majeure as a reason to cancel their contract with the hotel? What if it were the bride and groom themselves who could not travel to their dream destination wedding?

These intervening governmental acts add an important objective component to the situation. Even without the governmental acts, if we look at the criteria above, it seems clear that the existence of the pandemic is beyond the control of the parties. The second criterion is more difficult. Could the parties avoid the effects of the pandemic? Could they have travelled to Canada earlier, or could they trim the guest list, or require that the guests wear personal protective equipment to avoid risk? The third criterion—that the event could not have been reasonably foreseeable—would seem to be met as well, as the requirement of foreseeability would not be met simply because epidemiologists have predicted that a coronavirus epidemic would eventually occur. The final question is also potentially tricky—is it possible to perform the obligation at all? Can the bride and groom get married? If they are in the same place as the hotel, can they not get married, even if their guests cannot attend? What amount of risk should the bride and groom be expected to tolerate to get married? If the hotel staff are prepared to work, should the bride and groom be expected to get married?

In a pandemic scenario, it is crucial for successful invocation of a force majeure defence that intervening governmental acts might themselves constitute force majeure, even if the pandemic itself does not. If the government of China forbade citizens of Wuhan to leave their apartment buildings, let alone fly to Canada, that act in and of itself might qualify as force majeure, thus obviating the need to decide whether the threat of exposure to a potentially lethal coronavirus would serve as an excuse for not following through with the wedding plans and the hotel contract. If the government forbade gatherings of more than 10, or more than 25, or more than 50 people, then at the very least the wedding would have to be smaller. Governmental acts might thus answer some of these questions, but not necessarily all, particularly when they take the form of suggestions or 'discouragement', but fall short of outright prohibitions.

Something that is hard to capture but is not unimportant is the sense of whether the party seeking to avoid the obligation is using the alleged force majeure event as a convenient reason to avoid an obligation. This type of consideration is not explicitly part of the analysis, although it might come into the consideration of whether performance is really impossible, or simply undesirable.

This question of foreseeability is in essence a question of risk allocation—how do we expect the parties to have allocated the risks that the contract could not be performed, and in particular the risk that this particular event occurred? All of these requirements—and correlatively, the ability to invoke force majeure successfully—are highly fact-intensive. Note also that they also change over time. The COVID-19 pandemic might reasonably have been regarded as a force majeure event for contracts concluded before January 2020, and possibly even before 11 March. After that, it is much more difficult to say that the drafters of a contract should not have foreseen, and bargained around, not just the pandemic itself but potential factual and legal consequences of the pandemic.

The above discussion addresses force majeure and provides some rather broad-brush sketches of its application in the common and civil law traditions. Private international law principles come into play, for example, in the event that a court is asked to apply a law that is not the law of the forum—for example, when a French court is asked to apply English law, or vice versa. This might arise when you have a cross-border transaction, with one party in each jurisdiction, and they choose to have their contract governed by the law of one of the jurisdiction. As we see from the above discussion about differences between the common and civil law, an English court would be capable of applying French doctrine of force majeure, but would the English court really embrace the French approach of rewriting the contract for the parties, or would it instead permit the parties to terminate their contracts, leaving the losses to fall as they lay? Private international law also governs the enforcement of judgments give in one court by another court. Thus, if a French court ordered an English entity to perform its contract, would an English court enforce that order for specific performance? It might be clear that the English court would have enforced a pecuniary judgment, but orders for performance are less easily transferable across jurisdictions.

Cases tend to take time to wend their way through the courts. The time at which a case is heard could conceivably have an effect on the outcome; as one commentator noted about the December 2020 case *JN Contemporary Art*, '[T]he *JN* court's exceedingly liberal interpretation and application of the parties' force majeure provision is driven by the current direct circumstances that for many have made it impossible to perform their contracts' (Farren 4). The implication is that cases decided after a crisis has receded and performance becomes possible might result in a different interpretation.

As the above discussion should have illustrated, even for something as pervasive as a pandemic, the doctrine of force majeure provides somewhat limited, and possibly unpredictable, redress for those seeking to avoid their contracts. In the first instance, it should be noted that the notion of permitting parties to avoid their contractual obligations goes contrary to the fundamental principle of sanctity of contract. The four elements of the defence are thus deliberately difficult to satisfy. Each of them is quite fact-dependent; thus, different factual scenarios might well lead to different outcomes regarding liability. The timing of the suit, and of the potential violation, also matters—the duration of the pandemic, and the different factual and legal situations that apply at different times, mean that predicting the success of force majeure defence is difficult. It might notably be even more difficult in the next pandemic, depending on when that hits—given what we have learned from COVID-19, it might be hard for parties to argue that the pandemic was not reasonably foreseeable. Scientists had been expecting something like the COVID-19 pandemic for many years; the general public, including those who enter into legal contracts, might now be expected to foresee something like it as well. For how long from now (2021) will it be the case that another pandemic is not reasonably foreseeable?

Furthermore, the nature of the remedy might well depend on the applicable law, and on the court that is applying that law. It is thus not surprising that the British Institute of International and Comparative Law (BIICL) (2020) has proposed that the encouragement of negotiated solutions for international commercial contracts should performance be difficult because of the COVID-19 pandemic. After canvassing a number of potential defences (in addition to force majeure), BIICL's concept note suggests that alternative dispute resolution practices should be made available to contracting parties who are seeking to ascertain the effect that the pandemic ought to have on their relationship, and that the law should be applied (and possibly adapted) to encourage and support negotiated outcomes, and to encourage the maintenance of contractual obligations whenever possible.

Force Majeure in Public International Law

Public international law traditionally addresses the relationships between states, though in recent years non-state entities, such as foreign investors, have played a more active role in public international law than they had previously done. Force majeure is a principle found in public international law as well as in municipal law. A force majeure event can be raised as a defence by public entities as well as by private individuals.

Thus, force majeure is one of the circumstances excluding wrongfulness by which a state can temporarily relieve itself of its obligations. Because international obligations, whether they be based in a treaty or in general international law, are meant to be binding, the criteria that permit breaching those obligations are stringent and extremely hard to satisfy (Bjorklund 2008: 520). The philosophical backdrop to force majeure is thus quite similar to what is found in municipal law, as are the requirements for its invocation.

A sustainable force majeure claim requires the occurrence of an irresistible force or of an event beyond the control of the state, which makes performance of its obligations materially impossible. (ILC 2001: Article 23) Here again, you see the idea of an event that is beyond the control of the entity seeking to use it. The idea of irresistible force suggests that the state has no element of free choice. Force majeure should be compared with its related obligation, 'necessity', a doctrine that excuses a state from responsibility for acts necessary to safeguard an essential interest against a grave and imminent peril. The difference between force majeure and necessity boils down to the element of volition—has the state had a choice about which obligation to breach (albeit one that is justified and reasonable), or was there simply no choice at all (Bjorklund 2008: 472)? If it is the latter, then you might have a force majeure event; if the former, then the elements of necessity would apply.

As is the case with domestic law, the force majeure event must be beyond the control of the state concerned. This might best be thought of as an obligation to engage in due diligence. If the state should have prevented it from occurring, for example, then the state cannot use the event as an excuse. This has come up more often in the context of riots or insurrection, but this quote is of interest in the pandemic context: 'The Government is liable, however, where it fails to show due diligence in preventing or suppressing the riot, or where the circumstances indicate an insufficiency of protective measures or a complicity of government officers or agents in the disorder' (UN) 1978: 215). Related to the idea of due diligence is the notion of foreseeability. Could, or should, the state have foreseen that the problem was likely to occur? If so, its obligation to prevent it would be greater.

Think about how these first variables might arise in the context of a pandemic. The COVID-19 virus is believed to have originated in China. It seems relatively uncontroversial that the virus can be viewed as an irresistible force or event. That would be true whether the entity seeking to raise a force majeure defence was China or another country. What about the follow-on questions? What obligation, if any, did China have to stop the pandemic, or to prevent its escape beyond its borders? Could it have done so? Was it reasonable for it not to have done so? Could China try to excuse itself from liability on the grounds of the virus, or would the viral contagion be regarded as having been within China's control? Another country might not have the same problem of failing in its due diligence obligations, at least early on in the crisis, but later still one sees that governmental actions might have had effects on the country's ability to fulfil its own obligations. Did governments act properly? Was there a problem of 'underreach'—of failing to do enough—to prevent the crisis, or to prevent its spread (Pozen and Scheppele: 2020)?

Another requirement for the successful invocation of a force majeure defence at public international law is that performance of the obligation be 'materially' impossible; indeed, the irresistible force or unseen event must be causally linked to the situation of material impossibility (Crawford 2002: 170). This material impossibility criterion is something short of absolute impossibility, but it is clear that difficulty, or the fact that performance is burdensome, is not adequate. If a country is experiencing an economic crisis as a result of a pandemic, for example, the fact that it would be difficult for it to pay its debts is unlikely to be sufficient grounds on which to resist payment. A classic case from the Permanent Court of International Justice illustrates what is likely still a salient view of impossibility. In the *Serbian Loans* case, Serbia claimed in the aftermath of the First World War that it was not obligated to repay its debts to French nationals on grounds of force majeure. The loan instrument said that Serbia's obligation was to pay either in gold francs or in paper francs. Though the sum was large, it was not absolutely impossible for Serbia to pay. The tribunal implicitly suggested that if the requirement had been actual payment in gold francs, material impossibility would have intervened (because they were simply not available) (ILC 2001b: para. 23).

The force majeure situation must not be caused by the state in question. If the force majeure event is itself attributable to the state, the state cannot rely on it. To go back to the *Serbian Loans* case, for example, if the Serbian government had instituted currency controls that forbade the export of currency, and then said it could not pay the debt because it could not export any currency, that argument must fail, since Serbia itself created the problem. Note here the difference from the private law context, in which a private Serbian entity might be able to invoke those currency controls as force majeure preventing payment of a debt outside the country.

The final consideration in a public international law defence of force majeure is whether the state had itself assumed the risk of the event occurring. This would generally arise in the context of a treaty in which, analogous to the contractual situation outlined above, the parties might have anticipated the problem and, in their agreement, assumed the risk of the event's occurrence and the ensuing consequences. This provision does not seem particularly likely to be relevant in a pandemic context—or at least, not any more relevant in a pandemic context than in any other context.

This chapter has focused on force majeure, but the related doctrine of necessity is likely to be at issue in many cases as well. Necessity is perhaps even harder to invoke than force majeure. Because the difference between them is the element of volition—that a state is choosing to violate its obligation, albeit in a situation of extreme gravity, the standard is that much higher. Necessity excuses wrongfulness in cases of grave and imminent peril to the essential security interests of a state. In the case of a pandemic, it is quite easy to imagine circumstances in which it is extremely difficult to honour one's obligations, or perhaps very attractive not to do so. Imagine, perhaps, the incentive for a country to bar exports of a vaccine in order for them to made use of at home. It would not be impossible for the state to permit the export; the state would be choosing to violate its General Agreement on Tariffs and Trade (GATT) 1994 obligation to permit the export of the vaccine (for these circumstances, I am assuming that one of the exceptions to Article XI of GATT 1994 does not apply). It is unlikely that the state would be able to invoke necessity, especially as currently conceived, but that does not mean that it would not try.

A pandemic might be called upon by states as an excuse for violating any of their obligations, yet it seems especially likely that it could play a role in international economic law, notably in trade (as in the hypothetical border closure above), and in investment law. Investment treaties permit foreign investors to submit claims for breaches of the treaty, such as breaches of the national treatment obligation (non-discrimination on the basis of nationality) or the obligation to accord fair and equitable treatment. The border closure question is not altogether hypothetical; reportedly, the United States stopped the transit of personal protective equipment destined for Canada at the border during the early stages of the COVID-19 crisis (Abedi 2020).

To return to a slight variation on the wedding example, and to introduce the element of investment law, what if the hotel in Quebec is owned by a Mexican investor? What if Quebec forbade guests to stay in hotels and forbade gatherings in hotels, but continued to permit small religious services, in-person student attendance in schools, and study hubs in libraries? Would Quebec's acts, for which Canada would be responsible under international law, violate the fair and equitable treatment obligation, thereby violating its obligation under the Comprehensive and Progressive Trans-Pacific Partnership? Would the decisions to permit certain gatherings, whilst excusing others, be regarded as arbitrary? Would Canada be able to claim force majeure, or necessity, to excuse its violation (assuming that the violation exists)? Given that the virus, and governmental responses to it, are likely to shift over time and to endure for many months, does the defence likely shift from force majeure to necessity? What are the implications of that shift for the success of the defence and for the implications arising from it (compensation payments, etc.)? These are not easy questions to answer, and they might be answered in many different ways. Each of those small differences could potentially have an effect on the outcome of a case, making it difficult to predict with any degree of certainty what the result would be.

The duration of a pandemic—its starting point *and* its ending point—is relevant for public international law as well as for municipal law (Paddeu and Waibel 2020: 698). The doctrine of force majeure assumes an ending date—a time when the catastrophe is over, as does the doctrine of necessity. For something like a pandemic, that is exceptionally hard to ascertain. It also might not be the same date in all places. As Paddeu and Waibel explain, 'Pandemics are biological events, but they are also social events …' (Paddeu and Waibel 2020: 699). The biological and social aspects of a pandemic might end at different times. The ending point might have an effect both on liability and on any obligations to pay reparations—the obligation is excused only so long as the pandemic is in force. Once the obligation reappears, so might the question of compensation. The ILC articles say that invocation of a circumstance precluding wrongfulness is 'without prejudice to ... the question of compensation for any material loss caused by the act in question' (ILC 2001a, 2001b). Whether compensation is unnecessary for damage that arose during the crisis, or whether it is simply postponed, has not been definitely answered (Bjorklund 2008: 510–16). This complication provides yet another layer of uncertainty, on top of that introduced by the difference that factual variations might make as to liability.

As was the case with municipal law, these issues might be solved practically, by negotiation, rather than legally, by a court or other tribunal. States might hesitate to submit cases on the 'glass houses' theory—if they do make claims, then claims might come back against them as well (Arato et al. 2020: 631). Imagine attempting to charge China with having violated international law by failing to exercise due diligence to prevent the escape of the virus. What about the decisions taken (and not taken) by other countries? The messiness of the attempts to overcome issues such as a causal link between the initial steps taken to downplay the threat of the virus, not just in China but in other countries as well, might be seen as intervening factors. A long investigative article in the *New Yorker* magazine illustrates the multiple missed opportunities for the spread of the coronavirus to have been arrested in multiple jurisdictions (Wright 2021: 20–59). One might be able to trace initial culpability to one country, but actually attributing every single infection to initial failures to warn would strain principles of legal causation.

Conclusion

This discussion about well-developed legal doctrines and the difficulties that are likely to be encountered should a respondent try to invoke them might be seen as overly legalistic quibbles, and to avoid the bigger questions about responsibility for, and consequences of, a virus that unleashes a pandemic. For example, frail health systems starved for funds for decades played a role in the expansion of the COVID-19 crisis, as did the overarching philosophy prioritizing open markets and freedom of movement for goods and people (Quintana and Uriburu 2020: 690–1). Quintana and Uburu argue that 'from the perspective that not even the COVID-19 pandemic is an entirely natural or contingent crisis, one can identify limits and, crucially, complicities of international law in the reproduction of injustice in and through crises' (Quintana and Uriburu 2020: 693).

Reservations about the use of force majeure in either the private or public context arise from the principle of *pacta sunt servanda* and the law's devotion to the sanctity of contract. Yet creating a regime where exceptions are the norm, or are too easily invoked, might not be beneficial in the long term. Arato and his co-authors point out that force majeure might be regarded as a generalized exception to a state's international law obligations, particularly in international economic law, but there might be some dangers in this approach because it suggests that international law cannot itself accommodate crises, but must somehow be got round or avoided in light of the pandemic (Arato et al. 2020: 629). Finding flexibility within the law, rather than outside it, might serve the purpose of ensuring that the law can respond to crises such as the pandemic and avoiding charges of illegitimacy on the grounds that 'regular' law is so draconian that it must needs be avoided by an equally draconian exception.

It is early days yet regarding legal responses to the COVID-19 pandemic, even as the days during which regular activities have been interrupted seem increasingly long. The myriad ways that this particular pandemic will affect both public and private international law have only just begun to emerge. Thus, in addition to applying the doctrine of force majeure to the pandemic, one also has to consider whether the pandemic itself might affect general international law. Indeed, Paparinskis has suggested that the pandemic will be found to be sufficiently widespread, representative, and consistent to alter customary international law as it currently stands, particularly with respect to matters such as fault and the obligation to comply with international obligations (Paparinskis 2020: 620–1). It will be some time before we can assess whether or not that is true.

References

Abedi, Maham. 2020. 'Coronavirus: Trump Asks Medical Supply Firm 3M to Stop Selling N95 Respirators to Canada'. *Global News*, 3 April.

Arato, Julian, Kathleen Claussen, and J. Benton Heath. 2020. 'The Perils of Pandemic Exceptionalism'. *American Journal of International Law 114* (4): p. 627.

Atamer, Yesim M. 2011. 'Article 79'. In *UN Convention on Contracts for the International Sale of Goods (CISG) Commentary*, edited by Stefan Kröll, Loukas A. Mistelis, and Maria del Pilar Perales Viscasillas, pp. 1039–1079. Munich, Germany: Verlag C. H. Beck.

Berger, Klaus Peter, and Daniel Behn. 2020. 'Force Majeure and Hardship in the Age of Corona: A Historical and Comparative Study'. *McGill Journal of Dispute Resolution 6* (4): p. 79.

Bjorklund, Andrea K. 2008. 'State of Necessity and Force Majeure'. In *The Oxford Handbook of International Investment Law*, edited by Peter Muchlinski, Federico Ortino, and Christoph Schreuer, p. 459. Oxford: Oxford University Press.

Bradley, Curtis, and Laurence R. Helfer. 2020. 'Introduction to "The International Legal Order and the Global Pandemic"'. *American Journal of International Law 114*: p. 571.

Braun, Tillmann Rudolf. 2021. 'State Responsibility and Investment Protection in the Time of Pandemic'. In *Investment Protection, Human Rights, and International Arbitration in Extraordinary Times*, edited by Rainer Hofmann, Julian Scheu, Stephan Schill, et al., (forthcoming). Germany: Nomos.

British Institute of International and Comparative Law. 2020. 'Concept Note 2 on the Effect of the 2020 Pandemic on Commercial Contracts'. September. https://www.biicl.org/documents/10423_revised_concept_note_2_004wb_21.pdf.

Cordero-Moss, Guiditta. 2020. 'Covid-19 and Force Majeure under the Vienna Convention on Sales and In Civil Law'. *New York Dispute Resolution Lawyer 13* (2): p. 50.

Crawford, James. 2002. *The International Law Commission's Articles on State Responsibility: Introduction, Text and Commentaries*. Cambridge: Cambridge University Press.

Farren, David. 2021. 'Force Majeure and the Coronavirus Pandemic: A Case Law Update'. *JDSupra*, 12 February. https://www.jdsupra.com/post/contentViewerEmbed.aspx?fid=63487763-fe45-4f84-95c4-ed373f801fd3.

Heldrich, Andreas, and Beghard M. Rehm. 2005. 'Modernisation of the German Law of Obligations: Harmonisation of Civil Law and Common Law in the Recent Reform of the German Civil Code'. In *Comparative Remedies for Breach of Contract*, edited by Nili Cohen and Ewan McKendrick, p. 123. Oxford: Hart Publishing.

Holmes, Oliver Wendell. 1897. 'The Path of the Law'. *Harvard Law Review 10*: p. 457.

Hyland, Richard. 1994. 'Pacta Sunt Servanda: A Meditation'. *Virginia Journal of International Law 34*: p. 405.

International Institute for the Unification of Private Law (UNIDROIT). 2016. 'Principles on International Commercial Contracts'. https://www.unidroit.org/instruments/commercial-contracts/unidroit-principles-2016.

International Law Commission (ILC). 2001a. 'Draft Articles on Responsibility of States for Internationally Wrongful Acts, with Commentaries'. United Nations. https://legal.un.org/ilc/texts/instruments/english/commentaries/9_6_2001.pdf.

ILC. 2001b. 'Commentary to Text of Draft Articles Provisionally Adopted by the Commission on Second Reading'. UN Doc A/CN.4/515 and Add. 1–3.

Joshi, Riddhi. 2020. 'Force Majeure under the ILC Draft Articles on State Responsibility: Assessing Its Viability against COVID-19 Claims'. *ASIL Insights*, 17 September.

Lando, Henrik, and Caspar Rose. 2004. 'On the Enforcement of Specific Performance in Civil Law Countries'. *International Review of Law and Economics 24*: p. 473.

Lando, Ole. 2005. 'CISG and Its Followers: A Proposal to Adopt Some International Principles of Contract Law'. *American Journal of Comparative Law 53*: p. 379.

Nicholas, Barry. 1992. *The French Law of Contract* (2nd edn). Oxford: Clarendon Press.

Paddeu, Federica, and Freya Jephcott. 2020. 'COVID-19 and Defences in the Law of State Responsibility'. *EJIL:Talk!*, 17 March. https://www.ejiltalk.org/covid-19-and-defences-in-the-law-of-state-responsibility-part-i.

Paddeu, Federica, and Michael Waibel. 2020. 'The Final Act: Exploring the End of Pandemics'. *American Journal of International Law 114*: p. 698.

Paparinskis, Martins. 2020. 'The Once and Future Law of State Responsibility'. *American Journal of International Law 114*: p. 618.

Perillo, Joseph. 1997. 'Force Majeure and Hardship under the UNIDROIT Principles of International Commercial Contracts'. *Tulane Journal of International and Comparative Law 5*: p. 5.

Pozen, David E., and Kim Lane Scheppele. 2020. 'Executive Underreach, in Pandemics and Otherwise'. *American Journal of International Law 114* (4): p. 608.

Quintana, Francisco-José, and Justina Uriburu. 2020. 'Modes International Law: COVID-19, International Legal Responses, and Depoliticization'. *American Journal of International Law 114*: p. 687.

UN. 1978. '"Force Majeure" and "Fortuitious Event" as Circumstances Precluding Wrongfulness: Survey of State Practice, International Judicial Decisions and Doctrine'. *Yearbook of the International Law Commission 2* (1).

UN. 1980. 'Convention on Contracts for the International Sale of Goods'. 11 April, 1489 UNTS 3.
Wajs, Jordan. 2020. 'Common Law in a Pandemic: Spanish Flu of 1918'. *The Lawyers' Daily*, 1 May.
Weidemaier, Mark C. W., and Mitu Gulati. 2020. 'Necessity and the COVID-19 Pandemic'. 13 May. *Capital Markets Law Journal*. https://ssrn.com/abstract=3599503.
Wright, Lawrence. 2021. 'The Plague Year'. *The New Yorker*, 4 and 11 January.

Index